Sexual Medicine
in
Primary Care

Sexual Medicine *in* Primary Care

William L. Maurice, M.D., F.R.C.P.(C)

Associate Professor
Division of Sexual Medicine
Department of Psychiatry
University of British Columbia
Vancouver British Columbia
Canada

in consultation with Marjorie A. Bowman, M.D., M.P.A.
Chair, Department of Family Practice and Community Medicine
University of Pennsylvania, Philadelphia, Pennsylvania

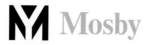

Mosby

St. Louis Baltimore Boston Carlsbad Chicago Naples New York Philadelphia Portland
London Madrid Mexico City Singapore Sydney Tokyo Toronto Wiesbaden

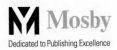

Mosby
Dedicated to Publishing Excellence

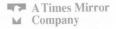

A Times Mirror
Company

Editor: Elizabeth M. Fathman
Developmental Editor: Ellen Baker Geisel
Project Manager: Carol Sullivan Weis
Production Editor: Florence Achenbach
Designer: Jen Marmarinos
Manufacturing Supervisor: David Graybill

Composition by Clarinda Company
Printing/binding by R.R. Donnelley & Sons Company

Mosby, Inc.
11830 Westline Industrial Drive
St. Louis, Missouri 64146

Library of Congress Cataloging in Publication Data
Maurice, W.
    Sexual medicine in primary care / William L. Maurice
        p.   cm.
    Includes bibliographical references and index.
    ISBN 0-8151-2797-9
    1. Sexual Disorders.   2. Primary care (Medicine)   I. Title
    [DNLM: 1. Sexual Disorders.   2. Sexual Dysfunctions.   3. Primary
Health Care.   WM 611M455s   1998]
RA427.9.M384   1998
616.85'83—dc21
DNLM/DLC
for Library of Congress   98-39997
                                                                        CIP

99 00 01 02 03   /   9 8 7 6 5 4 3 2 1

To my loving wife, Rosamund, who has been enormously supportive, accepting, patient (as is usual for her), and tolerant over the missed times together and missed holidays (not to mention the papers strewn about in my office and elsewhere).

FOREWORD

Rarely has a book been so timely! With the advent of Viagra and the resulting interest in female sexuality, questions, concerns, and discussion about sexual function and dysfunction have come to dominate the media in explicit and sometimes colorful language. Grandparents and their grandchildren both are suddenly equally interested in what their genitals are capable of and neither group is willing to settle for anything less than their "personal best." The interest in drugs to provoke desire, speed up (or slow down) arousal, facilitate orgasm, and reduce sexual discomfort has never been greater, and the pharmaceutical industry is working overtime to meet the demand. Physicians are in the vanguard of this fever, because patients request and expect sound advice, thoughtful recommendations, and effective interventions from their primary care providers — whether covered by managed care or not!

It is certainly the case that the HIV/AIDS epidemic served as the "wake-up call" to health professionals to begin explicit discussion of sexual behavior in routine office practice. The recognition that heterosexual and homosexual individuals were often unwittingly engaging in unsafe sex prompted the introduction of sexual history taking and sexual education as a means of disease prevention. It is only in the last decade that physicians have been called upon to initiate sexual inquiry to prevent illness and to enhance pleasure for their patients. There has been growing recognition that sexuality plays a significant role in quality of life, that sexual problems cause both emotional and physical distress, and that sexual inquiry and education are essential components of responsible and comprehensive health care.

It is also true that many physicians feel inadequately trained or prepared for dealing with the sexual concerns of their patients. Medical schools have not routinely included courses in human sexuality in their curriculum, and, in fact, educators are often uncertain of how best to teach the necessary skills. Even as ubiquitous a subject as physical examination diagnosis has caused consternation as educators debate whether or not to use live patients or paid actors for teaching genital examination. In many programs, the curriculum dealing with the review of systems deals with sexual matters, if it deals with it at all, in a fairly cursory and perfunctory fashion.

It is not surprising, then, that primary care physicians faced with time constraints, managed care demands, and inadequate training often feel unprepared to tackle the topic of sexual health in the detail and with the sensitivity it deserves. Concerns about offending (or embarrassing) patients, crossing boundaries, and risking legal repercussions have also contributed to the unwillingness of many physicians to open this particular "can of worms."

And yet, patients are clamoring for information and guidance in dealing with sexual problems and complaints. Questions about the impact of medication on sexual response, safe and unsafe sexual practices, unreliable erections and inadequate lubrication, and even talking to children about sex have become regular currency in physician offices. Most patients expect their health care provider to be an expert in all aspects of sexual health, even if their provider feels ill prepared and leary of the job.

It is for this reason that *Sexual Medicine in Primary Care* is such a timely and welcome volume. All the issues, questions, and concerns that physicians may encounter in dealing with the sexual concerns of their patients are addressed, including how to initiate and conduct sexual inquiry, and how to do so in a fashion that respects the privacy and enhances the comfort of their patients. It deals with such neglected topics as how to modify questions to include sensitivity to the age, gender, sexual orientation, and activity level of patients. The inclusion of sample dialogue between physician and patient illustrates the words to be used and the detail necessary to obtain an accurate picture of the patient's sexual behavior and concerns.

This book addresses topics that are often neglected: the distinction between sexual complaints and sexual dysfunctions, the difference between crossing boundaries and actual sexual violations, the need to avoid pigeonholing patients as either exclusively heterosexual or homosexual. It reviews the impact of physical illness and disability on sexual function and helps clarify how and whether sexual problems are the result of physical illness or exacerbated by it. Also included are such topics as nonparaphiliac and paraphiliac sexually compulsive behavior, an increasingly common source of concern among patients (and their partners), gender identity disorders, and child and adult sexual abuse.

Clinical vignettes highlight the enormous array of problems and issues that patients bring to their primary care physician. Dr. Maurice provides suggestions and recommendations as to how to deal with the myriad of issues presented. Moreover, in each and every chapter, the available clinical and research literature on the topic under discussion is reviewed and summarized. The chapters on the assessment and treatment of male and female sexual dysfunctions provide an outstanding review of common but often complex problems.

It is unusual to find so much practical information on such a long-neglected topic in one volume. *Sexual Medicine in Primary Care* is likely to become one of the books that primary care physicians not only purchase but actually use in their daily practice. It is a book that is well worth reading and one that is an excellent source book for consultation on a subject that touches the lives of all patients.

Sandra R. Leiblum, Ph.D.

Professor of Psychiatry
Co-Director, Center for Sexual and Marital Health
UMDNJ-Robert Wood Johnson Medical School
Piscataway, New Jersey

FOREWORD

Most primary care physicians lack formal education in the diagnosis and management of sexual problems, yet patients with concerns about sex visit primary care physicians regularly. Every day patients seek information and explicit help for sexual concerns, others hope the doctor will ask them about these personal issues, and still others seek, with their physician's collusion of avoidance, explanations for their symptoms other than a sexual disorder.

Medical schools include courses in human sexuality during the first or second years. Medical students learn the biology of the sexual response cycle, the endocrinology of reproduction, and even some psychology and sociology of sexuality. These valuable courses prepare the student to enter clinical training with a solid factual foundation about sex. Additionally, courses in medical ethics, physical diagnosis, and medical interviewing transform the student from a layman to a budding professional. As such, the student learns that all patient concerns may be respectfully and confidentially explored, all body parts and cavities examined while the doctor-to-be's response remains genuinely human, caring, therapeutic and altruistic. This delicate integration of human responsiveness and clinical acumen challenges professional development most when the topic turns to sex. Usually, the young doctor's knowledge is academic and experience is intensely personal, not professional. To be fully human in such circumstances risks, at best one's acting unprofessionally, and at worst, one's offending by appearing to cross a sexual boundary. It is not surprising that the medical profession remains slow to learn how to help patients with sexual problems, and why so many doctors simply avoid the topic entirely.

It is easy to understand how training in the clinical skills of interviewing, counseling, and physical examination applied to sexual problems may not occur during clinical education. One fortunate outcome of the HIV epidemic has been the systematic education of physicians to use screening interviews to ask patients about potentially risky sexual behaviors. Additionally, educational programs now teach primary care physicians how to counsel patients about safer sex practices. Unfortunately, when it comes to other sex problems, most physicians, whether in residency training or it practice, give them glib and superficial focus, a rapid referral, or a quick change in the subject. The 1998 meteoric rise of Viagra in the pharmaceutical sky empowered physicians, with a flick of the pen, to help patients with impotence. No interview was needed, both patient and physician understood "the problem" and believed there was a safe, quick fix. For the American public, the magnitude of mail erectile dysfunction became the constant focus for jokes, news stories, and commentaries.

Sexual Medicine in Primary Care could not have been published at a better time. It combines common sense wisdom and medical facts with an extensive review of a literature not easily found by the physician-reader. Sexual problem diagnosis, treatment reports, and scientific studies are uncommonly published in medical literature. Instead, they are the topics for journals in psychology, social work, and sex therapy. Dr. William Maurice deftly brings an extensive academic and practical knowledge base within reach of the average physician and medical student.

Talking about sex is difficult and Dr. Maurice provides model dialogues that guide the physician between possibly offensive common language of sexual experience and the jargon of medical physiology. Furthermore, his approach to interviewing a patient about sex demonstrates the necessary balance between direct questions and open-ended facilitation. With medical dialogue about sex, he advises to first ask permission, then to pose direct screening questions before proceeding to open-ended questions or facilitation of a patient's discourse.

The clear description of the medical conditions that interfere with sexual health provide guidance in diagnostic decision making and treatment. Although it is unlikely many primary care physicians will learn some of the sex education and counseling techniques described, the new advances in the use of medications and simple patient education will vastly increase the physician's medical effectiveness. Furthermore, the clear recommendations for referral and the description of the many types of professionals who may be of service to patients will raise awareness for all physicians. Teachers of primary care medicine should find this readable text full of useful interview tips, algorithms for diagnosis and treatment, and models for counseling and referral. The Appendix V is particularly useful, because it provides an extensive table of the multiple medications that interfere with sexual function.

As medical care moves increasingly into arenas of health maintenance and even to health enhancement, the patient's sexual health will continue to move into the domain of the primary care physician. The health care professional will need the knowledge, communication skill, and network of professional specialists to help patients achieve their desired level of sexual health. *Sexual Medicine in Primary Care* will certainly contribute by providing the information and suggestions for physicians' interaction with their patients about these problems.

F. Daniel Duffy, M.D., F.A.C.P.

Senior Vice President
General Internal Medicine
American Board of Internal Medicine

PREFACE

When, as a young man, I began listening to people talk about sexual problems, I had a very limited frame of reference, namely, my own personal life experiences, fantasies, and attractions. Listening for the past twenty-eight years to the sexual stories of thousands of men and women (individuals and couples, people who were otherwise physically and mentally healthy, well people and those who were unwell, people of different ages and from many cultures other than my own) I learned that the panorama of what is sexual for people extended far beyond my own personal boundaries.

The element that allowed me the privilege of entering this private sanctuary of patients* has been the evolving capacity to listen to others talk about sexual difficulties and developing the ability of speaking to others about this subject in a manner as neutral as talking about the weather. Use of these listening and talking skills provoked both greater patient trust ('here was a person who know what he was talking about') and greater interest on my part (evident before, but socially constrained). My personal curiosity was only satisfied, in turn, by more reading and listening.

Listening and talking skills in relation to sexual issues did not arise (unfortunately) from my medical school education or my specialty training in Psychiatry. Instructors in both settings were tongue-tied when considering anything sexual, but then again, this was the rule rather than the exception during those years. (One wonders how much has really changed since then beyond the surface. For example, health professionals can often now talk of "sexual abuse" but many seem unable to go beyond this phrase, or "chapter title", to ask about the details). I am thus deeply grateful to Masters and Johnson for allowing me a unique (literally at that time) opportunity to be in their clinic and for their generosity in letting a naive psychiatry resident into their midst for a research and clinical elective. One could not ask for more hospitality, generosity, and wisdom than I received from them. They helped me in getting my "feet wet" and I have not looked back since.

Over the years, I've learned from patients that sexual desires and actions are a source of great pleasure, but they may also entail much private pain when a problem exists. This is the central rationale for the incorporation of questions by a health professional about this otherwise private area into whatever else is being discussed with that patient. In my opinion, questions about sexual matters are a necessity for almost all patients. Those questions are part of the job.

---

*The word "patient" is used throughout this book simply because that is what I am used to calling people who consult me for professional reasons. However the content of this book has equal relevance to health professionals who use some words differently than I do. Some (including some physicians) are used to using the words "client" or "consumer," and these words could easily be used as substitutes for "patient" in most areas of this book.

The pain experienced by patients with sexual difficulties extends in a variety of different directions — from a fear of becoming infected with HIV, to having erection problems with a new partner after thirty-five years of monogamous sexual activity with another who recently died; from having been sexually attacked as a child to a fear of death during "sex" after a heart attack; and from thinking that one has been born into the wrong body from a gender viewpoint, to an irresistible impulse to expose one's genitalia in public. Those who are professionally engaged in talking to individuals about these difficulties know that when the inhibitions lift, they are often told of private thoughts, experiences, and fantasies that have never been revealed to anyone else, not even a loved sexual partner. Ironically, two people may engage in what is almost universally acknowledged as potentially the most intimate of human connections, and at the same time, have trouble talking about what just occurred. As curious as it might seem, it often seems easier to talk about sexual difficulties with a stranger, such as a health professional. Whatever the reasons (e.g., trust and no expectation of being judged), health professionals are in a particularly advantageous position to hear about those troubles.

Given this unique position of the health professional, one might wonder how medical and other health professional schools have responded in providing the necessary educational experiences to their students. The professional school that I know best is the one to which I'm attached, The University of British Columbia. Judging by informal conversations with teachers in other medical schools, our program seems to be not typical. We have an intricate lecture program in Sexual Medicine for our students, lectures that are integrated into preexisting courses. This is capped by clinical opportunities for students to practice sex history-taking and interviewing skills with other students and with simulated patients and for some to participate in the process of talking to a person or couple referred to a sex-specialty clinic because of a sexual concern. Residents (physicians in specialty training) in a variety of disciplines have similar experiences. This book is partly the result of requests from medical students and residents for a greater degree of preparation before actually being confronted with the unfamiliar task of talking to a patient about sexual matters.

The main impetus, however, for this book has been my clinical practice. Primary care physicians have been the source of over ninety percent of the thousands of clinical referrals that I've received over the years. Most commonly, I was sent a brief letter stating the main sexual problem with some other information about the patient's health and physical status. On some occasions, I was able to be extremely helpful in one or two visits. On other occasions, while the patients indeed had sexual difficulties, I've puzzled over why they were referred to anyone who focuses on sexual issues, since this seemed quite subsidiary to some other set of difficulties (medical, relational, or intrapersonal). On yet other occasions, the clinical situation proved more complex in that the sexual problem turned out to be plural (i.e., problems). In all these situations, I was repeatedly struck by how much I thought could have been accomplished on a primary care level with a bit more time and a few more questions. A given patient may never have had to see me because, for example, the problem was quickly solved or the initial assessment resulted in a conclusion that the patient should be referred for some other kind of care, or I might have seen the patient but for a shorter period of time because of preparatory work that had gone before.

PART I of this book is the result of requests from clinicians, medical students, and residents for written information on issues of sex history-taking. Topics include what questions to ask and words to use, how to ask the questions, and what paths to follow in clarifying some particular concern. However, there is a paradox inherent in the notion of learning skills from a book. Such phenomena are usually learned in the manner of an apprentice (see quote from Aaron Copland at the beginning of the Introduction to Part I). In fact, as helpful as a book might be (and I obviously hope this one will prove substantially so), nothing substitutes for hearing *directly* from people about their sexual thoughts, dreams, fantasies, and hopes; their sexual activities when alone or with others; their sexual worries, fears, dread, or even terror; and, most of all, the pain of not feeling like a "normal" woman or man.

Sometimes, the main concern of a patient in a primary care setting is sexual. Most other times, talking about sexual issues usually involves grafting this topic onto an interview that is already taking place on some other topic. An assumption made here is that the reader is familiar with the literature on interviewing in health care generally, so that little attempt has been made to review this subject in detail. The rationale for this particular book is that, usually, little is said in general texts on the subject of talking to patients about sexual matters. One can easily obtain a list of references to general texts on interviewing by consulting one of the available books.[1]

As much as one might promote the notion of encouraging discussions with patients on sexual matters, many primary care clinicians declare unease at raising this issue without knowing what to do with the answers and without being able to provide some level of treatment. Caring for patients with sexual difficulties is the purpose of Part II of this book — the treatment of common sexual dysfunction in primary care. Although some of the suggestions made may seem mechanistic and cook-bookish, that is not what is intended. In no other area of human enterprise is there such intricate connections between mind and body as is the case with anything sexual. It seems so much easier to write about sexual toys or gizmos than about the human relations part of the treatment of sexual problems, but there are no therapeutic circumstances in which the latter do not play a prominent part.

It should not surprise readers that this book is written from a physician's perspective, since it represents my own professional background. However, when considering the care of people with sexual difficulties, physicians may be in a minority. Many sex-experts have been educated in a variety of health care disciplines apart from medicine, especially psychology, social work, and nursing. Physicians tend to specialize in particular areas such as STDs and HIV/AIDS, erectile dysfunction, and gender identity disorders. Since professional attention to sexual problems is inherently interdisciplinary, this book was written with much consideration given to clinicians and students in *all* of the health sciences. Hence the phrases "primary care clinicians" or "primary care health professionals" have been used throughout this book.

Finally, I would like to add a comment about the word "sex." Multiple meanings for this word is the usual reason for placing it in quotation marks in the text. It would be a gross understatement to say that defining the word is difficult. When used in a clinical setting, "sex" generally has two meanings: the nature of the patient as male or female (although the word "gender" is increasingly being used for this purpose), and as a synonym for the specific practice of intercourse. When used to describe one particular sexual practice such as intercourse, it takes little reflection to agree that the word "sex" really encompasses so much more. When, for example, a man and woman engage in sexual activity that involves "everything but," almost everyone still considers the activity to be sexual. Likewise, when a man and a woman are passionately kissing and both people experience the physical manifestation of sexual arousal (erection and vaginal lubrication among other things) who would not also call that sexual? And when a man or woman masturbates alone and is orgasmic, isn't that also "sexual"?

What about the definition of the seemingly broader term, *sexuality*? Is it the same as "sex" and "sexual"? Of "sexuality" (and it probably could be said of all three words), "everyone either grasps the definition from contextual cues, assigns it a private meaning, or simply pretends to understand".[2] "Sexuality" involves physiological capabilities, sexual behavior, and sexual identity — among other things.[2] (pp. 3-4). The reader will find the word "sexuality" infrequently used here because its meaning seems even less precise than "sex" and "sexual." The word "sexual" seems most comfortable and is used most often, perhaps because being an adjective rather than a noun or verb, it modifies another word.

REFERENCES

1. Morrison J: *The first interview: revised for DSM-IV*, New York, 1995, The Guilford Press.
2. Levine SB: *Sexual life: a clinician's guide*, New York, 1992, Plenum Press.

W. Maurice

Vancouver, BC

ACKNOWLEDGMENTS

I am profoundly indebted to the many patients with sexual problems (who, to preserve confidentiality, must remain anonymous) that I have treated over the past 28 years. This is more than ritual intellectual appreciation. The emotional part of my gratitude was "brought home" to me by a phone call I recently received from a woman asking to see me because of a sexual concern. She explained that her parents consulted me about 25 years ago, that her call now was on their suggestion, and that, in turn, was because of their thankfulness at my having been so helpful to them many years before in preserving their marriage! As appreciative as her parents evidently were, I was touched and even beholden to them because of what they gave to me.

I am particularly grateful to Marjorie Bowman for having worked as a consultant on this book, and for the care that she took in scrutinizing what I had written. She provided the perspective of someone on the "front lines" of family practice, which I, as a specialist, was obviously unable to do. When I began searching for a consultant, I felt strongly that whoever filled this position should be a woman in order to provide balance to the perspective I would inevitably present as a man. I also thought that she should be an American to provide balance to the cultural perspective that I would inevitably present as a Canadian. On all three counts, I (and readers) have been generously rewarded. Above all, her sensitivity to patient needs was repeatedly made obvious to me, as was her passionate concern for the way women patients, in particular, should be treated.

Some friends and colleagues read and critiqued parts of the manuscript, and while no one apart from myself bears responsibility for the finished product, this review process was particularly valuable to me. My psychiatrist friends and colleagues, Jon Fleming and Sheldon Zipursky, gave me their considerable wisdom and time. Irv Binik, Phillis Carr, Sandra Leiblum, Jamie Powers, Ray Rosen, and Ruth Simpkin, provided detailed and useful comments. Others, Eli Coleman, Bill Coleman, Christine Harrison, Mike Myers, Oliver Robinow, Tim Rowe, Bianca Rucker, Roy O'Shaughnessy, and Noelle Vogel, either advised me on specific issues or offered important general observations on this, or an earlier version of the manuscript. Many medical students and psychiatry residents offered substantial ideas over the past years and many of these have been incorporated into the manuscript.

George Szasz (now retired) was a colleague for 20 years, and over that period of time, we shared so many ideas that it sometimes became difficult to know the source. I have known my other colleagues in the UBC Division of Sexual Medicine for fewer years and yet their contributions to my education and this book have also been substantial. Stacy Elliott was particularly helpful in reading part of the manuscript and advising me about ejaculatory disorders involving reproduction. As well, Rosemary Basson, Donna Hendrickson, and Ron Stevenson have all given me useful ideas, more so than they may even realize.

Laura Hanson, a student in the PhD Psychology program at the University of British Columbia, provided organized and very helpful work as a research assistant. The high quality of work and good humor of my secretaries (plural because my office moved while the manuscript was in preparation) Maureen Piper, Judy Wrinskelle, and Francesca Wilson made my life immeasurably easier in the process of preparing this manuscript.

My editors at Mosby have been extremely responsive from the beginning of this project. Mike Brown as Acquisitions Editor (although not presently working for Mosby) immediately and impressively responded to my initial proposal and was eventually responsible for the connection between Mosby and myself. Besides advising me in many useful ways, he was ultimately helpful in locating Marjorie Bowman. Ellen Baker Geisel, Development Editor, has been my principal contact at Mosby. Her sense of humor, good cheer, and helpful advice has been crucial in seeing this project through to fruition. Florence Achenbach and Jen Marmarinos were invaluable as production editor and designer, respectively. They brought my manuscript to life.

Finally, the Lady Davis Fellowship Trust allowed me to contemplate and plan much of the foundation for this book during my treasured sabbatical in Jerusalem and that debt is one that I cannot ever repay.

Bill Maurice

CONTENTS

PART III APPENDICES

DETAILED CONTENTS

PART II SEXUAL DYSFUNCTIONS IN PRIMARY CARE: DIAGNOSIS, TREATMENT, AND REFERRAL

PART III APPENDICES

Part I

SEX HISTORY-TAKING, INTERVIEWING, AND ASSESSMENT

*If you want to understand music better you can do nothing more important than listen to it . . . every-
thing that I have to say in this book is said about an experience that you can only get outside this book.*

AARON COPLAND, 1957[1]

In the era in which we live, public sexual speech sometimes seems everywhere, from prime-time
TV drama where a "call girl" explains to a private detective that her client usually shouts the
name of his wife when he "comes,"[2] to a magazine ad for women's shoes that depicts an actress
reading a newspaper while sitting on a toilet with her underpants just above her ankles,[3] to
everyday radio and TV talk shows on which people seem to compete in verbally exhibiting the
most intimate details of their sexual problems.

At the same time that the media have become more tolerant concerning private sexual behavior and public sexual speech, conservative political forces demonstrate considerable opposing
strength. This social ambivalence was the background against which Laumann and his colleagues
planned and executed their landmark "sex" survey in 1992 (The National health and Social Life
Survey [NHSLS]) on a nationally based random sample of the United States population. Results
of the study—referred to frequently in this book—were published in the form of two volumes.
The first volume is titled *The Social Organization of Sexuality: Sexual Practices in the United States* and
was written for medical and social scientists. The second volume is a distillation of the first, titled
Sex in America: A Definitive Survey, and was written for a public audience.[4,5]

In spite of the enormity of the HIV/AIDS crisis and the desire of all to have more and better
information with which to combat HIV/AIDS, the description of the United States government's
failure to support the Laumann et al. project is sobering (see pp. 35-42 in *"The Social Organization
of Sexuality"*). The unacceptability of broaching particular topics (e.g., masturbation) with study
subjects, government rejection of the project, and the ultimate support of a consortium of private funding sources are additional demonstrations (if more are needed) of jumbled social attitudes toward sexual issues.

In the study by Laumann et al, almost 80% of 3432 adults between ages 18 and 59
answered detailed questions about their sexual behavior, thoughts, and feelings in face-to-face
interviews that lasted about 90 minutes and were conducted by interviewers who were

complete strangers.[4] The interviewers were *not* health professionals but lay people working for the National Opinion Research Center (NORC). Although most had previous experience in public survey interviewing, an additional *short* training program was designed for this particular survey.

If lay interviewers who received only brief extra training can talk with ordinary people for a lengthy period of time about the minutiae of one of the most intimate and private areas of their lives, health professionals certainly could do the same. Laumann et al. concluded, in fact, that adults are quite willing to talk about their sexual behavior, providing that the "interview is conducted in a respectful, confidential, and professional manner"[4] (p. 602).

While the "sexual revolution" of previous decades brought changes in private sexual behavior, these changes did not necessarily extend into the consulting rooms of health professionals. *Talking about "sex"* is what begins this process. *Talk* is the key to the search for understanding sexual thoughts, sexual feelings, and sexual actions—ultimately it is the key to helping patients. Talk is the focus of Part I of this book. Before the past decade or so, only health professionals with a special interest in sexual problems would talk to patients about sexual issues. Today, the greater degree of societal openness about sexual matters has resulted in greater patient acceptance and understanding that questions about sexual issues are legitimately related to health.

A woman in her mid-30s and a man in his mid-40s lived together for five years. They were seen because of a problem with "intimacy." In talking about their sexual activity, it quickly became evident that none had occurred between the two of them (or anyone else) in three years. Neither had previously talked with a health professional about these issues, apart from a recent discussion with their family doctor who referred the couple. When asked why they were seeking help now rather than at some time previously, the woman explained the following:

- She and her husband recently changed family doctors and the new physician asked her about birth control
- Their previous family doctor had not discussed birth control. If the previous physician had asked, the woman would have said that she was not using any form of birth control. If asked why, she would have said that birth control was not necessary, since no sexual activity had occurred in years

The woman was unwilling (or unable) to volunteer the above information but had no difficulty explaining her status to her current family doctor when pertinent questions were asked.

In addition to the greater appreciation of connection between sexual issues and health, the advent of HIV/AIDS and child sexual abuse has markedly changed attitudes toward talking about sexual issues in health settings. Professionals who work in such areas might be regarded as negligent (or even unethical) if they bypass sex-related questions in the process of their investigations.

A married man underwent cardiac surgery in a Canadian hospital on several occasions. The last occasion was six years before his death at the age of 59. He received a blood transfusion during his last operation, and one year later the blood donor tested positive for HIV when attempting to donate blood a second time. Two years passed before the Red Cross Society traced the blood donation to the hospital where the patient had his surgery. Another two years transpired before the hospital traced the unit of blood to the transfusion given five years earlier.

At that point, the family physician was informed that the blood transfusion given to his patient might have been contaminated by HIV. Parenthetically, the physician was prominent and well regarded in his community and, at the time his patient's cardiac surgery occurred, he held a significant position in the medical licensing body of the Province. The physician chose not to tell the patient of the possibility that he (the patient) was infected with HIV and therefore was unable to test for this infection, since patient consent was required. One of the reasons given by the physician for not disclosing the patient's HIV status to him was that the patient was sexually inactive and therefore of no risk to his wife.

Evidence for the patient's sexual inactivity was based on a review of the chart. The patient had seen a cardiologist one year before his surgery and the report of the specialist noted that the patient experienced "impotence." In addition, in a functional inquiry performed by the family doctor earlier in the year of the cardiac surgery, there was a notation saying that the patient's libido was "slightly decreased." Also, on two other occasions (two and four years after the surgery), the physician's notes indicated that the patient's libido was "none." There was no elaboration in the notes of the meanings of the words, "impotence" and "libido." The physician evidently assumed that "impotence" and the absence of sexual desire were equivalent to the cessation of sexual activity. In fact, the couple had been sexually active (including intercourse) at varying levels for much of the time after the patient's surgery.

Six years after his cardiac surgery, the patient again entered the hospital, was tested for HIV antibodies, and was found to be positive. He died during this hospitalization of AIDS-related pneumonia. Within weeks after the patient's death, his wife was notified that her husband had been HIV positive. She was immediately tested, and six weeks later she was told that she was positive as well.

The medical licensing body in that jurisdiction penalized the physician by suspending (albeit temporarily) his license to practice medicine.[6] In addition, the estate of the patient, his wife, and his children, sued the hospital, the Red Cross, and the family physician for damages for personal injuries. After a trial that lasted for more than one year, the three defendants were deemed negligent. Liability of damages of over $500,000 was apportioned[7]:

Hospital	30%
Red Cross	30%
Physician	40%

> Neither the licensing body nor the court explicitly acknowledged in their judgements the crucial role of the physician's evident inability to talk candidly with his patient about sexual matters despite the great potential significance of this factor to his health and that of his wife.

The physician in this true case history is testimony to the pitfalls involved in avoiding sexual issues, since he lost his license to practice medicine and also suffered social disgrace on a national level. Once thought of as elective in health care, the notion of inquiring into sexual function and practices is now commonplace within the mainstream of public and health professional expectations.

At least two elements explain the reluctance to talk about sexual issues in a clinical heath care setting (there are others—see Box 1-1 in Chapter 1):

- If the health professional introduces the issue of sexual difficulties and the patient says that "yes, a problem exists," the health professional has to know what the *next* question should be (or, in other words, the health professional must know what to do with the answers). Without thinking of the implications, many health professionals seem to conclude (by inaction) that it may be better to omit questions about sexual issues rather than face the hazard of not having prepared follow-up questions.
- After the nature of a problem is thoroughly investigated by a health professional, what does one do about it? Again, many health professionals appear to conclude that it is better not to ask if one can not bring about some change. (This topic is the focus of PART II.)

How does one inquire and what questions does one ask? Regardless of which of the urgent health/social themes is being discussed—HIV/AIDS, sexual assault, paraphilias, teen pregnancy, or sexual dysfunctions—talk is the means by which information is acquired. Theoretical issues involving history-taking (including the inquiry into sexual matters) and the circumstances governing such an exploration (see Chapter 1. Sets the stage for the remainder of the book.)

Consideration of special interviewing techniques used in asking sex-related questions (Chapter 2) implies that the subject of "sex" is different from other subjects in health care, a correct notion that reflects a social situation in which health professionals are no less victims than everyone else in the community. That specialness of the topic governs the content of questions in two ways:

- The nature of the general screening questions that are asked (Chapter 3)
- The specialized questions which elicit more detailed information of a person with a particular sexual dysfunction (Chapter 4)

Given the setting of health care, an assumption is made that investigation of a sexual concern is grafted onto a basic health assessment that includes essential medical information. Added to this is an etiological inquiry into the recent sexual experiences and sex-developmental history of the individual (Chapter 5). Chapter 6 provides a detailed description of the process involved in the investigation of the most common sexual complaint, namely, a sexual dysfunction.

When talking about any sexual issue within a health care setting, two previous, omnipresent, and nonpathological factors must always be considered: the gender and sexual orientation (1) of the patient and (2) of the health professional. These two issues are discussed in Chapter 7. Neither gender nor sexual orientation of the health professional has any necessary connection to the care of the patient, which after all, is the central objective in health care. Nevertheless, one or both factors may influence the process, since patients may have views that pull or push them from, for example, women or gay health professionals.

The gender of each party is obvious and therefore can affect the health professional/patient relationship. In contrast, sexual orientation is hidden and becomes apparent only when one or both parties choose to disclose it.

Chapter 8 reviews the many issues and questions that an interviewer must address concerning medical, psychiatric, and sexual disorders (apart from dysfunctions). Chapter 8 completes the PART I focus on general aspects of talking to people about sexual matters.

REFERENCES

1. Copland A: *What to listen for in music*, New York, 1967, McGraw-Hill.
2. Chandler & Co: *PBS/KCTS*, April 11, 1996.
3. *The Globe and Mail*, Adacity, C 1, June 7,1997.
4. Laumann et al: *The social organization of sexuality: sexual practices in the United States*, Chicago, 1994, The University of Chicago Press.
5. Michael RT et al: *Sex in America: a definitive survey*, Boston, 1994, Little, Brown and Company.
6. *Members' Dialogue*, College of Physicians and Surgeons of Ontario, September 1993.
7. Pittman estate v Bain: 112 D.L.R. (4th) 257 (Ont Gen Div 1994).

CHAPTER 1

TALKING ABOUT SEXUAL ISSUES: HISTORY-TAKING AND INTERVIEWING

Significant obstacles exist between the clinician's capacity to ask a question and the patient's capacity to respond. Whereas comprehensive knowledge is required of the cardiovascular system to cover all the symptom bases, these questions are typically asked without anxiety or inhibition once the questions are memorized and their rationale understood. Similarly, the patient experiences little or no hesitancy in responding truthfully to these paths of inquiry. The same milieu does not generally exist with sexual history taking.

GREEN, 1979[1]

O ther than descriptions of interviewing methods used by researchers[2] and opinions of specialist-clinicians who treat people with sexual difficulties,[3] health professionals have little guidance on the subject of talking to patients about sexual issues. Less still is any direction given to primary care clinicians for integrating this topic into their practices. For guidance on sex-related interviewing specifically, the primary care clinician may want to begin by examining clinical research in the general area of interviewing, as well as the observations of those who have written about their personal general interviewing ideas and practices.[4]

SOME RESEARCH ON GENERAL ASPECTS OF HEALTH-RELATED INTERVIEWING AND HISTORY-TAKING

As Rutter and Cox stated, "many practitioners have advocated a variety of approaches and methods on the basis of their personal experience and preferences. . . [but]. . . there has been surprisingly little systematic study of . . .interviewing techniques for clinical assessment purposes."[5] Only a few items from the research literature in the area of health-related interviewing are described here.

Direct Clinical Feedback

One interviewing-research question has been the value of direct clinical supervision in the development of interviewing skills generally. While this form of supervision makes sense intuitively, the process has been subject to little research. One study compared the value of direct clinical feedback to medical students using four different techniques: three of them (audio replay, video replay, and discussion of rating forms) were compared to a fourth whereby a student interviewed a patient and subsequently discussed findings (indirectly) with a supervisor.[6] The students who received any of the three *direct* clinical feedback methods did much better. The same individuals were assessed five years later as physicians and strikingly (since long-term follow-up studies in health education are quite unusual) those who received feedback "maintained their superiority in the skills associated with accurate diagnosis."[7]

In another study, two groups of medical students were videotaped on three different occasions during the school year while performing a history and physical examination.[8] Both groups viewed their own tapes but one group received additional evaluative comments by a faculty member. By the end of the year, those in the latter group performed significantly better in the following:

- Their interviewing verbal performance
- The content of the medical history they obtained
- Their use of physical examination skills

Teaching Interviewing Skills

One might conclude from the findings of both studies that if direct supervision proved superior in the process of learning interviewing skills generally, the same conclusion might be drawn for interviewing a patient about a specific subject such as "sex." The importance of this conclusion can not be exaggerated when one considers the dearth of questions about sexual issues in ordinary health histories. One way to change this situation is to deliberately teach the skill of sex history-taking and interviewing in health professional schools instead of (as now often seems to be the case) seemingly expecting clinicians to absorb this skill in the course of developing their clinical practices.

It may be instructive to also consider a series of studies of interviewing styles that were based on talks with mothers who were taking their children to a child psychiatry clinic.[5,9-14] These interviews were conducted by experienced health professionals. Four experimental interviewing styles were compared for their efficacy in eliciting factual information and feelings. The four were given the following names:

- Sounding board
- Active psychotherapy
- Structured
- Systematic exploratory

The research group concluded that good-quality factual information required detailed questioning and probing, that several approaches were successful in eliciting feelings, and that these two issues were compatible in the sense that attending to one did not detract from the other. Although their findings were related more to the process of interviewing and not specific to any particular topic, their conclusions seemed as applicable to the area of "sex" as with any other. The clinically apparent need for the health professional to initiate sex-related questions when talking with patients (see "Interviewer Initiative" in Chapter 2) echoes the conclusion of these studies that asking detailed questions is more productive. In extrapolating from these studies and insofar as "sex" can legitimately be seen as psychosomatic, there should be no incompatibility in the attention that a clinician might give to the acquisition of information that is factual and related to feelings when talking to a patient about sexual matters.[15]

Another study that examined the proficiency in history-taking generally in second-year medical students also may have implications for sex history-taking.[16] Two methods of measurement were used:

- The Objective Structured Clinical Examination (OSCE)
- A written test

The authors believed that patient information could be divided into three domains:

1. Information required to make a diagnosis
2. Information to determine risk for future disease
3. Information to assess the patient's available support system

The study found that students concentrated on obtaining diagnostic information on both of the tests used and that, unless modeled by faculty, information on risk factors and psychosocial data was omitted. Since sex-related problems are often relegated to the psychosocial arena, an assumption that one might derive from this study is that unless a sexual problem is given by the patient as a chief complaint (and therefore in the "diagnostic" arena) it is unlikely to be detected—unless faculty modeling occurs.

Extrapolations from all of these studies in interviewing and history-taking as far as "sex" is concerned imply the following:

1. Teaching of skills by direct supervision should be included in health science educational programs
2. Direct questions are more productive
3. There is no difficulty in attending to factual information and feelings
4. Faculty modeling is a significant element in the learning process

Extrapolations from studies in interviewing and sex history taking imply:

1. Teaching of skills by direct supervision should be included in health science educational programs
2. Direct questions are more productive
3. There is no difficulty in attending to factual information and feelings
4. Faculty modeling is a significant element in the learning process

INTEGRATING SEX-RELATED QUESTIONS INTO A GENERAL HEALTH HISTORY

Texts on general aspects of health-related history-taking and interviewing reveal great inconsistency in the definition of a "sexual history" and consequently in what is expected of the health professional. Some texts contain little or no information on the subject[17]; others include a separate chapter [1,18-22] or portion of a chapter.[4,23] Complete or partial chapters are usually brief and the information is so concentrated that the content is difficult to use in a practical sense. Some authors focus on "sex" as it relates to a particular psychiatric or medical disorder, for example:

1. Sexual desire in depression[24]
2. Sexual abuse as it relates to dissociation, posttraumatic stress disorder, and somatization disorder[25]
3. The "hysterical" patient[26]
4. Sexually transmitted diseases[27]

Others focus special attention on a particular sexual problem.[21] Some authors recommend asking about the patient's past sexual development[28]; others suggest a focus on current problems.[20] Specific suggested questions are offered by some,[19] and others may also include a brief rationale for these questions.[29] When questions are suggested, little guidance is usually given on when they should be asked.

"Human Sexuality" textbooks are also of limited help. Some may include a chapter on "assessment" or "sex" history-taking and interviewing.[30-32] Although the quality of information in these chapters may be high, the amount that is squeezed into this one section results in "information overload" and therefore becomes of minimal practical use to the frontline clinician.

Journal articles on sex history-taking provide a similar variety of opinions about what should be included. The advent of HIV/AIDS has pushed physicians into promoting the need for taking a sex history.[33,34] So, too, is the effect on health professionals of the recognition of the frequency of child sexual abuse in the history of adults.[35] Sometimes, history-taking suggestions are in the form of topics to be covered rather than specific questions to be asked.[36]

Among the more informative sources of information on sex-related interviewing and history-taking (but still of limited value to primary care clinicians) are the comments about interviewing that are attached to some of the community based research reports on sexual behavior. Kinsey and his colleagues included a chapter on the subject of interviewing in their volume *Sexual Behavior in the Human Male*.[37] More recently, large-scale "sex" surveys in the United States[38] (see introduction to PART I), the United Kingdom,[39] and France[40] included reports about the interviewing process when outlining their study design (see Table 1-1 for a comparison of some aspects of the three surveys).

Table 1-1   Comparison of Three Major "Sex" Surveys Published in the 1990s

Survey Aspects	United States	United Kingdom	France
Government Opposition	Yes	Yes	No
Financial support	Private	Private	Government
Random survey Method	Yes	Yes	Yes
Principal Interview Method	Face-to-face	Face-to-face	Telephone
Completed Interviews	3432	18,876	20,055 (Short: 15,253) (Long: 4820)
Response rate (%)*	79	63.3-71.5	65.5-72
Population age Range	18-59	16-59	18-69
Interviewers Specially trained	Yes	No	Yes
Duration of Interview (minutes)	90	46-60	Short interview: 15 Long interview: 45

*Range depends on method of calculation.

Thus health-related interviewing texts, specialty books on "Human Sexuality," and journal articles are enormously variable in their content when considering sex history-taking and tend to be disappointing in that they provide little aid to clinicians.

STUDIES IN MEDICAL EDUCATION THAT RELATE TO GENERAL ASPECTS OF SEX HISTORY-TAKING

In the 1960s and 1970s, sex education in medical schools concentrated on providing information about "sex" and helping people to be more at ease with the subject. Beginning in the 1980s, some schools added a focus on skills, that is, interviewing and history-taking, or, to put it differently, they added focus on the practical issue of how physicians and patients actually talk about the subject of sex. Attitudes and practices of sex history-taking have been examined from a research viewpoint, and understanding conclusions from these studies may provide some practical direction.

Comfort and Preparedness

Comfort and preparedness in "taking a sexual history" was studied in a group of first-year medical students.[41,42] The idea of including this topic in a medical history, as well as facilitating factors and obstacles, was examined. The authors found that the sexual orientation of the patient seemed an important variable in that students expected to be most comfortable with heterosexual patients of the same sex and least comfortable with an (presumably gay) AIDS patient. The authors also found that "the most consistent predictor of both knowledge and attitudes about sexual history-taking was a student's personal sexual experience." The kinds of experiences that were particularly linked with comfort and preparedness in taking a sexual history were:

1. Having taken a sexual history in the past
2. Having spoken to a health professional oneself about a sexual concern
3. Having a homosexual friend

Age seemed related only to the extent that older students expected to be more comfortable with an AIDS patient.

Practice

The importance of practice was seen in a study of medical students who were involved in different sexuality curricula at two different schools.[43] In one, students were not expected to be involved in sex history-taking. In the other, students conducted a sex history with a volunteer or observed one taking place. The curricula were otherwise similar. The three groups (no interview, conducting an interview, and observing an interview) were assessed regarding knowledge about:

- Sexual issues
- The propriety of including sex-related information in a medical history
- Self-confidence in the ability to conduct the interview

The students who previously conducted a sex-related interview did significantly better than those who were neither participants nor observers. However, findings relating to students who were in the observer group were intermediate on measures of knowledge and perceived personal skill.

The reasons, "why other doctors fail to take adequate sex histories," were determined in another study[44] and include the following:

1. Embarrassment of the physicians
2. A belief that the sex history is not relevant to the patient's chief complaint
3. Belief that they (the subjects) were not adequately trained

A large majority of senior medical students thought that knowledge by a physician of a patient's sexual practices was an important part of the medical history but only half were confident in their ability to actually acquire this information from a patient.

> A large majority of senior medical students thought that knowledge by a physician of a patient's sexual practices was an important part of the medical history but only half were confident in their ability to actually acquire this information from a patient.

Social and Cultural Factors

Social and cultural factors relating to the patient also seem to influence whether or not a sex history is taken. Sixty emergency room medical records of adolescent girls who complained of abdominal pain that required hospitalization were reviewed.[45] The authors found that asking about sexual issues in the context of an emergency room occurred a great deal more with individuals from minority groups than with white adolescents with the same complaint. They concluded that racial stereotyping was an important factor in asking questions about sexual experiences. Although they supported the inclusion of such questions in an assessment, the authors argued that histories in an emergency room should be characterized by efficiency and a minimum of irrelevant questioning, and that, in spite of the pertinence of questions about sexual experiences to the complaint of abdominal pain in an adolescent girl, such questions were more often omitted in those who were white.

Skills Versus Self-awareness

In a demonstration of the sex history-taking usefulness of direct teaching of skills compared to sexual self-awareness, family practice residents were randomly allocated to two groups emphasizing one or the other of these approaches.[46] Each group received two hours of training. The first hour was common to both groups and involved general counseling skills and information about sexual dysfunctions. In the second hour, the two groups were separated and concentrated on sexual history-taking issues or the comfort and sexual self-awareness of the resident. One week later, residents conducted a videotaped interview with a simulated "patient" with sexual and other problems but who was also instructed to reveal sex-related information only if asked directly. Almost all subjects (11/12) in the skills-oriented group asked the "patient" about the nature of her sexual difficulty, compared to 25% (3/12) of the awareness-oriented group.

Clinical Practice

Physicians in clinical practice (versus medical students and residents in educational programs) also have been studied. In a widely quoted and well-conceived study, a group of primary care internists were taught to ask a set of specific sex-related questions of all new patients attending an out-patient clinic.[47] These physicians were then compared to nontrained colleagues. After the visit, physicians completed a questionnaire and patients were interviewed concerning their encounter with the physician. The following results were noteworthy and instructive:

1. More than half of the patients had one or more sexual problems or areas of concern
2. Age and sex did not influence the prevalence of sexual problems
3. Many more patients (82%) who saw trained physicians were asked about sexual functioning than those who saw untrained physicians (32%)
4. Among both groups of physicians, discussions about sexual issues were more likely if the patient was less than 44 years old
5. Ninety one percent of the entire group of patients thought that a discussion about sexual issues was, or would be, appropriate in a medical context and approval was almost unanimous (98%) among patients whose physician had, in fact, included a sex history
6. Age of the patient was not a factor in the determination of appropriateness
7. Thirty eight percent of the entire patient group thought that follow-up for sexual problems would be helpful
8. Physicians found that, in many instances, the sex history was helpful in ways other than simply as a means to identify sexual problems or concerns

In summary, medical students, family practice residents, and physicians in clinical practice in the community have all been studied on the issue of sex history-taking. The following factors appear to influence the learning process:

1. Having talked to patients about sexual issues in the past
2. Having a sexual problem oneself and having discussed it with a health professional
3. The sexual orientation of the patient
4. Having a homosexual friend
5. The belief that asking about sexual issues is relevant to the patient's concerns
6. Having received specific training
7. Social and cultural issues

STUDIES IN MEDICAL EDUCATION ON SEX HISTORY-TAKING IN RELATION TO HIV/AIDS

There is little question that HIV/AIDS is the major impetus for the recent teaching of sex history-taking in medical schools and the promotion of sex history-taking among practicing physicians. This development results from the knowledge that sexual activity represents the prime method of viral transmission. Many agree with the statement "that the taking of a candid and nonjudgmental sexual history is the cornerstone of HIV preventive education. . ."[48] Recognition of the crucial position of physicians in HIV prevention has resulted in several studies of physician sex history-taking practices.

In general, studies of physicians with different levels of medical education and experience (e.g., internal medicine residents, primary care clinicians) and using various research techniques (e.g., standardized patients, telephone interviews) indicate the infrequency and/or inadequacy of history-taking around vulnerability to HIV/AIDS infection and the consequent inability to take preventive measures.[48,49-52] One of these surveys demonstrated that in spite of the finding that 68% of 768 respondents said they had received "human sexuality training" in medical school, only a small minority of primary care physicians routinely screened patients for high-risk sexual behavior.[51] "Sexuality Training" was evidently helpful *after the fact*, since physicians who received this training in their medical education "felt more comfortable in caring for patients known to be infected. . ." with HIV. Another study showed that while self-reports of questions concerning homosexuality doubled and questions about the number of sexual partners tripled, questions concerning sexual practices increased by only 50% over the five years of the project (1984-89).[53] Yet another study demonstrated that only 35% of primary care physicians reported that they routinely (100%) or often (75%) took a sex history from their patients. Less than 20% of those who took histories reported asking questions regarding sexual activities that increase the risk of acquiring HIV/AIDS.[54]

> In spite of the finding that 68% of 768 respondents said they received "human sexuality training" in medical school, only a small minority of primary care physicians routinely screened patients for high-risk sexual behavior.

Two particularly revealing projects involved a visit to primary care clinicians by a simulated patient. In the first study, physicians agreed to participate after being told that a simulated patient would appear in their practice.[55] The "patient" was female in order to include obstetrician-gynecologists. Other than obtaining prior agreement, the "patient" was unannounced. She revealed the following information:

- That she had been exposed to *Chlamydia* by a previous partner
- She expressed interest in engaging in sexual activities with a new partner
- She wanted to talk about concerns regarding STDs generally and HIV in particular

Comparisons were subsequently made between the report of the "patient" and the self-report of the physician on several issues, including risk assessment and counseling recommendations. The greatest discrepancies (all of which involved physicians overestimating their history-taking skills in the opinion of the "patient") occurred with the following topics:

- STD history
- Patient use of IV drugs
- Patient sexual orientation
- Condom use
- Counseling concerning anal intercourse and use of a condom
- Safe alternatives to intercourse

In the second simulated-patient study, the "patient" had a history of engaging in sexual activities that made her vulnerable to HIV/AIDS infection.[56] Physicians were provided with educational materials before the visit. Whether these materials were used or not did not alter the finding that the questions least frequently asked of the "patient" were about oral or anal sex practices, sexual orientation, and the use of condoms. The authors concluded that there was a need for prevention training.

From these HIV/AIDS-related studies, one might conclude that the generic form of "Human Sexuality" training in medical schools seems to result in greater acceptance toward those who *already have* HIV/AIDS but it is insufficient in *preventing* transmission. Effective preventive behavior by physicians evidently requires more specific curricular intervention that addresses history-taking skills and, in particular, inquiry about patient sexual practices.

> The generic form of "Human Sexuality" training in medical schools seems to result in greater acceptance toward those who already have HIV/AIDS but it is insufficient in *preventing transmission.* Effective preventive behavior by physicians evidently requires more specific curricular intervention that addresses history-taking skills and, in particular, inquiry about patient sexual practices.

What, Then , Is the Definition of a Sex (or Sexual) History?

Is taking a sex history by a family physician who has only a few minutes to ask questions about sexual issues and wants to concentrate on, for example, STDs and HIV/AIDS-related sexual behavior the same as for a forensic psychiatrist who is evaluating a patient referred because of pedophilia? Is it the same (in time and content) for a health professional asking questions about child sexual abuse as for an interviewer involved in a population survey in which each interview might take hours to complete? Is it the same for a clinical psychologist or psychiatrist who asks a few screening questions as part of the assessment of a patient who is depressed as it is for a clinical sexologist who is evaluating a couple referred specifically because of erectile problems?

The answer to these questions is obviously "no." In all these situations, the result might be called a "sex history" but the time involved and the questions asked would be quite different. Rather than use the singular, it might be more reasonable to talk in the plural, that is, of sex histories—inquiries that are sexual in nature but differ because of the diverse requirements of the situations. In fact, instead of considering a "sex history" or "sex histories," it may be easier to simply think about the task of talking to a patient about sexual matters.

> Instead of considering a sex history or sex histories, it may be easier to simply think about the task of talking to a patient about sexual matters

A primary care clinician must therefore be skilled in talking to patients about a variety of sexual issues, depending, among other things, on the patient, the problem presented, the amount of time available for questioning, and the context in which the patient is seen.

Practical Aspects of Introducing Sexual Questions Into a Health-related History

Practical aspects of talking to patients about sexual matters can be viewed in the context of the familiar format of why, who, where, when, how, and what. This conceptual arrangement has been used elsewhere in dissecting this subject but the content here is different.[1] So is the order. Issues that involve the manner in which questions are phrased (how) are considered in Chapter 2, and which questions to ask (what) are discussed in Chapters 3, 4, and 5.

Why Discussion May Not Occur (Box 1-1)

The following may be reasons why discussions of sexual topics in a health care setting do not occur:

1. Not knowing what to do with the answers is the most common reason given by physicians in particular for avoiding the topic of "sex" in medical history-taking. When investigating what this explanation means, two factors become evident:

   > Not knowing what to do with the answer is the most common reason given by physicians for avoiding the topic of sex.

   - Uncertainty about what the next question should be
   - Perplexity regarding what to offer the patient after all the questions are asked and "Pandora's box" is opened

2. Worry that patients might be offended by an inquiry into this area is a recurrent theme of medical students. In spite of the almost uninhibited media display of sexuality, many people (including medical students and physicians) continue to regard sexual issues as "personal" and are concerned that questions in this area might be regarded as intrusive.

3. Lack of justification is a common explanation given by medical students for the frequent omission of sexual topics from medical histories. However, when some medical problems are presented to a physician, specific aspects of a person's sexual life experience are often the subjects of inquiry (e.g., issues that may be medically relevant). Examples include:

   - Sexual dysfunctions associated with diabetes mellitus[57]
   - Sexual sequelae of child sexual abuse[35]

   Thus it seems as if an association between "sex" and a medical disorder must be *demonstrated* before there is sufficient rationale to include sex-related questions in a medical history. A closely related issue is doubt among some health professionals about the acceptability of sexual issues in health care apart from disorders that affect others (such as STDs).

4. Talking with older patients about sexual matters appears difficult for health professional students. The age of the student may be relevant, since many are much younger than their patients. The student may find that this situation resembles talking with their parents about the subject (an experience that most would not have had and that may be thought of as highly embarrassing if it did occur). Avoidance of discussing sexual issues with older patients is particularly unfortunate because some sexual difficulties clearly become more common with increasing age. For example, menopause in women can result in discomfort with intercourse, which, in turn, is explained by decreased estrogen, resulting in diminished vaginal lubrication.[58] Menopausal women will obviously not be well served by the medical establishment if they are not asked about discomfort or pain with intercourse. Not surprisingly, when women in general are surveyed on the acceptability of talking to a physician about sexual concerns, almost three fourths think that it is appropriate to do so. Moreover, the response seems to be age related in that approval *increases* with age.[59]

Box 1-1

Why 'Sex' Questions Are Not Asked

1. Unclear what to do with the answers
   Unfamiliarity with treatment approaches
   • Uncertainty about the next question
2. Fear of offending patient
3. Lack of obvious justification
4. Generational obstacles
5. Fear of sexual misconduct charge
6. Sometimes perceived irrelevant
7. Unfamiliarity with some sexual practices

---

5. Magnified concerns about professional sexual misconduct and consequent licensure problems result in reluctance by some health professionals to initiate conversations with patients about sexual issues. The primary organization responsible for medical malpractice insurance in Canada has, in an exaggerated way, cautioned their clients about discussions with patients on the subject of sex and has thereby magnified the already difficult problem of health professional restraint.[60]

6. The appropriateness of sex-related questions in the acute stage of an illness may be viewed by the health professional as a dubious focus because of more pressing patient concerns. An example is when the patient has little opportunity for sexual experiences with a partner (e.g., a situation that occurs when a patient is in hospital). In this illustration, sex is defined narrowly as related only to the function of the genitalia.

7. Unfamiliarity with some sexual practices (e.g., gay patients talking to a heterosexual physician) may restrain the health professional from introducing the topic.

Why Discussion Should Occur (Box 1-2)

Reasons why discussions should occur in a health care setting include the following:

1. HIV/AIDS, as everyone knows, is a *sexually* transmitted disease that is also lethal. It has become a powerful (perhaps, *the* most convincing) stimulus for sex history-taking by health professionals (see introduction to Part I).[61] Considering HIV/AIDS, prevention is, at the moment, the best deterrent. This, in turn, means talking to patients about their sexual practices. As used here, the term *sexual practices* refers to:

> Considering HIV/AIDS, prevention is the best deterrent. This means talking to patients about their sexual practices.

   • The types of sexual *activities* engaged in by the patient, as well as the nature of *relationships* with sexual partners
   • The characteristics of sexual *partners*
   • The *"toys"* (mechanical adjuncts such as vibrators) used in sexual activities
   • Methods used to prevent STD transmission and conception

In the words of Hearst: "Responsible primary care physicians no longer have the option of deciding whether to do AIDS prevention; the question today is how to do it. . . ."[62] Health professionals are simply not fulfilling their role if inquiry is not made about sexual practices, and if, in the process, the opportunity for dispensing preventive sexual advice is lost. Physicians, in particular, are thought to be in a unique position to prevent HIV infection, since 70% of adults in the United States visit a physician at least once each year and 90% do so at least once in five years.[51]

> Physicians are thought to be in a unique position to prevent HIV infection, since 70 percent of adults in the United States visit a physician at least once each year and 90% do so at least once in five years

2. Many medical disorders such as depression[63] and diabetes[57] are known to disrupt sexual function. A comprehensive view of such disorders is plainly impossible without also asking how a patient's sexual function is affected (see Chapter 8).

3. Treatments such as surgery[64] or drugs[65] can interrupt sexual function. A health professional should inquire about drug side effects (see Chapter 8 and Appendix III).

4. Inquiry into past sexual events may be essential to understand the nature of a disorder in the present. Such is the case with lack of sexual desire after sexual assault as an adult or child (See Chapters 8 and 9).[66]

5. The observation that ". . .sexual function is a lifelong capacity, not normally diminished by middle or older age" represents a change in social attitudes.[67] The aging of the population translates into increasing expectations by many patients regarding sexual function. These hopes may conflict with the difficulty that many young health professionals experience in discussing sexual matters with older people.

6. Sexual dysfunctions are common, at least on an objective level.[68] So, too, are sexual difficulties. Intuitively, it seems reasonable for a health professional to ask particularly about problems that occur most frequently (sexual dysfunctions and difficulties) as compared to problems that are unusual.

7. On the topic of sex as well as others, health professionals tend to be problem oriented. This book and many others on the same subject admittedly "focus on the darker side. . .more than on its brighter side"[38] (p. 351). However, the "other side" is what happens when "things go right." Laumann and colleagues (see introduction to PART I) addressed this side of sex in their chapter (brief by their own admission) on the association between sex, and health and happiness (pp. 351-375).

Sexual activity and good health are related. Of patients in the Laumann et al. study who had no sexual partners in the past 12 months, most (6% versus 2% of the entire sample) were in poor health.[38] Sexual activity and happiness were correlated. Of those who considered themselves "extremely or very happy" (compared to those who were "generally satisfied" or "unhappy"), three groups of respondents were most prominent:

- Those who had one sexual partner
- Those who had "sex" two to three times per week
- Women who "always" or "usually" experienced orgasm in partnered sex (p. 358)

The association between "sex," emotional satisfaction, and physical pleasure was examined also in the Laumann et al. study[38] (pp. 363-368). Those who found their relationships "extremely or very" pleasurable or satisfying were more often the people who had one (versus more than one) sex partner, especially if the partner was a spouse or there was a cohabitational relationship (p. 364). The authors commented that while "association is not causation (p. 364)," "the quality of the sex is higher and the skill in achieving satisfaction and pleasure is greater when one's limited capacity to please is focused on one partner in the context of a monogamous, long-term partnership"(p. 365).

8. Why not? Masters and Johnson asked this question (still germane more than 25 years later) in a medical journal editorial that did not receive the attention that it seemingly deserved.[69] They were critical of the opinion that physicians apparently needed special justification for asking "sex" questions while paradoxically being taught to ask questions about everything else in the course of a general medical examination. "The biologic and behavioral professions must accept the concept that sexual information should be as integral a part of the routine medical history as a discussion of bowel or bladder function."

9. Not including sexual matters in a health history can sometimes be considered negligent and possibly unethical. An example is the second case history provided in the introduction to PART I. In that instance, the physician (in a "sin" of omission rather than commission) clearly failed the medical dictum of "do no harm."

Who (which patients) Should Be Asked About Sexual Issues?

Almost all patients should be given the *opportunity* to talk about a sexual concern in a health professional setting. Providing such an opportunity does not mean asking a "sex" question but rather using a method that involves asking if it's OK to ask a "sex" question (see "Permission" in Chapter 2 and an example of a specific permission question in Chapter 3).

> Almost all patients should be given the opportunity to talk about a sexual concern in a health professional setting.

Common sense dictates at least two exceptions to routinely giving everyone an opportunity to talk about sexual issues. First, it obviously

---

Box 1-2

Why Ask Questions About "Sex"?

1. Morbidity and mortality—STDs and HIV/AIDS
2. Symptoms of illness
3. Treatment side effects
4. Past may explain present problems
5. Function potentially lifelong
6. Dysfunctions and difficulties are common
7. Association with health and happiness
8. Why not?
9. May be negligent if ignored

does not apply to an emergency setting (unless, for example, the emergency is sexual in nature, such as sexual asphyxia [see Chapter 8 for definition]). Rather it applies to situations such as the first few visits of an "intake" procedure. Second, when applied to physicians, the idea of routinely giving everyone this opportunity relates more to generalists, that is, primary care specialists (e.g., in medicine: family physicians, pediatricians, gynecologists, and internists) and medical specialists whose area of work is directly related to sexual function (e.g., urologists). Providing an opportunity to talk about sexual issues on a routine basis rather than a selective basis does not apply to medical specialty areas such as Ophthalmology and ENT (ear, nose, and throat).

Where (in a health professional history) Should Questions Be Asked About Sex?

Sometimes, a patient spontaneously indicates that a sexual concern is the principal reason for the visit. When this occurs, the sexual problem obviously has priority. However, such information usually has to be elicited carefully. In a medical setting, three different circumstances (not mutually exclusive) exist in which this could happen:

1. The prime location in a medical history for asking about sex-related information is within a Review of Systems (ROS [sometimes referred to as a Functional Inquiry]; see "Permission" in Chapter 2 for an example). A ROS consists of a few questions about each body system to ensure that nothing is wrong with a patient other than the initial complaint(s). In such a context, a few additional questions about sexual concerns could be easily included.

2. Another possibility for the introduction of questions about sexual issues is within a Personal and Social History. For example, in the process of asking about relationships, one could ask about sexual concerns.

3. A sex-related question could be asked during a physical examination (least desirable and an option that is, obviously, unavailable to nonphysicians). For example, one could ask about genital function in the process of examining genitalia. In one sense, this situation is easier for physicians, since it seems that psychological defenses of patients are diminished when their clothes are off. However, the lowering of defenses during a physical examination can be hazardous to the patient because questions about sexual issues can be misinterpreted as a physician's sexual invitation and the patient's misconception could provoke a charge of sexual harassment or misconduct. Although sex-related questions during a physical examination may represent a more efficient use of professional time, the potential for misunderstanding is sufficiently great that this method should be avoided.

> The lowering of defenses during a physical examination can be hazardous to the patient because questions about sexual issues can be misinterpreted as a sexual invitation by the physician and the patient's misconception could provoke a charge of sexual harassment or misconduct. Although sex-related questions during a physical examination may represent a more efficient use of professional time, the potential for misunderstanding is sufficiently great that this method should be avoided.

When Should Questions About Sex Be Asked?

Green offered a clear and sensible opinion on when questions should be asked about sexual issues: "The optimal time. . .is not when a patient's initial visit has been prompted by influenza, otitis media and bronchitis. Nor is the appropriate time the anniversary of the physician-patient relationship. . .Delay in approaching the topic communicates discomfort. The effect when 'the subject' is finally broached is comparable to the painfully familiar scene of a father who initiates discussion of the 'facts of life' with his son on his 13th birthday."[1] Generally speaking, the aphorism of 'the earlier the better' should be applied. Screening questions (see Chapter 3) can be introduced after the acute problem that initially led the patient to the health professional has disappeared or is under control.

If a problem is introduced in the process of screening, more detailed diagnostically oriented questions can be asked on a subsequent occasion (see Chapter 4). The diagnostic process may involve a physical examination (see Chapter 6) and the use of laboratory tests (see PART II).

SUMMARY

Extrapolations from studies on general aspects of health- related interviewing and history-taking imply the following:

1. Concerning sexual issues, teaching of skills by direct supervision and feedback should be included in health science educational programs
2. An interviewer can attend to both factual information and feelings
3. Faculty modeling in obtaining information about the patient's psychosocial status and risk factors is a significant element in the learning process

When considering the integration of sex-related questions into a general health history, interviewing texts, books on "Human Sexuality," and journal articles appear to be of limited practical help.

Studies in sex history-taking have involved medical students, residents, and practicing physicians. The studies can be separated into ones that considered sex history-taking in general and those that focused on the specific subject of STDs. In the former group, factors found to be associated with positive attitudes toward sex history-taking and conducting such a history were:

1. Personal sexual experience
2. The belief that such questions were relevant to the patient's chief complaint
3. Feeling adequately trained
4. Confidence in taking a sex history
5. Having previously taken a sex history
6. Having spoken to a health professional oneself about a sexual concern
7. Having a homosexual friend
8. Social and cultural factors
9. Skill training (as compared to personal comfort and self-awareness)

Studies that focused on "sex" history-taking as it applies to HIV/AIDS prevention indicate that relevant questions occur infrequently and inadequately. Previous "sexuality training" appeared to be helpful to physicians in caring for those already infected with HIV but it was insufficient in the process of preventing transmission, which, in turn, required an inquiry into the sexual practices of the patient.

Rather than attempting to define a "sex" history (there are many such definitions), it might be more productive to simply talk about asking questions of patients about sexual matters. One might consider the introduction of such questions under the headings of Who, What, When, Where, Why, and How.

Reasons why "sex" history-taking does *not* regularly occur include:

1. Not knowing what to do with the answers
2. Concern that patients might regard "sex" questions as intrusive
3. Lack of a sense of justification
4. Difficulty in talking to older patients about this subject
5. Concern about accusations of sexual misconduct
6. The sense that such questions are inappropriate in the context of other difficulties manifested by the patient
7. Lack of familiarity with some sexual practices

Reasons why "sex" questions *should* occur in a health history include finding that:

1. Such questions provide an opportunity to introduce HIV/AIDS prevention information
2. Disrupted sexual function may be a symptom of a medical disorder or it may be a side effect of its treatment
3. Past sexual history may help explain the present
4. Sexual issues are important at all stages of the life cycle
5. Sexual dysfunctions in particular are quite common
6. Sexual function is related to general health
7. There is no explanation for not asking questions of a sexual nature
8. Not asking "sex" questions may constitute negligence from a legal point of view

The problem of who should be asked questions about sexual issues can be resolved by saying that almost everyone should have the *opportunity* to talk about sexual concerns if they so choose. Other than situations in which a sexual problem is the main issue that brought the patient to the health professional, questions can be asked in the context of a medical review of systems (ROS) or a personal and social history. Physicians may also ask questions during a physical examination but caution should be exercised because of the possibility of misinterpretation of the intent and consequent accusations of sexual misconduct. It may be easier to say when the time to ask such questions is not optimal than when it is.

"Sex" questions are improper in the midst of concern over some other issue that brought the patient to the attention of the health professional. (Questions about many topics are reasonably omitted in such situations). The context for "sex" questions is after the acute problem subsides and the professional is reviewing general aspects of the patient's health history.

The "how" (or methods used) of asking "sex" questions is considered in detail in Chapter 2 and is therefore not included here. Similarly, the "what" (content) did not form part of Chapter 1, since it forms the content of Chapters 3, 4, and 5 and subsequent portions of the book.

REFERENCES

1. Green R: Taking a sexual history. In Green R (editor): *Human sexuality: a health practitioner's text*, ed 2, Baltimore and London, 1979, Williams and Wilkins, pp 22-30.
2. Pomeroy WB, Flax CC, Wheeler CC: *Taking a sex history: interviewing and recording*, New York, 1982, The Free Press.
3. Risen CB: A guide to taking a sexual history, *Psychiatr Clin North Am* 18(1):39-53, 1995.
4. Morrison J: *The first interview: revised for DSM-IV*, New York, 1995, The Guilford Press.
5. Rutter M, Cox A: Psychiatric interviewing techniques: 1. methods and measures, *Br J Psychiatry* 138:273-282, 1981.
6. Maguire P et al: The value of feedback in teaching interviewing skills to medical students, *Psychol Med* 8:695- 704, 1978.
7. Maguire P, Fairbairn S, Fletcher C: Consultation skills of young doctors: 1—benefits of feedback training in interviewing as students persist, *Br Med J* 292:1573-1576, 1986.
8. Stone H, Angevine M, Sivertson S: A model for evaluating the history taking and physical examination skills of medical students, *Med Teach* 11:75-80, 1989.
9. Cox A, Holbrook D, Rutter M: Psychiatric interviewing techniques VI. Experimental study: eliciting feelings, *Br J Psychiatry* 139:144-152, 1981.
10. Hopkinson K, Cox A, Rutter M: Psychiatric interviewing techniques III. Naturalistic study: eliciting feelings, *Br J Psychiatry* 139:406-415, 1981.
11. Rutter M et al: Psychiatric interviewing techniques IV. Experimental study: four contrasting styles, *Br J Psychiatry* 138:456-465, 1981.
12. Cox A, Rutter M, Holbrook D: Psychiatric interviewing techniques V. Experimental study: eliciting factual information, *Br J Psychiatry* 139:29-37, 1981.
13. Cox A, Holbrook D, Rutter M: Psychiatric interviewing techniques VI. Experimental study: eliciting feelings, *Br J Psychiatry* 139:144-152, 1981.
14. Cox A, Rutter M, Holbrook D: Psychiatric interviewing techniques—a second experimental study: eliciting feelings, *Br J Psychiatry* 152:64-72, 1988.
15. Kaplan HS: Sex is psychosomatic (editorial), *J Sex Marital Ther* 1:275-276, 1975.
16. Rezler AG, Woolliscroft JA, Kalishman SG: What is missing from patient histories? *Med Teach* 13:245-252, 1991.
17. Newell R: *Interviewing skills for nurses and other health care professionals*, London, 1994, Routledge.
18. Attarian P: The sexual history. In Levinson D (editor): *A guide to the clinical interview*, Philadelphia, 1987, W.B. Saunders Company, pp 226-234.
19. Long LG, Higgins PG, Brady D: *Psychosocial assessment: a pocket guide for data collection*, Norwalk, 1988, Appleton & Lange, pp 105-117.
20. Turnbull J: Interviewing the patient with a sexual problem. In Leon RL: *Psychiatric interviewing: a primer*, ed 2, New York, 1989, Elsevier Science Publishing Co., Inc., pp 151-155.
21. Kraytman M: *The complete patient history*, ed 2, New York, 1991, McGraw-Hill, pp 468-470.
22. Lloyd M, Bor R: *Communication skills for medicine*, Edinburgh, 1996, Churchill Livingstone, pp 73-84.
23. Coulehan JL, Block MR: *The medical interview: a primer for students of the art*, ed 2, Philadelphia, 1992, F.A. Davis Company, pp 217-224.
24. Shea SC: *Psychiatric interviewing: the art of understanding*, Philadelphia, 1988, W.B. Saunders Company.
25. Othmer EO, Othmer SC: *The clinical interview using DSM-IV*, vol 1, *Fundamentals* and vol 2, *The difficult patient*, Washington, 1994, American Psychiatric Press, Inc.
26. Mackinnon RA: *The psychiatric interview in clinical practice*, Philadelphia, 1971, W.B. Saunders Company, pp 115- 117.
27. Cohen-Cole SA: *The medical interview: the three-function approach*, St. Louis, 1991, Mosby-Year Book, Inc., p 82.
28. MacKinnon RA, Yudofsky SC: *Principles of the psychiatric evaluation*, Philadelphia, 1991, J.B. Lippincott Company, pp 53-54.

29. Aldrich CK: *The medical interview: gateway to the doctor- patient relationship*, New York, 1993, The Parthenon Publishing Group, pp 102-104.

30. Semmens JP, Semmens FJ: The sexual history and physical examination. In Barnard MU, Clancy BJ, Krantz KE (editors): *Human sexuality for health professionals*, Philadelphia, 1978, W.B. Saunders Company, pp 27-43.

31. Marcotte DB: Sexual history taking. In Nadelson CC, Marcotte DB (editors): *Treatment interventions in human sexuality*, New York, 1983, Plenum Press, pp 1-9.

32. Hogan RM: *Human sexuality: a nursing perspective*, ed 2, Norwalk, 1985, Appleton-Century-Crofts, pp 161-173.

33. Lewis CE: Sexual practices: are physicians addressing the issues? *J Gen Intern Med* 5(5 suppl):S78-81, 1990.

34. Gabel LL, Pearsol JA: Taking an effective sexual and drug history: a first step in HIV/AIDS prevention, *J Fam Prac* 37:185-187, 1993.

35. Wyatt G: Child sexual abuse and its effects on sexual functioning, *Annual Review of Sex Research* 2:249-266, 1991.

36. Alexander B: Taking the sexual history, *Am Fam Physician* 23:147, 1981.

37. Kinsey AC, Pomeroy WB, Martin CE: *Sexual behavior in the human male*, Philadelphia and London, 1949, W.B. Saunders.

38. Laumann EO et al: *The social organization of sexuality: sexual practices in the United States*, Chicago, 1994, The University of Chicago Press.

39. Johnson AM et al: *Sexual attitudes and lifestyles*, Oxford, 1994, Blackwell Scientific Publications.

40. Spira A, Bajos N, and the ACSF group: *Sexual behavior and AIDS*, Brookfield, 1994, Ashgate Publishing Company.

41. Vollmer SA, Wells KB: How comfortable do first-year medical students expect to be when taking sexual histories? *Med Educ* 22:418-425, 1988.

42. Vollmer SA, Wells KB: The preparedness of freshman medical students for taking sexual histories, *Arch Sex Behav* 18:167-177, 1989.

43. Vollmer SA et al: Improving the preparation of preclinical students for taking sexual histories, *Acad Med* 64:474-479, 1989.

44. Merrill JM, Laux LF, Thornby JI: Why doctors have difficulty with sex histories, *South Med J* 83:613-617, 1990.

45. Hunt AD, Litt IF, Loebner M: Obtaining a sexual history from adolescent girls: a preliminary report of the influence of age and ethnicity, *J Adolesc Health Care* 9:52-54, 1988.

46. Liese BS et al: An experimental study of two methods for teaching sexual history taking skills, *Fam Med* 21:21-24, 1989.

47. Ende JE, Rockwell S, Glasgow M: The sexual history in general medicine practice, *Arch Intern Med* 144:558-561, 1984.

48. Calabrese LH et al: Physicians' attitudes, beliefs, and practices regarding AIDS health-care promotion, *Arch Intern Med* 151:1157-1160, 1991.

49. Bresolin LB et al: Attitudes of U.S. primary care physicians about HIV disease and AIDS, *AIDS Care* 2:117-125, 1990.

50. Boekeloo BO et al: Frequency and thoroughness of STD/HIV risk assessment by physicians in a high-risk metropolitan area, *Am J Public Health* 81:1645-1648, 1991.

51. Ferguson KJ, Stapleton JT, Helms CM: Physicians' effectiveness in assessing risk for human immunodeficiency virus infections, *Arch Intern Med* 151:561-564, 1991.

52. Curtis JR et al: Internal medicine residents' skills at identification of HIV-risk behavior and HIV-related disease, *Acad Med* 69:S45-47, 1994.

53. Lewis CE, Montgomery K: The AIDS-related experiences and practices of primary care physicians in Los Angeles: 1984-89, *Am J Public Health* 80:1511-1513, 1990.

54. McCance KL, Moser R Jr., Smith KR: A survey of physicians' knowledge and application of AIDS prevention capabilities, *Am J Prev Med* 7(3):141-145, 1991.

55. Russell NK et al: Extending the skills measured with standardized patient examinations: using unannounced simulated patients to evaluate sexual risk assessment and risk reduction skills of practicing physicians, *Acad Med* 66 (Sept Suppl), S37-S39, 1991.

56. Bowman MA et al: The effect of educational preparation on physician performance with a sexually transmitted disease-simulated patient, *Arch Intern Med* 152:1823-1828, 1992.

57. Schiavi RC et al: Diabetes mellitus and male sexual function, *Diabetologia* 36:745-751, 1993.

58. Masters WH, Johnson VE: *Human sexual response*, Boston, 1966, Little, Brown and Company, p 240.

59. Maurice WL, Sheps SB, Schechter MT: *Physician sexual contact with patients: 2. A public survey of women in British Columbia*. Paper presented at the meeting of the Society for Sex Therapy and Research, New York, March 1995.

60. *Information letter, Can Med Protect Assoc* 7:2, 1992.

61. Canadian AIDS Society. *Safer sex guidelines: health sexuality and HIV*, Ottawa, 1994, *Can AIDS Society*.

62. Hearst N: AIDS risk assessment in primary care, *J Am Board Fam* Pract 7(1):44-48, 1994.

63. Nofzinger EA et al: Sexual function in depressed men, *Arch Gen Psychiatry* 50:24-30, 1993.

64. Yavetz H et al: Retrograde ejaculation, *Hum Reprod* 93:381-386, 1994.

65. Barnes TRE, Harvey CA: *Psychiatric drugs and sexuality*. In Riley AJ, Peet M, Wilson C (editors): *Sexual pharmacology*, New York, 1993, Oxford University Press.

66. Becker JV et al: Level of postassault sexual functioning in rape and incest victims, *Arch Sex Behav* 15:37-49, 1986.

67. Tiefer L, Melman A: Comprehensive evaluation of erectile dysfunction and medical treatments. In Leiblum SR, Rosen RC (editors): *Principles and practice of sex therapy: update for the 1990s*, ed 2, New York, 1989, The Guilford Press, p 208.

68. Frank E, Anderson C, Rubenstein D: Frequency of sexual dysfunction in normal couples, *N Engl J Med* 299:111-115, 1978.

69. Masters WH, Johnson VE: Undue distinction of sex, *N Engl J Med* 281:1422-1423, 1969.

CHAPTER 2

TALKING ABOUT SEXUAL ISSUES: INTERVIEWING METHODS

. . . with respect to discourse on sexuality there is major discontinuity between the sensibilities of politicians and other self-appointed guardians of the moral order and those of the public at large, who, on the whole, display few hang-ups in discussing sexual issues in appropriately structured circumstances.

LAUMANN ET AL, 1994[1]

Clinicians experienced in talking to people about their sexual difficulties would not question the above quote. When the "appropriately structured circumstances" represent a health setting, patients display little hesitation in talking about sexual matters if they are talking with a health professional who knows what questions to ask and shows no embarrassment. A polished interviewer can often accommodate patient sensitivity with the topic of "sex" but an awkward interviewer presents a predicament for the patient. Some patients decide not to continue when they experience obvious interviewer discomfort and simply find someone else with whom to talk. However, in relation to sexual worries, a lengthy period of time may (and often does) intervene. Years (rather than months or weeks) typically transpire between one unsuccessful effort and a subsequent attempt to talk with a health professional about a sexual problem.

A married couple, both 37 years old, were distressed about their inability to have intercourse. The man had erection difficulties. While the couple developed mutually gratifying sexual experiences apart from intercourse, they were unable to conceive. In the past, they were referred to a physician because of the physician's expertise in the treatment of infertility. Both partners described the physician's impatient attitude that was directed toward the woman. The physician indicated bluntly that she could not find anything wrong during the examination and displayed little feeling for the woman's obvious fear of vaginal entry. The physician suggested that surgery would make the vaginal opening larger. Both partners were uncomfortable with this idea and with the physician's abrupt manner. They stopped seeing her after two visits.

Although they thought about consulting a health professional who was experienced in the treatment of sexual and reproductive difficulties, they were concerned about a repetition of the experience with the first physician. It was another two years before they talked with someone else. The new physician's sensitivity, patience, and skill in treating vaginismus allowed the couple to eventually have intercourse, and conception occurred.

PRELIMINARY ISSUES

Rapport

"Rapport" is one aspect of the health professional/patient encounter that governs other elements of the interview. Like an umbrella, it covers the way *all* information is collected, rather than one specific issue. Rapport means the development of a physician/patient relationship based on trust and respect and within which information can be readily obtained. Developing rapport involves interviewing (the manner in which information is acquired) more than history-taking (the content of the information itself). A health professional engenders rapport in ways that include the following:

1. Demonstration of a caring attitude
2. Respect for the patient and the concerns voiced
3. The manner used in asking questions

Rapport seems more fragile around the topic of "sex" than around other issues. The explanations for this sensitivity are not difficult to find. In talking about sex, the patient:

1. Trustingly reveals something very personal to a health professional
2. Hopes for an empathic and knowledgeable response
3. Really doesn't know what to expect

> An interviewer's lack of familiarity with a sexual word or sexual practice can be declared candidly with a minimum loss of respect from the patient, or even the opposite—enhanced regard because of the willingness to acknowledge one's limits.

If the patient encounters embarrassment, rapport (regarding this subject) is diminished. Yet, some uneasiness is to be expected from anyone who is a novice in talking to patients about sexual issues. (With experience—it is surprising how little is needed—one learns to be more composed). If discomfort is obvious, candor and honesty by the interviewer will minimize the loss of rapport. Lack of familiarity with a sexual word or a sexual practice can be declared candidly with a minimum loss of respect from the patient, or even the opposite—enhanced regard because of the willingness to acknowledge one's limits.

Interviewing Versus History-taking

What appears to be missing from interviewing books directed toward health professionals are suggestions about *how* to ask sex-related questions (interviewing), quite apart from *what* to ask (history-taking). The nature of questions may be less disconcerting to patients than the way in which questions are asked.

How, rather than *what*, to ask involves interviewing techniques, some of which are particularly advantageous when talking specifically about sexual issues. There are at least ten such methods (Box 2-1). The use of some of the ten methods are illustrated in Appendices I and II.

INTERVIEWING METHODS

Permission

It is not unusual for "sex experts" to explain the absence of sex-related questions in an interview on the "hang-ups" of the interviewer. Health professionals, however, tend to "blame" the patient for the sex-information gap by saying that to have asked about this

---

Box 2-1

Interviewing Methods

1. Ask patient's PERMISSION
2. Interviewer takes INITIATIVE
3. LANGUAGE: MEDICAL/TECHNICAL versus slang
4. STATEMENT/QUESTION TECHNIQUE
5. PRIVACY/CONFIDENTIALITY/SECURITY
6. DELAY SENSITIVE QUESTIONS
7. Display NONJUDGMENTAL attitude
8. Provide EXPLANATION
9. Discuss FEELINGS
10. Promote OPTIMISTIC ATTITUDE

---

subject would have risked alienating the person being interviewed. One way to eliminate blame entirely is for the interviewer to simply request the patient's permission to ask a question about this topic.

The permission technique accomplishes the following objectives:

1. It erases the health professional's worries about being intrusive, since it becomes the patient's responsibility to decide on the acceptability of the topic
2. The interviewer shows respect for the patient and sensitivity toward the patient's feelings
3. Control is explicitly given to the patient by offering the possibility of saying "no"

Chapter 3 offers some suggested responses if, indeed, a patient declines the invitation. Some *will* refuse but most will not. Many actually want to discuss sexual concerns with a health professional. This was illustrated in a random sample survey of 6000 women in the Canadian province of British Columbia.[2] The study pertained to the subject of physician's sexual involvement with patients. Among other things, subjects were asked to respond to the statement that it is "OK for the doctor to ask a question about sexual problems as part of a general check-up on an adult patient." The majority (73.6%) of the 2079 respondents agreed. This opinion was *positively correlated with the age respondent*, a finding that was enlightening in view of the particular difficulty that many young interviewers seem to have when talking about sexual issues with older people (especially older women).

Of course, asking permission to talk about sex makes this topic different in any health setting. Some physicians object to asking permission for this very reason, that is, because one does not ask permission to talk with a patient, for example, about liver function or depression. However, tradition seems to allow physicians to ask about, for example, liver function and depression, whereas talking about the subject of sex in a medical context is to be viewed favor-

> Asking permission may perpetuate the idea that this topic is something special. Little appreciation is thus given to the fact that for many people "sex" is a special subject. Community attitudes dictate this distinction rather than health professional behavior.

ably only when the justification is proven (as in relation to, for example, diabetes or HIV/AIDS). Asking permission may perpetuate the idea that this topic is something special. Little appreciation is thus given to the fact that for many people "sex" *is* a special subject. Community attitudes dictate this distinction rather than health professional behavior. The concept of asking permission reflects a need to be sensitive to popular feeling and thus becomes a practical (rather than ideological) matter for the interviewer.

The permission technique can be used effectively in an interview in two ways: (1) entering the field of "sex" generally and (2) asking about a particular and potentially sensitive aspect of "sex":

A 54-year-old man went to see his family physician because of shortness of breath associated with exertion. The physician conducted a thorough history, during which he included a "review of systems" (ROS). The physician routinely included sexual matters in his ROS and used the permission technique to initiate a discussion on this subject. He typically did this with men after asking about urinary function:

Q: Do you have any pain when you urinate?

A: *No*

Q: Do you notice any blood when you urinate?

A: *No*

Q: Is it OK if I ask you some questions about your sexual function?

A: *No problem*

Obviously, the health professional may ask further questions when a positive reply is given. In the occasional instance when the response is negative, the professional might say something like (see Chapter 3) "it's certainly OK with me if we don't talk about this now but if you change your mind at any time in the future, we could talk then."

Interviewer Initiative

Only occasionally do patients volunteer information about sexual matters to health professionals, especially if a problem exists. Patients have mixed feelings about this apparent paradox. Health problems are the very reason for consulting a health professional but to not divulge information is patently counterproductive. Talking about sexual problems can be so embarrassing that it could paralyze any desire to ask for help. When secrecy exists, it is obviously deliberate. However, when a person does not tell all of the truth, it is not the same as lieing. Patients withhold information only when questions are not asked. Replies are usually truthful when questions *are* asked. (There are also other reasons for a person's lack of candor, such as being concerned about giving the "right" answer to a

> When secrecy exists, it is obviously deliberate. However, when a person does not tell all of the truth, it is not the same as stating a lie. Patients withhold information only when questions are not asked. Replies are usually truthful when patients are asked.

question, but this is less important than questions not being asked.) Therefore to discover the presence of problems, the onus is very much on the interviewer to ask pertinent questions.

Laumann et al. ". . . discovered that respondents found it very difficult to come up with language of their own to talk specifically about sexual practices. It was much easier for them to answer direct, simple questions we posed that asked for yes or no answers or simple indications of the frequency with which some behavior had occurred."[1]

Many mental health professionals use a nondirective method of acquiring information from patients. This technique involves relative silence by the professional and spontaneity by the patient in talking about concerns, whatever they might be. Such an approach directly conflicts with the notion of interviewer initiative. In a nondirective environment, frankness in talking about sexual issues rarely occurs, especially detailed descriptions of problems. Although one reasonably *begins* the inquiry process with an open-ended style of questioning ("Tell me about . . ."), *direct and explicit follow up questions are obligatory when sexual issues are being discussed.*

Kinsey and his colleagues cited two possible reasons for the nondisclosure of sexual information[3]:

- Judgmental attitude on the part of the interviewer
- Illegality of the sexual behavior

A third factor should be added, namely, not asking questions. By taking the initiative, the interviewer is in a position similar to the poker player who is asked to show his or her cards first to prove a winning position. It is as if the patient is saying, "prove to me that you're not going to tell me that I'm abnormal or that you won't think less of me for what I've done." This is apparent in entering the field of "sex," as well as asking questions about the details of "who does what to whom" (often called by patients: "nitty gritty").

A man in his late 20s and married for one year talked with his new family doctor about his erectile difficulties. Although embarrassed, the patient welcomed the physician's questions about this problem. Unknown to the patient's previous physician, and in response to direct inquiry from his current physician, the patient reported that he had never experienced intercourse with his wife or anyone else. Moreover, he described erections that were full at all times until the point of attempted vaginal entry, when he would ejaculate. His erection would then promptly disappear. Since his erectile difficulties seemed to result from his rapid ejaculation, the treatment focus shifted away from his concern about erections to the problem of his ejaculation. Using medications to control the timing of his ejaculation, his virtual panic over anticipated erectile loss diminished greatly. The conjoined use of sex therapy techniques allowed the patient and his wife to consummate their marriage within several weeks.

Language

The subject of "sex" is unique in medicine in that there are two languages used to describe the same phenomena: medical/technical language and slang. When health professionals talk about the sexual thoughts, feelings, or behavior of their patients, this usually occurs in the idiom of medical/technical jargon. Such words are almost always safer than slang in preserving the relationship with the patient. Safety is important in protecting the patient from the unwitting imposition of unacceptable values by the interviewer and the subsequent risk of losing that person as a patient.

The following are four potential problems that can arise as a result of using medical/technical terms; all are related to the element of comprehension.

1. One cannot assume that a patient understands medical/technical jargon. In clinical practice, problems related to understanding are more likely to arise when talking to someone from a different linguistic or cultural group. Patients usually don't ask for explanations or definitions of words for fear of appearing ignorant. Men seem more concerned about this than women, especially men from a third world culture where gender role expectations render embarrassment as a result of having "lost face" because of "not knowing." It is diplomatic for the health professional in this situation to begin by assuming lack of understanding of medical/technical terms and to take the initiative in providing definitions.

2. A comprehension problem may result from embarrassment or discomfort with the topic of "sex" on the part of the health professional with the consequent inclination to avoid anything but the most superficial reference to the subject.

A 24-year-old man was referred because of an inability to ejaculate when awake. The family physician who referred the patient had completed an investigation of the man's physical status, blood tests (including a hormonal profile), referral to a urologist, and urological tests that involved a testicular biopsy. The family physician suggested previously to the patient that he "masturbate," since this was not part of the patient's sexual experience in the past. The patient reported that this was ineffective. Referral to a specialty clinic occurred because all the tests were reported as negative. As the discussion proceeded with the patient about the details of his attempts at masturbating (number of times, duration of attempts, where stimulation was applied), he revealed his complete lack of understanding of how men masturbate and his consequent inability to implement the suggestions of his family doctor. Permission was then asked of the patient to demonstrate male masturbation techniques on a rubber model of an erect penis. This was done, and that evening the patient ejaculated while awake for the first time in his life.

---

3. Slang (rather than medical/technical words) may help as an alternative form of communication when comprehension is in doubt but this has to be balanced

against the risk that the health professional may alienate the patient in the process. If slang is contemplated, a safer method is by the conjoined use of the permission technique described previously.

A 35-year-old married woman was referred because of her lack of sexual interest and her husband's threats to leave the marriage unless this changed. In talking with her about her sexual desire under various circumstances, it seemed that she did not understand the nuances of some of the questions. She was consequently asked permission to use another word for "desire" or "interest"—a word (so it was explained) that some people find offensive but which everyone seems to understand. She was told that if she disliked the word, she should indicate this to the interviewer so that it would not be used again. She agreed to his arrangement. She was then told that the word was "horny." She replied that the word was certainly familiar to her and that she understood what it meant. She proceeded to describe when she had, in fact, felt this way during her lifetime. However, she added, rather pointedly, that the word "horny" was frequently used by her husband and that she herself found it "disgusting" and preferred that it not be used again.

---

4. Patients sometimes stumble in their attempts to use medical/technical terms. An example is the use of the word "organism" instead of orgasm. An approach to this situation is to allow the patient to learn a more accurate sexual vocabulary simply by the interviewer using the correct word repeatedly. The challenge to the health professional is to find a way of adjusting what the patient says without being condescending in the process.

Statement/Question Technique

When talking to people about their sexual thoughts, feelings, and behavior, Kinsey et al. realized that many forms of sexual activity occurred far more often than had been previously assumed.[3] Using the same example and armed with the knowledge that the vast majority of American men had this experience, Kinsey phrased inquiries to convey that ". . . everyone has engaged in every type of activity." This became known as the *ubiquity technique*.[4] The use of the ubiquity technique avoided the necessity of asking men: "have you ever masturbated?" and instead proceeded to the next question, namely, "how old were you when you began to masturbate?" Apart from the "ubiquity" approach specifically, other methods for asking questions about sensitive issues in general have also been suggested.[5]

A variation or alternative to the "ubiquity" technique is not to make assumptions but to preface a question by a statement phrased in such a way that the interviewer is talking of "most" or "many" people rather than everyone. Furthermore, this preliminary statement outlines the subject of the subsequent question. The interviewer then asks the person if their personal experience includes what was just described.

A couple in their mid-20s was referred because the woman was nonorgasmic in sexual activity with her husband. When seen alone, the woman revealed that she regularly came to orgasm through masturbation and that her husband was unaware of this. The fact that "many" women had difficulty in giving explicit directions to a sexual partner was mentioned, and the interviewer asked whether this conformed to the woman's own experience. She answered by saying that she also found it awkward to be completely candid in spite of the fact that her husband was receptive and, in fact, had asked her on many occasions what she "wanted." (What she wanted was to be able to tell him what she wanted.) She felt reassured in knowing that the problem of "communication" was not only hers. She was encouraged to discuss her masturbation experiences with her husband and was told that men usually appreciate such information. As a result of very explicit discussions with her husband she developed a considerably higher level of arousal with him than ever before.

This method of stating something factual followed by a question about the person's own experience seems extremely useful in talking about "sex" for several reasons. First, many people seem to be perennially hungry for sex-related information, especially about the minutiae of what people "do," think, and feel. Since people generally do not talk candidly about these subjects or read the many relevant books and magazine articles available, *the statement part of this technique provides a way of disseminating information.* Second, the initial information statement indicates to the patient that if the description is part of their own personal experience, they should not feel alone, since "many" others are "in the same boat."

However, "many" or "most" does not mean "all," and what is being discussed may *not* have been part of the life experience of the person interviewed. In that situation, the person could say so without feeling deviant and could also know that they, too, had lots of company. In other words, the interviewer "normalizes" the patient's sexual behavior. This approach provides a "win-win" opportunity for the patient.

Privacy, Confidentiality, and Security

- *Privacy:* the property of the individual; a right to control the disclosure of information about oneself
- *Confidentiality:* the extent to which information is disclosed to a third party
- *Security:* the physical property of the system used to process and store information[6]

In the medical system, privacy relates to the patient, confidentiality relates to the behavior of the health professional, and security relates to the method of protecting the information obtained. All are associated with keeping information secret (expected in any health system but secrecy and "sex" are particularly linked).

An example in which the privacy of sex-related information becomes problematic is when a patient is well known to a health professional because of a long association between the two but the subject of "sex" was never discussed. This circumstance some-times results in a patient consulting with another health professional solely for the purpose of obtaining a referral to a sex-specialist and doing so without the embarrassment of talking about this subject with his or her usual doctor.

A 35-year-old woman with multiple sclerosis (MS) was referred because of orgasm difficulties that had begun recently. Symptoms of MS began seven years earlier. The patient experienced two episodes of illness, neither of which resulted in any permanent disability. She was married and never previously experienced sexual difficulties. Two months earlier, she found it progressively more difficult to come to orgasm. She was a patient of her family doctor since her teens. She became socially friendly after they met at a swimming pool. Neither her family doctor nor her neurologist ever talked with her about her sexual function. When sexual problems appeared, she found it impossible to discuss the problems with either. As a result, she went to the medical clinic at the university where she worked and asked for a referral to the "sex clinic."

Clinical problems in relation to confidentiality generally arise when one partner does not want information given to the other. Most often this pertains to sexual activity with another person or atypical sexual behavior. In this situation, it is not unusual for patients to ask for an explicit statement of assurance of confidentiality when divulging information that is regarded as potentially damaging. (In providing such reassurance to a patient, health professionals must consider any legal reporting obligation that may exist in their jurisdiction such as a child in need of protection and serious risk of harm to another person or to oneself.)

A couple was referred because of the woman's lack of sexual interest. They both were 28 years old. They were married three years ago and had known each other for two years before their marriage. Her sexual interest lessened in the last year.

In talking with her separately, she was asked questions that attempted to clarify whether her diminished sexual interest related to her husband specifically or was more general. She specifically asked if the conversation was just between the interviewer and herself or whether the information revealed would be given to her husband. She was reassured that anything discussed would be strictly confidential. Two other statements were added. First, the "right" was reserved to tell her that if what she was about to explain was something that her husband should probably know this opinion would be given directly to her rather than her husband. Secondly, she was informed that in the legal jurisdiction in which the interview was taking place, courts had the power to subpoena medical records and that she should be aware of that in case she was about to reveal something that was illegal.

She then proceeded to disclose the following:

- She had fallen in love with another man
- Sexual disinterest was not a problem with her new partner
- She wanted to separate but was concerned about her husband's anger and wanted to tell him in the presence of a health professional present

They were subsequently seen together and when she revealed this information to her husband, he was neither angry nor surprised (although upset), and indicated that for several months, he wondered whether she had become interested in someone else.

Security of medical records represents a special problem that has legal and ethical ramifications. The fact that medical records can be subpoenaed by the courts or medical licensing authorities in many legal jurisdictions can place a very real restraint on the ethical obligation of the health professional to maintain patient confidentiality. Because written documents remain in files for long periods of time and medical records can become legal evidence, the health professional may be justified in keeping skimpy notes. However, when records are not complete and thorough, the interviewer may be handicapped by forgotten information and imprecise memories. Also, information omitted from a medical record is, obviously, unavailable to other health professionals in an emergency situation. If a secret *is* recorded, the special nature of the revelation should be noted in the record. Some clinicians, especially those working in hospital in-patient settings where many people have access to the medical record, keep a second set of records available only to themselves. A second set of notes preserves security in a medical, but not a legal, sense. While charts remain the property of the clinician, recent regulations enacted in many jurisdictions in North America allow patients to have legal access to their medical records. Presumably, this access applies to a second set of records as well.

> A second set of records preserves security in a medical, but not a legal, sense. While charts remain the property of the clinician, recent regulations enacted in many jurisdictions in North American allow patients to have legal access to their medical records. Presumably, this access applies to a second set of records as well.

A married couple in their early 30s with two young children was seen in consultation because of an impending separation, due, according to the referral source, to sexual difficulties. When the husband was seen alone, he spontaneously talked about having long-standing and frequent sexual fantasies involving men, occasional sexual experiences with men, and a desire to develop a sexual relationship with a particular man with whom he worked. In talking with his wife by herself, she was obviously aware of her husband's wish to form a relationship with a male work-colleague but felt that it was unacceptable for him to have any sexual relationship outside of their marriage. She recalled that before their marriage, he said something (she could not remember the details) about having sexual desires for men as well as women. She thought then that his interest in men was unimportant and not something that would interfere with their development as a couple.

The interviewer puzzled about what to record in the chart, since he recognized the possibility that he might have to account for what he had written if there was a legal contest between the two partners in the future over, for example, custody of their children. In view of the explicit discussion between the two about the husband's current interest in developing another relationship (which was thus not private information) the interviewer concluded that he could incorporate this into the record without problem. However, the interviewer also believed that, since the husband was given assurance of confidentiality when he was seen alone, the husband may have revealed aspects of his history that might otherwise not have emerged. Therefore the interviewer felt that it would not be proper to record details of the man's past sexual history and wrote only brief notes about what his wife already knew concerning his sexual interest in men.

Delaying Sensitive Questions

In an ordinary medical history, the *sensitivity* of patients to particular *questions is* often not of primary concern to the interviewer. For example, in asking about abdominal discomfort, one is not ordinarily concerned about how the person is going to react to the question. However, in a "sex" history, some topics elicit an almost predictably hesitant response from people. In the interest of preserving the relationship with the patient, questions concerning such subjects need to be approached with tact and sensitivity. One method for obtaining the required information while simultaneously maintaining rapport is to delay asking questions about a delicate topic until later in an interview or in a subsequent interview after a greater degree of trust is established. (Although waiting before asking "sensitive" questions is intuitively appealing, research support is inconsistent.)[7]

One example of delaying sensitive questions is in talking to people about the details of a sexual experience. Doing so is quite unlike simply telling someone about the presence of a particular problem, such as ejaculating quickly or not experiencing orgasm. Describing the events of a sexual encounter, however helpful that may be to an interviewer in understanding a problem, is quite alien to most people. Sexual partners may even find it painful to talk so explicitly with one another, in spite of the fact they were both there when the events occurred! In reviewing the dynamics of a sexual circumstance, it is infinitely easier to describe, for example, the preliminary courtship invitations or initial sexual signals than the later circumstances in bed, such as which part of a man's penis his partner usually stimulates with her fingers. While talking about sexual minutiae is never easy, it is less stressful when a greater degree of trust is established between patient and interviewer.

A couple in their early 30s was referred because the woman was nonorgasmic. They were reluctant to discuss this, as well as details of their sexual experiences as a couple, pleading lack of experience in talking with others about their personal experiences and not expecting to have to talk so explicitly during the appointment. The interviewer felt it unwise to pressure them into revealing detailed information before they were comfortable. Discussion initially concentrated on nonsexual relationship issues.

On the second visit, the couple was only slightly more forthcoming. When they realized their concerns were not being addressed, they became more receptive to explicit questions about their lovemaking. Discussion took place about their "signal system," what would happen before vaginal entry, and aspects of intercourse. They revealed that she was regularly orgasmic with clitoral stimulation when masturbating or when her husband was stimulating her with his fingers. They also explained that he would regularly ejaculate quickly, often before entry. He was particularly embarrassed about this and had told his wife not to reveal information about his ejaculation to the interviewer. She felt that she simply did not have enough time to come to orgasm before he ejaculated.

Another example of the need to delay sensitive questions is when there is the possibility that someone has engaged in an atypical form of sexual behavior.

A couple, married for 10 years and each 39 years old, was referred to a "sex" clinic because of the man's sexual disinterest. His wife discovered a cache of sexually explicit magazines in the trunk of their car one year earlier and, since then, sexual experiences between the two partners had been almost nonexistent. When subsequently seen alone, the husband described an interest in such magazines extending back to his teens, but he did not consider this to be a problem since it hadn't interfered with his sexual experiences with his wife in the past. The magazines were heterosexually oriented and his chief interest was in looking at pictures of women undressed. He spent several hours each week looking for such magazines and about $500 each month in purchases. He masturbated almost every day while looking at the pictures. His wife was unaware of these details.

The interviewer wanted to inquire about other atypical forms of sexual interest but felt that his relationship with the man was tentative, particularly since the referral was initiated by the man's wife. On the next visit, the man was asked about some paraphilic behaviors. It emerged that since his teens he had sometimes privately dressed in women's clothes and stole women's undergarments from clotheslines at night. He was not sexually interested in children, had never exhibited his genitalia in public, and had not engaged in any sexually violent behavior toward others. He never discussed any of his sexual behavior with anyone before and, while he was concerned about his wife discovering his private sexual interests, he felt relieved at being able to discuss these issues with another person. On the fourth visit, and in response to specific questions, he described (with palpable hesitation) having tied a ligature around his neck on several occasions in his life to become more sexually aroused. The last time was several years ago but he was concerned that this might happen again and that there might be life-threatening consequences. He was immediately admitted to hospital and referred to a psychiatrist who was expert in the assessment and treatment of paraphilias.

Nonjudgmental Attitude

The injection of personal values into discussions about sexual behavior was a major issue for Kinsey and his co-workers.[3] Their interviewing observations concentrated on two issues: (1) confidentiality and trust and (2) the interviewer's attitude. They displayed particular sensitivity toward the intrusion of the interviewer's values into the process of questioning when they wrote that ". . .there are always things which seem esthetically repulsive, provokingly petty, foolish, unprofitable, senseless, unintelligent, dishonorable, contemptible, or socially destructive. Gradually one learns to forego judgment on these things, and to accept them merely as facts for the record. If one fails in his acceptance, he will know of it by the. . .quick conclusion of the story."[3]

Patients who describe their private sexual thoughts or experiences and who are also in psychological pain as a result are not usually asking others for an opinion or approval. Rather, such a person is seeking a listener rather than a judge, someone to assist in the process of change. If the patient wanted a right/wrong opinion, they would have consulted a clergyman instead of a health professional. If the interviewer cannot function in a helpful way and without judgment, the patient should be referred elsewhere. The meeting between health professional and patient is not the place for proselytizing. The problem is not a matter of the nature of one's personal values. Indeed every health care professional operates within a personal value system. The problem is one of imposing these values on a patient and, in particular, doing so in a covert manner. In a welcome departure from tradition, Bancroft included a statement of his personal values within the introduction to his text *"Human Sexuality and Its Problems."*[8] Health professionals who have strong beliefs that make it impossible for them to be dispassionate in caring for patients with sex-related concerns should make their philosophical position known beforehand.

> Health professionals who have strong beliefs that make it impossible for them to be dispassionate in caring for patients with sex-related concerns should make their philosophical position known beforehand.

Occasionally, patients ask for an opinion about the propriety of sexual experiences or relationships. One can be precise in answering without simultaneously telling patients how they should manage their lives.

A 22-year-old man was referred because of an inability to ejaculate in attempts at intercourse. His current sexual partner was his first intercourse partner. He experienced noncoital sexual activities with her in the previous three years during which he had no difficulty with ejaculation. The same was true with masturbation.

In the course of talking with him, he revealed, with much reluctance, an event when he (the patient) was 15 years old in which his brother stimulated him to ejaculation. He regarded this as evidence of homosexuality, about which he was persistently distressed. All his subsequent sexual experiences were with women and his sexual fantasies consistently related to women. He described himself as repulsed by the notion of homosexual behavior. He asked the interviewer if his (the patient's) earlier life experience was an indication of homosexuality and the interviewer's opinion about the "decency" of homosexual behavior. The interviewer reassured him by placing the sexual event with his brother in the context of the sexual evolution of a heterosexual adolescent boy; the event seemingly had little or no relevance to the issue of his sexual orientation as an adult. To that was added a statement that the determinants of homosexual and heterosexual behavior were unclear but that, in any case, the "job" of a health professional was to assist in helping to understand and solve problems rather than to give opinions about the correctness of a person's actions. The latter was described as being more a matter for the clergy. An offer was made to help find a priest (the patient was Catholic). The suggestion was accepted.

Explanation

Health professionals, especially physicians, are not renown for giving jargon-free explanations to patients about their difficulties. The impact on patients of information about the nature of a disease varies. However, when talking about sexual disorders in particular the impact can be immense, since lack of information, or misinformation, can be a critical factor in the origin of the problem. Tiefer observed that "the major source of information for the young has been the mass media, both because of parents' silence and because of the dearth of sex education . . . advice in the nonfiction media reinforces the impression that sex is very important without providing the kind of information that ordinary readers or viewers can actually use."[9] Given these circumstances, the provision of information by a health professional can be therapeutically valuable.

A 57-year-old man was referred because he repeatedly delayed the prostate surgery that was recommended by his family doctor and urologist. He had symptoms of prostate gland enlargement and was diagnosed as having "benign prostatic hypertrophy." He previously had used an oral medication to diminish the size of his prostate and found that it helped initially but that his symptoms were worsening. The suggested treatment at this point was transurethral surgery (TURP), which involved the removal of prostatic tissue obstructing the flow of urine through his urethra. The patient was concerned about possible impairment of sexual function as a result of surgery and was not reassured by what he perceived to be bland encouragement by his physicians.

He had been divorced for three years and was sexually active with a woman in her early 40s. They had talked seriously about marriage. He saw, on a TV talk show, information about the use of a penile prosthesis as a treatment for "impotence" after prostate surgery and wanted assurance that this would be available to him after his operation. In a specifically structured visit involving the interviewer and the patient's urologist, the details of the surgery were reviewed with the patient. This was done with the help of a rubber model of the male genitalia, which showed internal and external organs. The mechanism of expected impairment of ejaculation with a TURP procedure was explained, as well as the method by which erections occurred. The reasons for not expecting erectile impairment were also explained. The patient underwent surgery and experienced retrograde ejaculation as a result, without associated erectile difficulties. Neither he nor his partner perceived this as a major interruption of their sexual experiences and did not ask for further treatment.

Feelings

Health-related histories generally contain questions about experiences or behavior, not about feelings. However, sexual disorders often require an understanding of all three. Feelings surrounding sexual issues may be etiologically, diagnostically, or therapeutically prominent. In a developmental history, it may be useful to determine when a particular event occurred and also how the person felt about that experience. Feelings may provide a crucial link between the past and the present.

A couple in their early 40s was referred on the initiative of the husband and because of a lack of sexual desire on the part of the wife. This extended to a time shortly after their marriage and began in relation to her first pregnancy about 15 years earlier.

In the course of talking to the woman alone and in the context of a developmental history, she was asked about her intercourse experiences during each of her three pregnancies. She described diminishing sexual interest as her first pregnancy evolved. This was the opposite of her prior sexual enthusiasm. She related that her disinterest was the result of the prolonged morning sickness and bloating associated with the pregnancy. She denied particular feelings connected to specific sexual experiences that occurred at that time. However, at the end of the interview and in response to a question about whether there was anything else of importance in relation to her sexual concerns, she tearfully recalled the last time she and her husband had intercourse prior to her first delivery. This occurred hours before her "water broke" and the delivery of a stillborn child. Since that time, she believed that "sex" was the main cause of the death of her child but had only recently stated this to her family doctor. Before the current visit, she had not seen the possibility of a connection between feeling responsible for the death of the baby and the disappearance of her sexual desire. She accepted the suggestion of exploring this idea in psychotherapy.

The interviewer must consider feelings from the past as well as feelings in the present, including during the interview itself. In any discussion of sexual matters, it is reasonable to assume that the patient is uncomfortable (in a psychological sense). To suppose otherwise is to not acknowledge the strangeness of talking to someone else about something usually considered private. Embarrassment is to be expected. Indeed, if there is no embarrassment, the interviewer must ask why—at least to him or herself, if not to the patient as well. One way of assessing the patient's feelings about the interview is simply to ask, and to reassure the patient about the usualness of uneasy feelings. The need to do this may extend beyond the first visit. Patients often return on a second visit and say that when thinking about the first visit they could not believe they said "those things."

Optimism

Life problems often seem worse than they actually are. Hope is one of the most powerful weapons in the armamentarium of any health professional.[10] Changing the patient's perspective on a problem can be a mechanism for engendering optimism. This is the basis of the proverbial story of the man who cried because he had no shoes, until he saw another who had no feet.

> People often perceive a sexual difficulty (especially something that impedes intercourse) in a global way rather than as a limited disorder. Sexual problems thus become reflections of masculinity or femininity. The impact of a health professional's optimism can extend far beyond the sexual problem to the entire view of oneself.

On the surface, sexual problems are no different. However, patients tend to think of themselves as not simply having a sexual problem; they also think they are less of a man or woman in the process. That is, people often perceive a sexual difficulty (especially something that impedes intercourse) in a global way rather than as a limited disorder. Sexual problems thus become reflections of masculinity or femininity. Therefore the impact of a health professional's optimism can extend far beyond the sexual problem to the entire view of oneself.

Patients also tend to magnify the extent of a sexual disability and not to balance this with positive thoughts. Men and women seem to share this inclination equally. This negative point of view is apparent when a problem is first revealed and is also seen repeatedly when treatment benefits are quickly "taken for granted" and put aside in favor of worry over remaining problems. Patients seem to be concerned that they may be prematurely "dismissed," or perhaps, fear that the leftover troubles may be insoluble. Optimism of the health professional may be the major factor that keeps the patient in the treatment process.

A couple in their early 30s described a problem of nonconsummation of their five-year marriage. They both wanted children. This reproductive "agenda" was the main motivation for seeking medical care. Intercourse for the purpose of bonding or cementing their relationship was of secondary importance—at least initially. The sexual diagnoses were vaginismus and retarded ejaculation, both of which were life-long. He ejaculated with "wet dreams" but not otherwise. The vaginismus was treated with the classic Masters and Johnson method, which relies heavily on vaginal "dilators."[11] Over a period of two months, the woman became increasingly confident about inserting dilators into her vagina. Fear of "objects" in her vagina and pain with insertion of the dilators gradually disappeared. Eventually, she was able to introduce her husband's penis into her vagina. They were impassive when it finally occurred. In discussing this attitude, they talked regretfully of the fact that he had not yet ejaculated inside. The clear implication was that perhaps he never would. They were reassured that this would likely happen soon. They remained skeptical until ejaculation did, in fact, occur several weeks later.

SUMMARY

Talking to people about "sex" requires knowing the questions to ask and consideration of the ways in which to discuss the subject. In other areas of talk between patients and health professionals, methods of asking questions can affect the quality of information obtained. In relation to sexual issues, techniques of inquiry may affect the quality and the quantity of the information gathered. In this chapter the methods suggested for use in asking sex-related questions have the potential to enhance both.

The following interviewing methods have particular application to the topic of "sex":

1. Ask permission
2. Assume the initiative
3. Use "language" that fits a particular situation
4. Convey a sense of trust and confidentiality
5. Use a form of questioning that involves providing information followed by a question
6. Display an attitude of nonjudgmentalism
7. Delay inquiry into obviously sensitive areas
8. Provide information by way of explanation
9. Ask questions about feelings in addition to experiences
10. Promote an optimistic attitude

These ten techniques may be useful when interviewing patients generally; however, their use in talking about sexual issues specifically may critically alter the quantity and quality of the sex-related information obtained.

REFERENCES

1. Laumann EO et al: *The social organization of sexuality: sexual practices in the United States,* Chicago, 1994, The University of Chicago Press.
2. Maurice WL, Sheps SB, Schechter MT: Physician sexual contact with patients: 2. A public survey of women in British Columbia. Paper presented at the meeting of the Society for Sex Therapy and Research, New York, March 1995.
3. Kinsey AC, Pomeroy WB, Martin CE: *Sexual behavior in the human male,* Philadelphia and London, 1949, W.B. Saunders.
4. Green R: Taking a sexual history. In Green R (editor): *Human sexuality: a health practitioner's text,* ed 2, Baltimore/London, 1979, Williams and Wilkins, pp 22-30.
5. Sudman S, Bradburn NM: *Asking questions: a practical guide to questionnaire design,* San Francisco, 1982, Jossey-Bass Inc., Publishers.
6. Boruch RF: Resolving privacy problems in AIDS research. In Sechrest L, Freemen H, Mulley A: *Conference Proceedings: Health Sciences Research Methodology: a Focus on AIDS,* National Center for Health Services Research and Health Care Technology Assessment, Public Health Services, Rockville, 1989, Maryland.
7. DeLamater J, MacCorquodale P: The effects of interview schedule variations on reported sexual behavior, *Sociol Methods Res* 4:215-236, 1975.
8. Bancroft J: *Human sexuality and its problems,* ed 2, Edinburgh, 1989, Churchill Livingstone, pp 5-11.
9. Tiefer L: *Sex is not a natural act and other essays,* Boulder, 1995, Westview Press.
10. Frank J et al: Expectation and therapeutic outcome—the placebo effect and the role induction interview. In *Effective ingredients of successful psychotherapy,* New York, 1978, Brunner/Mazel.
11. Masters W, Johnson V: *Human sexual inadequacy,* Boston, 1970, Little, Brown and Company.

CHAPTER 3

SCREENING FOR SEXUAL PROBLEMS

The most basic, and also most difficult, aspect of studying sexuality is defining the subject matter. What is to be included? How much of the body is relevant? How much of the life span? Is sexuality an individual dimension or a dimension of a relationship? Which behaviors, thoughts, or feelings qualify as sexual—an unreturned glance? Any hug? Daydreams about celebrities? Fearful memories of abuse? When can we use similar language for animals and people, if at all?

TIEFER, 1995[1]

Defining the subject matter of "sex" is, indeed, difficult but nevertheless crucial, since its meaning will determine which difficulties one is searching for in the process of screening. The definition and the screening mechanism must be broad enough to encompass problems with sexual *function* and sexual *practices*. Problems with sexual function are reported by patients rather than observed by health professionals. In contrast, some sexual practices may be seen only as problematic by health professionals. In both instances, the onus remains on the health professional to elicit the information.

Problems with sexual function have been classified in DSM-IV[2]—a system heavily influenced by the research of Masters and Johnson[3] and Kaplan's revisions.[4] On the basis of direct observation of physiological changes associated with sexual arousal, Masters and Johnson described a *"sex response cycle"* that included four phases[3] (pp. 3-8) (Figures 3-1 and 3-2):

- Excitement
- Plateau
- Orgasm
- Resolution

Kaplan added a prior "interest" or motivational phase to Masters and Johnson's system[4] (pp. 3-7). In so doing, she reconceptualized the sex response cycle from four parts into three, which she renamed:

- Interest
- Response
- Orgasm

Kaplan referred to her revision as a *"triphasic model"* (Figure 3-3).

SCREENING CONTENT: DYSFUNCTIONS VERSUS DIFFICULTIES

While ideas based on the sex response cycle are widely used, they have not been universally accepted. One criticism is that when considering sexual function, the cycle seems to progress from one step to another but that this is not how sexual response is always ordered. For example, clinicians will sometimes encounter the occurrence of orgasm in a woman who does not feel any preexisting sexual desire. The reality of this

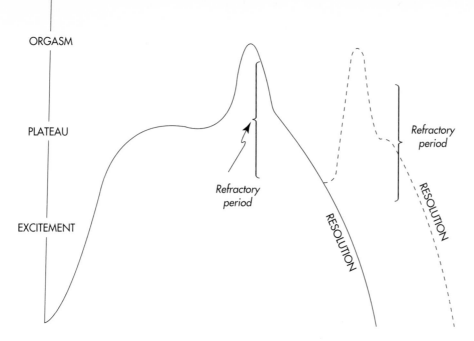

Figure 3-1 Male sexual response. (From Masters WH, Johnson VE: *Human sexual response*, Boston, 1966, Little, Brown and Company, p. 5.)

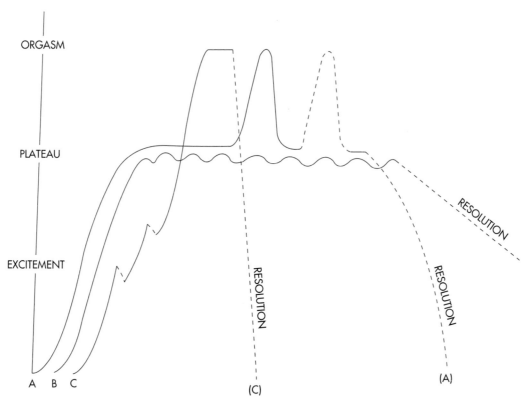

Figure 3-2 Female sexual response. (From Masters WH, Johnson VE: *Human sexual response*, Boston, 1966, Little, Brown and Company, p. 5.)

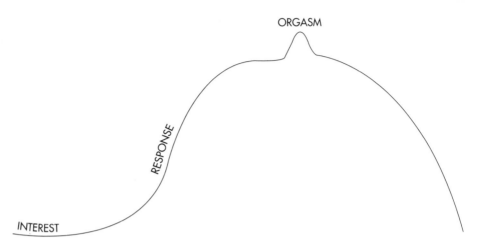

Figure 3-3   Triphasic model of human sexual response.

particular observation of the disconnection between desire and orgasm has been established in a research context.[5]

A second critique relates to gender and the different meanings of "sex" to men and women. In an exquisitely detailed and incisive analysis, Tiefer examined the entire concept of the sexual response cycle and the extent to which women have been absent in the formulation of sexual disorders in the various versions of the DSM[1] (pp. 41-58, 97-102). She faults the DSM classification system for the following:

1. Excessive "physiologizing"
2. Viewing sexual expression as consisting of reactions of body parts
3. Being "genitally focused"
4. Thinking of "heterosexual intercourse as the normative sexual activity, repeatedly defining dysfunctions as failures in coitus"

From Tiefer's perspective, the sexual concerns of women are different and have been sufficiently outlined in popular surveys, questionnaire studies, political writings, and fiction to include such issues as: intimacy, communication, emotion, commitment, pregnancy, conception, and getting old. ". . . women rate affection and emotional communication as more important than orgasm in a sexual relationship. . . "[1] (p. 56).

One well-executed, frequently quoted, and revealing questionnaire study referred to by Tiefer and which serves to buttress her argument was conducted by Frank and her colleagues.[6] One hundred predominantly white, well-educated, and "happily married" volunteer couples were questioned concerning the frequency of sexual problems. The authors found that in addition to the fact that 40% of the men and 63% of the women reported sexual dysfunctions, 50% of the men and 77% of the women reported *"difficulty that was not dysfunctional in nature."* The "difficulties" are outlined in Box 3-1. Most importantly from the point of view of screening, *the number of difficulties reported was more strongly and consistently related to overall sexual dissatisfaction than the num-*

Box 3-1

Sexual "Difficulties"

- Partner chooses inconvenient time
- Inability to relax
- Attraction(s) to persons other than mate
- Disinterest
- Attraction(s) to persons of the same sex
- Different sexual practices or habits
- "Turned off"
- Too little foreplay before intercourse
- Too little "tenderness" after intercourse

Adapted from Frank E et al: Frequency of sexual dysfunction in "normal" couples, *N Engl J Med* 299:111–115, 1998.

ber of "dysfunctions." If one therefore accepts the argument and evidence presented by Tiefer, a useful screening system must consider sexual problems to be impairments in physiology (sexual dysfunctions) *and* impairments in the "human relations" part of "sexual experiences" (i.e., difficulties or consequences of the ways people conduct themselves sexually).

EPIDEMIOLOGY OF SEXUAL PROBLEMS IN PRIMARY CARE

Apart from what one looks for in screening (sexual "dysfunctions" and/or "difficulties") a major rationale for the inquiry process is how common the detected phenomena are in general (epidemiological information about specific dysfunctions are included in Part II). The extent of sexual problems found in medical practices has been studied on several occasions.

One widely quoted study of sexual issues in general medicine practice was described in detail in Chapter 1.[7] Another study used a questionnaire (whose validity and reliability was previously tested) that contained items concerning dysfunctions and difficulties.[8] Of the 152 patients who were asked to complete the questionnaire, almost all did so (93%). The majority of patients (56%) identified at least one sexual problem on the questionnaire, and this compared to 22% having a marital or sexual problem found by simply examining the patient's medical record. Multiple reasons were cited for the discrepancy, including:

1. The physician did not ask relevant questions
2. The patient did not spontaneously report problems
3. The physician did not record the information in the patient's chart

Although identification of a problem by 56% of patients may appear to be an overwhelming number to a clinician, one must remember that not all people with sexual problems want treatment.[9]

> Although identification of a problem by 56% of patients may appear to be an overwhelming number to a clinician, one must remember that not all people with sexual problems want treatment.[9]

SCREENING CRITERIA

Given the immense numbers of patients with sexual problems, the need becomes obvious for a triage system whereby the nature of a problem and its impact can be evaluated and proper action taken: (1) further assessment and treatment or (2) referral. The beginning of this process requires a reasonable, respectful, and regular practice by which the presence of sexual problems can be identified with just a few questions. For reasons discussed in Chapter 1, it is a "given" that patients be provided the opportunity to discuss a sexual issue if they desire. To accomplish this goal, some sort of sex-screening question must be included in an assessment.

Other than considering specific sexual practice issues involved in STD and HIV/AIDS transmission, the idea of including general sex-screening in a health assessment has been considered only briefly by a few authors. Concepts vary from an elaborate "screening history" requiring 30 minutes[10] to a small number of specific screening questions.[11] The rationale for choosing particular questions was not always clear.

Useful screening questions in any area should observe at least four rules:

1. Screening questions should encompass a wide spectrum of common problems

A variety of sexual problems may exist in any community, ranging from frequent (concerns about genital function, sexual practices, or emotional communication) to unusual (confusion about one's status as a man or woman). A screening system must be sufficiently sensitive to at least "pick up" problems that are common. Freund's opinion is that "a problem must be sufficiently common to justify investigation of an entire population of patients."[12] Sexual dysfunctions and difficulties, as well as problems related to STDs and child sexual abuse, are far more numerous than other sexual disorders and these must be uncovered in any practical sex-screening process[13] (pp.43-55).

2. To be practical, screening questions should be few in number

> Realistically and reasonably, only a small amount of health professional time will be used to ask questions about sexual matters when the patient's major concern is elsewhere. Suggesting more than a few screening questions dooms the entire process from the start.

A small number of questions recognizes the limited amount of time that health professionals (especially nonpsychiatric physicians) spend with patients and the reticence that many patients have in spontaneously talking about sexual issues. Realistically and reasonably, only a small amount of health professional time will be used to ask questions about sexual matters when the patient's major concern is elsewhere. Suggesting more than a few screening questions dooms the entire process from the start.

3. The problem must be of sufficient severity to justify the effort of asking questions of the population[12]

The consequences of sexual problems must be considered from individual and social perspectives. In some instances, the severity of the impact on an individual is easy to discern (e.g., STDs) but in others the effect may be more subtle (e.g., repercussions on a relationship of a coexistent sexual dysfunction). Without "quality of life" information in the area of sexual problems, it becomes difficult to provide clear evidence about the effect of some problems on the individual. The existing literature on the effects of sexual dysfunctions on individuals and relationships, as well as clinical impression, suggest substantial repercussions[13] (pp. 52-55). The outcome of some sexual experiences such as child sexual abuse are well documented.[14] Newspapers have well reported the social disruption caused by STDs and HIV/AIDS, pedophilia, and child sexual abuse.

4. There must be effective treatment for problems that are common

The treatments of sexual dysfunctions and their usefulness are reviewed in Part II.

These four screening criteria can be applied, for example, to one of the screening systems commonly used in medical practice. Part of any medical evaluation includes asking a series of questions about the function of different parts of the body. This brief health questionnaire has been variously called the "Review of Systems" (ROS) or "Functional Inquiry" and includes a few questions about each body system. It is meant to accomplish two objectives, as follows:

- To provide more information about concerns not obviously connected to the patient's main complaint
- To uncover undiscussed problems that the patient may have thought to be irrelevant or unimportant

Until recently, questions about sexual issues were not usually part of a medical screening process. Questions relating to this subject were not asked or were buried in questions about other body systems. For example, questions about sexual function were included with questions about a man's urinary function.

There is no universally applicable sex-screening formula. Several approaches can be used, depending, for example, on such factors as the comfort and skill of the interviewer or the age of the patient. Screening questions asked of adolescents might well differ from questions asked of elders.

> There is no universally applicable sex-screening formula. Several approaches can be used.

With the understanding that *variety and flexibility* in sex screening are desirable, one general method is described below. This approach can be incorporated easily into the assessment of any patient whose main concern is not primarily sexual, specifically, into the medical "review of systems." (The ROS concentrates on body function or dysfunction; therefore sexual practice issues can be included easily.) When judging the usefulness of the proposed sex-screening process, one should recall the four criteria mentioned previously, that is, questions should:

- Cover a wide spectrum of common problems
- Be few in number
- Justify the severity criterion
- Be concerned with problems that have effective treatments

Questions should include an additional criterion as well, namely, practicality.

When health professionals choose sex-screening approaches, the selection is not usually between systems that are brief or lengthy. The choice is usually between (1) a system that is brief and comfortable to the clinician and inoffensive to the patient or (2) a complete *absence* of any sex-related screening questions whatsoever.

SEX-SCREENING FORMATS

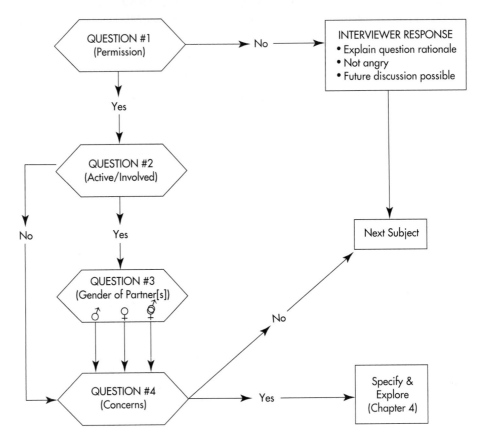

Figure 3-4   Flow chart for "sex" screening questions.

The older style sex-screening approach used to be: "How's your sex life?" While this fulfilled the wide spectrum and brevity criteria, it was also nebulous and indefinite. Being so general, it usually elicited an equally vague answer ("fine"), which was undoubtedly inaccurate on many occasions. In addition, the question potentially covered the whole of a patient's current sexual experience rather than concentrating on what was problematic and required attention.

A preferred approach (*Figure 3-4 and Box 3-2*) begins with the question: "CAN I ASK YOU A FEW QUESTIONS ABOUT SEXUAL MATTERS?"

This is not really a "sex" question but rather preliminary to other questions that might follow. Use of the permission technique was discussed in Chapter 2.

The answer to a permission question is usually "yes." After consent is given, the interviewer naturally continues to the next question. However, in the unusual situation that the patient says "no," the inter-

> The answer to a permission question is usually "yes." After consent is given, the interviewer naturally continues to the next question. However, in the unusual situation that the patients says "no," the interviewer has no ethical alternative but to respect the patient's decision and continue to the next subject.

viewer has no ethical alternative but to respect the patient's decision and continue to the next subject. Before proceeding, some of the implicit issues mentioned above should be made explicit. In particular, the interviewer should explain the rationale for asking the question in the first place. Reasons given may include the following:

- That this area is legitimate for discussion in a medical setting even if unconventional from the patient's point of view
- That the interviewer's response is one of understanding rather than anger
- That the patient is free to raise the topic at any time in the future

The second screening question asks the patient: "**ARE YOU SEXUALLY ACTIVE?**" This question is common especially in relation to HIV/AIDS prevention. The question could be made sharper if a time frame is added. For example, it might be phrased: "**HAVE YOU BEEN SEXUALLY ACTIVE IN THE LAST SIX MONTHS?**" This revision might be useful particularly in situations where sexual activity may be regular but not necessarily frequent, as for example, in the elderly.

The meaning of the phrase "sexually active" could be more specific if it included some definition of the word "active." "Active" might refer to actions with a partner, with oneself (masturbation), or both. If a patient has a partner, couple sexual activities should be the focus of this question, so that the question might be: "**HAVE YOU BEEN SEXUALLY ACTIVE WITH A PARTNER IN THE PAST SIX MONTHS?**" If the patient does not have a sexual partner, the definition of "active" might logically include solo sexual experiences. However, since the subject of masturbation is often a sensitive one for patients and clinicians and, since it is infrequently reported as a problem with sexual function or practice, one might reasonably refrain from asking about this specific subject in the context of screening questions.

There are two potential problems with the word "active":

- Teenagers may not understand what the word encompasses. Talking with teenagers may be one instance in which the word "sex" is useful, since teens (unlike adults) often have a broader definition than simply intercourse. In using this approach, the health professional must clarify what practices are entailed within the word "sex."
- Some people interpret the word "active" concretely and consider themselves "passive," so that even if sexually involved with another person they might answer the question in the negative. It might be better to

---

Box 3-2

Sex Screening Questions

1. Can I ask you a few questions about sexual matters?
2. Have you been sexually active with a partner in the past six months?
3. With women? men? both?
4. Do you or your partner have any sexual concerns?

use the word "involved" instead of "active" in such situations. (A strong counter argument is that the word "active" has become part of the English lexicon and that professionals and adult patients are adjusted to its use.)

The final version of the second sex-screening question might therefore be: "HAVE YOU BEEN SEXUALLY ACTIVE (OR INVOLVED) WITH A PARTNER IN THE PAST SIX MONTHS?"

A "yes" answer to the question of sexual activity results naturally in the interviewer proceeding to the next item, which may be about the gender of the partner—opposite or same sex. (Questions are formulated by using the words, "men" and "women," rather than "opposite" and "same"[see immediately below].) Acquiring information about sexual orientation is vital for reasons outlined in Chapter 7 (see "Sexual Orientation: Issues and Questions").

The third sex-screening question is actually an extension of the second and attempts to determine with whom the patient has been sexually active. The question is asked only if the patient says "yes" to the second question and can be phrased (e.g., when talking with a man): "HAVE YOU BEEN SEXUALLY ACTIVE WITH WOMEN, OTHER MEN, OR WITH BOTH?"

Following a "no" answer to the question of whether or not a patient is sexually active, an attempt should be made to discover whether or not the person's inactivity is a concern. If it is, this requires some exploration by the interviewer and an explanation from the patient. This, in turn, leads into a diagnostic process. If sexual inactivity is not a concern, the interviewer could naturally proceed to the fourth and last screening question, which is: "DO YOU OR YOUR PARTNER HAVE ANY SEXUAL CONCERNS?"

The utility of a question about "concerns" lies in the fact that it is open-ended and problem-oriented. However, one problem with this question is its subjectivity. A more direct, objective, and still open-ended and problem-oriented version would be, "DO YOU OR YOUR PARTNER HAVE ANY SEXUAL DIFFICULTIES?" A third possibility is the same question but with some added specific examples. The question could then become: "(for a man) DO YOU OR YOUR PARTNER HAVE ANY SEXUAL DIFFICULTIES, SUCH AS WITH YOUR INTEREST LEVEL, ERECTIONS, OR EJACULATION?" (For a woman) ". . . SUCH AS WITH YOUR INTEREST LEVEL, VAGINAL LUBRICATION, ORGASMS, OR INTERCOURSE PAIN?" These examples are of sexual dysfunctions. A clinician could, if desired, substitute other examples such as STDs.

Any of these four questions should fulfill the four criteria for screening questions described above. If the screening professional can ask only one question, the fourth is the most desirable.

CONCLUSION

A screening system for "sex" questions is a necessity for health professionals. The arrangement must be comprehensive (encompassing problems with sexual function and sexual practices), the questions few in number, and the problems sufficiently severe and treatable. Practicality also helps. There is not much use in proposing a system that no one will use.

Screening questions about sexual issues are a vital part of the health professional's intake procedure. However, screening questions cannot be definitive. The question inevitably arises: "What do you do if you get a positive answer?" One does, of course, the same as one would do with any other subject. In the practice of a health professional, this means allowing the patient to talk and ask more questions as part of a diagnostic process. This, in turn, leads to a conclusion and to a treatment plan. The next chapter discusses the first of these two steps.

REFERENCES

1. Tiefer L: *Sex is not a natural act and other essays*, Boulder, 1995, Westview Press.
2. *Diagnostic and statistical manual of mental disorders*, ed 4, Washington, 1994, American Psychiatric Association.
3. Masters WH, Johnson VE: *Human sexual inadequacy*, Boston, 1970, Little, Brown and Company.
4. Kaplan HS: *Disorders of sexual desire*, New York, 1979, Brunner/Mazel, Inc.
5. Rosen RC, Beck JG: *Patterns of sexual arousal: psychophysiological processes and clinical applications*, New York, 1988, The Guilford Press, pp 42-43.
6. Frank E, Anderson C, Rubenstein D: Frequency of sexual dysfunction in normal couples, *N Engl J Med* 299:111-115, 1978.
7. Ende JE, Rockwell S, Glasgow M: The sexual history in general medicine practice, *Arch Intern Med* 144:558-561, 1984.
8. Moore JT, Goldstein Y: Sexual problems among family medicine patients, *J Fam Prac* 10:243-247,1980.
9. Garde K, Lunde I: Female sexual behaviour. A study in a random sample of 40-year old women, *Maturitas* 2:225-240, 1980.
10. Munjak DJ, Oziel LJ: *Sexual medicine and counseling in office practice: a comprehensive treatment guide*, Boston, 1980, Little, Brown and Company, pp 3-10.
11. Kolodny RC, Masters WH, Johnson VJ: *Textbook of sexual medicine*, Boston, 1979, Little, Brown and Company, pp 587-588.
12. Freund K: Screening in primary care for women. In Carr PL, Freund KM, Somani S (editors): *The medical care of women*, Philadelphia, 1885, W.B. Saunders Company, pp 1-13.
13. Hawton K: *Sex therapy: a practical guide*. New York, 1985, Oxford University Press.
14. Browne A, Finkelhor D: Impact of child sexual abuse: a review of the research, *Psychol Bull* 99:66-77, 1986.

CHAPTER 4

SEXUAL DYSFUNCTIONS: DIAGNOSTIC TOPICS AND QUESTIONS

In the Brancacci Chapel of Florence's Carmine Church, Masaccio and Masolino painted (1427-1430) Adam and Eve without fig leaves. Fig leaves were added 225 years later to cover their genitalia. During the recent cleaning of these masterpieces, which signify the beginnings of Florentine renaissance art, fig leaves added in 1650 were removed in 1986-1989. The point . . . is that pictorially the church changed its position on what was morally acceptable. If the church which is not usually considered to be at the forefront of liberal thought, can be this flexible on sexuality, why are physicians still dragging their feet taking better sex histories?

MERRILL ET AL, 1990[1]

The thought that one is "opening a can of worms" is a central deterrent to asking sex-screening questions. Learning "what to do with the answers" is surprisingly not very difficult if one is willing to confront two obstacles:

- Overcoming the awkwardness of talking about this subject
- Learning about sexual disorders in a factual sense

After screening questions are asked and a problem surfaces (see Chapter 3), the next step in exploring the concern involves moving beyond the level of a "chief complaint." A "complaint" indicates only the area of trouble. Examples of referrals to a sex-specialty clinic can serve as illustrations. One form of referral provides virtually no information, as when a request is made to "please see this man for sexual counseling." In this case, the area is general, that is, "sex." Another and more common type of referral is, "This man has frequent trouble with erections. His physical examination is normal. Please assess." In this case the area is "sex" and penile function. This referral is more specific. Both are examples of a "complaint."

A clinical diagnosis is based on information about the complaint, the chronology of the disorder, and the "signs and symptoms" or the way it appears in the present. It can imply some knowledge about the genesis of the problem but this depends on the general level of knowledge of the disorder. A complaint is not enough to begin a treatment program because there is no separation of diagnoses that may appear with the same starting concern. For example, the complaint of a woman being nonorgasmic does not say whether this problem occurs in all situations or if it is limited to certain forms of sexual activity. The treatment approach in these two situations may be very different.

Diagnoses of sexual disorders often can be made on the basis of history-taking alone. Physicians, compared to other health professionals, may conduct physical examinations and use laboratory tests. In relation to sexual dysfunctions, these additional diagnostic procedures are of particular use in the following situations:

- When a woman complains about pain or discomfort with intercourse
- When a woman has disire or orgasmic dysfunctions or when a man has erectile difficulties that may be partly the result of a medical condition

---

Box 4-1

What to Determine in the Assessment of Sexual Dysfunctions

1. PATTERN OF SEXUAL FUNCTION (see Box 4-2, the principal content of this chapter
2. SEXUAL PRACTICES (see Chapter 5, The Present Context: Immediate Issues and Questions)
3. AFFECTIONATE BEHAVIOR (see Chapter 5, The Present Context: Immediate Issues and Questions)
4. RELATIONSHIP WITH PARTNER (see Chapter 6)
5. SEXUAL-DEVELOPMENT HISTORY (see Chapter 5, The Context of the Past: Remote Issues and Questions)
6. MEDICAL HISTORY (see Part II)
7. PHYSICAL AND LABORATORY EXAMINATIONS (applicable to physicians in selected instances, see Part II)

Otherwise, a physical examination may be *therapeutically* helpful from an educational point of view.

Preferably, to arrive at a clinical diagnosis of a sexual dysfunction, the clinician should have six types of information (seven [physical and laboratory examinations] if the health professional is a physician [Box 4-1]).

When considering the *pattern of sexual functioning* only, seven aspects (explained in the remainder of this chapter) should be investigated (Box 4-2). The application of these aspects is illustrated in Appendices I and II. Each aspect suggests one or more questions and they help answer the plea of the clinician: "What do I do with the answers?" Furthermore, asking about these topics can be done easily in the time frame that health professionals may spend with patients—especially physicians, where the duration of the visit may be ten to fifteen minutes.

Box 4-2

Pattern of a Sexual Dysfunction: What to Ask

1. DURATION of difficulty: lifelong or acquired
2. CIRCUMSTANCES in which difficulty appears: generalization or situational
3. DESCRIPTION of difficulty
4. PATIENT'S SEX RESPONSE CYCLE (desire, erection, ejaculation/orgasm if male; desire, vaginal lubrication, orgasm, absence of coital pain if female)
5. PARTNER'S SEX RESPONSE CYCLE (see #4)
6. PATIENT AND PARTNER'S REACTION to presence of difficulty
7. MOTIVATION FOR TREATMENT (when difficulty not chief complaint)

> Although specific words and phrases are suggested for each of the questions, interviewers must find their own ways of asking questions and using words with which they are comfortable.

For purposes of illustration, one particular problem is used, namely an erection complaint of a man who is 45 years old, heterosexual, married, with two children, and who has diabetes mellitus discovered five years ago. Although specific words and phrases are suggested for each of the questions, interviewers must find their own ways of asking questions and using words with which they are comfortable. The specific phraseology is less important than covering the topics.

PATTERN OF SEXUAL DYSFUNCTION

Diagnostic Topic #1: Lifelong or Acquired

> Acquired sexual dysfunctions always require a diligent search for an explanation of the change that has occurred.

A sexual disorder may have existed since the onset of adult sexual function (lifelong) or may have been preceded by a period of unimpaired function (acquired). The reason for separating the two is the clinical supposition that different factors may be responsible for the origins of each. In general, acquired sexual dysfunctions always require a diligent search for an explanation of the change that has occurred. One may want to look for the origin of a lifelong disorder as well but this investigation is not always therapeutically necessary.

An example of the importance of determining whether a disorder is lifelong or acquired and of the relative significance of explanatory factors in a patient's history is the problem of a woman being nonorgasmic. In this instance, a lifelong disorder can often be so successfully treated that the reasons for the problem may be of more intellectual than clinical interest. However, acquired orgasmic dysfunction may result, for example, from a large array of medical conditions that may be crucial to understand, especially from a treatment perspective. Thus the reason for the problem may be specific and, if so, the treatment should be specific as well. Hence, the lifelong/acquired differentiation is ultimately needed to give proper therapeutic direction.

Inherent in questions relating to this topic is also the duration of a concern.

An interview with the patient who has a chief complaint of an erection problem in our example may begin like this:

Q. Do you usually have erection difficulties?
A. Yes, as a matter of fact I do. I don't have erections anymore.
Q. Can I ask you some questions about that?
A. Sure.
Q. When did your erection troubles start?
A. About two years ago.
Q. What were your erections like before?
A. No problem.

The dialogue began with a screening question about erections. This was followed by a permission question (see "Permission" in Chapter 2 and Chapter 3) asking for the patient's consent to enter into the "territory" of the specific problem. Questions were then asked about duration and what the situation was like before the emergence of the trouble.

In this illustration, the man was discovered to be (1) open to questioning and (2) to have an acquired problem with his erections in that he had no difficulty until two years ago.

Diagnostic Topic #2: Generalized Or Situational

A sexual disorder may exist under all (generalized) or just some (situational) sexual circumstances. Discovering whether a problem is one or the other may be extremely valuable in speculating about its genesis. Generally, a problem that appears only sometimes (e.g., with one sexual partner but not with another) can be thought of as arising from psychosocial origins. (Important exceptions to this pattern are discussed in the introduction to Part II.) If, in contrast, a particular problem exists under all sexual circumstances, the interviewer should seriously consider the possibility of an impairment of one of the body systems controlling sexual function. The major categories of erection difficulties in most men can be successfully separated on the basis of sexual history alone.[2] A diagnostically oriented history can, obviously, be crucial in recommending a particular treatment approach.

> If a particular problem exists under all sexual circumstances, the interviewer should seriously consider the possibility of an impairment of one of the body systems controlling sexual function.

The interview with the man who has an acquired erectile problem could continue in the following way:

Q. What have you noticed during the past two years about the circumstances in which you have erection troubles?
A. What do you mean?
Q. Well, a man usually has an erection or swelling of his penis under three circumstances:

- Periodically during sleep (at night and when waking up in the morning)
- During sexual activity with a partner
- With masturbation

I'd like to ask you about the first of these. What is your penis like nowadays when you wake up in the morning?
A. I used to wake up hard because of a full bladder but that doesn't happen now.
Q. Actually, people used to think that morning erections had something to do with a full bladder but another explanation having to do with sleep cycles or patterns was discovered some years ago. You may not be aware of this but men who are healthy usually get erections three or four times a night when they are sleeping. Let me return to asking you some questions about your erection difficulties. What happens to your erections during sexual activity with your wife?

A. We try to have sex but I'm not usually hard enough to get in.

Q. I can see that is distressing and we'll discuss that in more detail in a moment. I also need to know what your penis is like when you're masturbating.

A. It's the same as when I'm with my wife. I don't get hard.

The first question was phrased in an open-ended manner. Although questions that are formulated in an open-ended way are generally promoted in health care settings, this approach may not have the same results when asking sex-related questions. Health professionals may begin with an open-ended question but very likely a patient will ask for more specific questions before answering. In the dialogue, the interviewer became more specific and in the process described something about expected erectile function. In an attempt to discover whether the erectile disturbances were generalized or situational, the interviewer asked separately about each of the circumstances in which a man is expected to experience an erection. The order of the questions was deliberate in that less provocative questions were asked before those that were more difficult to answer (see "Delaying Sensitive Questions" in Chapter 2). Morning erections were easier to discuss than erections with a partner. The topic of masturbation was last because it is a more sensitive subject. The patient's comment about erections with a full bladder provided an educational opportunity regarding normal male physiology (see "Explanation" in Chapter 2.) (Reflection on the distress of a patient was the focus of discussion of "feelings" in Chapter 2.)

> Health professionals may begin with an open-ended question but very likely the patient will ask for more specific questions before answering.

With the questions asked in relation to Diagnostic Topics #1 and #2, the interviewer ascertained that the man had an acquired form of erectile difficulty and that it existed when he woke up in the morning, when he attempted intercourse with his wife, and when he was masturbating. One can conclude, therefore, that his difficulties were acquired and also generalized.

Diagnostic Topic #3: Description

The interviewer must obtain a precise description of the problem as it exists in the present, the circumstances in which the problem arises. A description of pain with intercourse, for example, entails discovering such factors as location of the pain, what it feels like, and what makes it better or worse.

A description is a verbal picture. Although depending on words may be usual for many health professionals, this is not always the case for physicians. Medical doctors measure all sorts of physiological phenomena such as changes in blood pressure or breathing as part of the diagnostic process. They also examine sex-linked structures such as a penis or vagina but sexual complaints often relate to sexual *function* rather than *structure*. Ethical constraints prevent health care professionals from directly understanding changes in sexual function through direct observation. Hence the great dependence on words to help in comprehending sexual function that has gone awry.

> Ethical constraints prevent health care professionals from directly understanding changes in sexual function through direct observation. Hence the great dependence on words to help in comprehending sexual function that has gone awry.

To add descriptive information to what has already been discovered about the illustrated patient with acquired and generalized erectile dysfunction, the following questions could be added:

Q. If you were to compare the hardness of your penis when you wake up in the morning now to the time before you had troubles, what would it be like on a scale of 0 to 10 where 0 is completely soft, 10 is very hard and stiff, and 7 is required to enter a woman's vagina?
A. It varies a bit but it's usually about 5.
Q. How about when you're with your wife?
A. About the same.
Q. What is the hardness of your penis like when you're masturbating?
A. Not much different.

The first descriptive question was one that literally asked the patient what his penis looked like when erect, or rather, his definition of erection (or lack of it). The patient again asked for clarification of the question because he was not used to talking to anyone so explicitly about his erections. The interviewer asked for a precise description by presenting the patient with a quantitative method for providing this information. One can do this by using the 0 to 10 scale (as in the example) or by asking for a comparison on a percentage basis. Another alternative is to simply draw a penis in varying states of fullness and ask the patient to select the drawings that most closely resemble his in the past and the present.

In talking about sexual issues, it is often more useful to use simple English rather than jargon to avoid misinterpretation. For example, the question asking for a description included the words "hard" and "soft." If the question mentions only the word "erection," an incomplete erection might not be noted, since the definition of an "erection" for many men refers only to a penis that is fully hard and stiff.

The patient described a "partial" erection. That is, his penis was neither full nor completely flaccid at its largest but somewhere in-between. This same partial erection existed under all circumstances and had been this way for the past two years.

Diagnostic Topic #4: Patient's Sex Response Cycle

It is necessary to ask questions about the other two phases of the sex response cycle apart from the "response" portion, since the function of different parts of the cycle are, to some extent, interdependent, and consequently problems may exist in more than one area. For example, a man may experience erectile loss and continue to be sexually interested (the first phase) but also experience ejaculation difficulties (the third phase). To understand the sexual context for any patient's difficulty, information is necessary concerning all three phases of the patient's sex response cycle.

Using Kaplan's triphasic model, the interviewer initially asks about sexual interest or desire.[3] The problem that may exist for this phase is the *absence* of interest (referred to in DSM-IV-PC as "Hypoactive Sexual Desire Disorder").[4] This complaint manifests in men and women, although the appearance of the problem tends to be different in each (see Chapter 9).

> Specific questions about the patient's sex response cycle include the words "usually" and "often." This is deliberate, since the phenomena that are the subject of inquiry probably occur occasionally in everyone's sexual experience.

The specific questions about the patient's sex response cycle include the words "usually" or "often." This is deliberate, since the phenomena that are the subject of inquiry probably occur occasionally in everyone's sexual experience. Troubles that occur infrequently are not central to the interviewer's questions. *Persistent* and *frequent* problems should be the focus. In addition, the use of a word such as "usually" conveys an accurate but subtle message to a patient that occasional problems are to be expected.

The diagnostic interview with the man who has an acquired and generalized erectile dysfunction in which he consistently experiences partial erections could continue in the following way:

Q. What is your sexual desire or interest level usually like?

A. I think about it just as much as before but I worry about failing when I'm with my wife.

Q. I understand your concern about that but I also need to know what your ejaculation is usually like compared to the time before you had this problem.

A. It's weird. I can come when my penis is soft.

Q. That isn't abnormal. Erection and ejaculation are two separate events, although they usually work closely together. Do you have any problems with the timing of ejaculation such as being too fast or too slow?

A. No.

Q. Have you noticed any change in the intensity of your orgasm—the feeling that you get inside when you ejaculate?

A. It's not like it was when I was 20 but I haven't noticed any change in recent years.

Since the area of "response" (erection in a man) had been reviewed, the other two aspects of the sexual response cycle, namely, interest and ejaculation, became the main focus of inquiry. The words, "desire" and "interest," were used synonymously because in the opinion of the interviewer these words were less confusing than the more technical word, "libido." It was important to uncover whether the man's desire had diminished, since decreased desire may result in impaired erections.

The word, "interest," has several popular synonyms that a patient or interviewer might use. These include "desire," "drive," and "appetite."

Ejaculation, or the emission of semen, represents one of two components of the third phase (orgasm) of Kaplan's "triphasic model" in the male[3] (pp. 3-7). The other is the subjective feeling of orgasm itself. If it is difficult for men (or women) to describe the feeling of orgasm, one can, at least, ask whether the intensity of the experience has changed. In talking to a patient about ejaculation, one should ask about orgasm as well.

Ejaculation and orgasm are neurophysiologically distinct—a fact that is demonstrated by the prepubertal boy who can masturbate to the point of orgasm but who cannot ejaculate because the mechanism is not fully developed. Ejaculation is objective; orgasm is perceived as subjective but has biological correlates. Ejaculation problems are common in men (especially premature ejaculation); orgasm problems in men are unusual. A patient may be mystified by the differentiation of the terms, *ejaculation* and *orgasm,* since the two phenomena usually occur simultaneously. However, sometimes there is a problem with one and not the other. For example, in the syndrome of Anhedonic Orgasm (see Chapter 10), a man experiences the emission of semen without a powerful internal feeling at the same time.

The differentiation of ejaculation and orgasm also provides an opportunity for the interviewer to introduce some educational information into the discussion. In asking questions about ejaculation, patients may use a slang word such as "come." This word is so commonly used that for some it can substitute for a "technical" term. In the illustrated dialogue the patient used slang. Although this gave some level of permission to the interviewer to do the same, the interviewer continued to use the technical term, "ejaculation" (see "Language" in Chapter 2).

The patient had no evident impairment in the areas of "interest" except insofar as he worried about his "performance." He was puzzled by the ability to ejaculate when his penis was soft, since he was always hard in the past when this happened. Men tend to find this embarrassing and even think it to be "abnormal." Reassurance about the physiological normality of this process can be given through information. The patient did not have any problem with emission or with orgasm.

To summarize, this patient had acquired and generalized erectile difficulties. His erections were always partial and he had no additional trouble with his level of desire or with ejaculation.

Diagnostic Topic #5: Partner's Sex Response Cycle

As is the case with the patient (a man in this illustration), it is essential to ask questions about all phases of the sex response cycle in the partner (a woman in this illustration), since a problem may be confined to one area and not to others. For example, a woman with vaginismus may indicate sexual desire (the first phase), vaginal lubrication (the second phase), and orgasm (the third phase) but still experience significant vaginal discomfort with attempts at intercourse.

Sexual function involves a partner (except for masturbation) and thus sexual dysfunctions and "difficulties" are also partner-related. Although the partner can *sometimes* be implicated in the genesis of the dysfunction, the partner is *always* involved in terms of impact. Within a set of diagnostic questions, an interviewer thus needs to include information concerning the levels of interest, response, orgasm, and coital pain (if a woman) in the patient's partner.

> Although the partner can *sometimes* be implicated in the genesis of the dysfunction, the partner is *always* involved in terms of impact.

Obviously, the patient may not know the answers to such questions, may know only by inference, or may have to guess and therefore run the risk of being entirely inaccurate. The best method for obtaining this information is directly from the partner. Since many patients talk with health professionals alone (at least initially), the issue of a partner is included here even though the data obtained must be considered indirect and preliminary. In instances where partners are seen together, direct questions can be asked of each person.

The assessment or diagnostic interview with the patient with erectile troubles continues with questions about his wife's sex response cycle.

Q. What is your wife's interest in sexual activity usually like?

A. We've always been compatible except now she seems to want it more than me. I'm the one who turns her down. It wasn't like that before. It's not that I don't feel like it. I'm just not sure I can manage.

Q. When the two of you are touching each other and contemplating intercourse, does she often get wet in her vagina?

A. She sure does. She doesn't have any trouble. It's me with the problem.

Q. I understand what you mean but even if she wasn't involved in the generation of the problem, she's involved in the fact that things are not working the way they were before.

A. I suppose so. It's her problem too even if she didn't cause it.

Q. Let's go back to how she manages sexually. How about her coming to orgasm? Does that usually happen?

A. We don't have intercourse that often now but we . . . (pause) . . . have other ways to make that happen. I know she doesn't like other things as much as when I'm inside.

Q. Does she usually experience pain when you have intercourse nowadays, or did pain occur when intercourse was more frequent?

A. She certainly doesn't seem to nowadays. If she had this in the past, she never told me.

Sexual desire is subjective. Information obtained from a partner indirectly rather than from a sexually active person directly must be considered inferential unless the two people involved have had a very explicit discussion about this topic—an unusual event in the lives of many couples. In contrast, it is natural for people (as it was for this patient) to compare their own sexual interest level with that of their partner's and to comment particularly on changes that have occurred.

Problems with vaginal lubrication represent the second phase (response) of Kaplan's "triphasic model" in women.[3] Vaginal lubrication is, from a functional point of view, the equivalent of erection in a man in that both are evidence of pelvic vasocongestion and sexual arousal[5] (p. 279). Problems relating to lubrication in the absence of diminished desire are common in postmenopausal women but is not common at an earlier age. Such difficulties are most often the result of estrogen deficit or vaginal pathology (see Chapter 13).

The question about the patient's wife being sexually excited and vaginally wet involved asking two questions at one time. Generally, this is a confusing interviewing technique and one to be avoided. It was done here because becoming vaginally wet is so closely associated with excitement.

Orgasm is the third phase of Kaplan's "triphasic model" as applied to women[3] (pp.3-7). Although there are objective phenomena associated with orgasm in women, namely, vaginal and uterine contractions, the subjective experience is the focus of inquiry[5] (pp. 128-129).

Orgasm problems in women (in contrast to orgasm problems in men) are common. While the manner in which orgasm is experienced (for example, by masturbation or by vaginal intercourse) is *not* part of this question, it is phrased in such a way that concerns about this can be voiced if so wished by the patient.

Dyspareunia, or painful intercourse, does not easily fit into the "triphasic model." However, the fact that this is a frequent problem for women (although unusual in men) means that it should be included in "sex" questions relating to women.

The patient's wife was, apparently, sexually interested in spite of his troubles. Her response level was such that she became wet, or lubricated, when sexually excited. She seemed to be regularly orgasmic and painful intercourse was not obvious.

The patient with acquired and generalized erectile difficulties had partial erections at all times and no trouble with his level of sexual desire or ejaculation. His wife similarly had no disturbance with sexual desire (as far as he knew), becoming vaginally wet when sexually excited, being orgasmic, and not experiencing pain with intercourse.

Diagnostic Topic #6: Patient and Partner's Reaction to Problem

The reaction of a patient or partner to the existence of a sexual disorder is partly a result of the universal human search for explanations for unhappy life events. The response could also reflect the difficulty or its treatment. Worries about a sexual problem can become important as a perpetuating factor apart from the original cause. The psyche and soma are difficult to separate when trying to understand what has gone wrong, since there are so many connections between the two. Kaplan talked of "sex" being "psychosomatic."[6] Indeed, one can hardly provide a better example of the links between mind and body.

> The reaction of a patient or partner to the existence of a sexual disorder is partly a result of the universal human search for explanations for unhappy life events.

Reactions to sexual problems are heavily influenced by the virtually universal tendency of patients to blame themselves for the presence of sexual difficulties. Feelings of guilt are undoubtedly part of this process.

> Worries about a sexual problem can become important as a perpetuating factor apart from the original cause.

The interview with the patient with erectile dysfunction now concentrates on psychosocial issues:

Q. How do you feel about this problem?
A. Terrible. I feel like I'm not a man any more.
Q. Many people in your situation feel the same way. Has it affected your mood?
A. It's discouraging but I'm not really depressed if that's what you mean.
Q. How does your wife feel about what's happening?
A. I'm really not sure.
Q. Well what does she say?
A. She tells me not to worry so much. She says that it isn't such a big problem from her point of view.

The interviewer attempted to assess the feelings of the patient and the partner. As is the case with most men in this situation, the patient was clearly upset but was able to distinguish between being unhappy and feeling depressed. The interviewer empathically acknowledged the patient's feelings and the normality of his reaction (see "Feelings" in Chapter 2). The patient also connected his disturbance in sexual function to his sense of masculinity. There is, in fact, usually a great sense of loss of masculinity or femininity in the individual who is unable to have intercourse. The most dramatic examples of the impact of a sexual dysfunction on a patient's sense of gender completeness are in women with vaginismus who feel so incompetent as women that they sometimes suggest to their husbands that they "go elsewhere."

The patient in the illustration did not know what his partner thought, since she had not directly told him of her feelings. The interviewer pursued the subject by asking the patient to say something about his wife's reaction. Evidently, the wife's reaction did not reassure the patient.

This man with acquired and generalized erectile difficulty had partial erections but he didn't have trouble in the areas of sexual desire or ejaculation. His wife did not have problems with desire, lubrication, orgasm, or coital pain. This patient felt discouraged but his wife had been reassuring.

Diagnostic Topic #7: Motivation for Treatment

> Although sexual dysfunctions are extremely common, not every patient wants to change.

Although sexual dysfunctions are extremely common, not every patient wants to change. This observation is apparent clinically and has been made from a research viewpoint also.[7] Some may be unwilling to do whatever is required to bring about change. The "price" may be too high in terms of, for example, embarrassment in talking to a stranger about "sex" (even a health professional). Given the willingness of some patients to accommodate to the presence of a sexual problem, a health professional can not assume a desire for change, and therefore it becomes essential to ask someone with an apparent sexual dysfunction if, in fact, they want some assistance. Unwillingness to engage in the process of change may be especially evident when a sexual problem is uncovered in the course of history-taking around some other health issue. However, even if a patient rejects the offer of help in this situation, the problem is noted and may be addressed in the future. *Obviously, if a sexual problem is the patient's "chief complaint," motivation is self-evident and a question concerning the desire to change is superfluous.*

The brief diagnostic interview with the patient who has acquired and generalized erectile difficulties ends with the following dialogue (included only for the purpose of illustration rather than clinical need):

Q. Is this a problem that you want some help with in terms of change?
A. What would that involve?
Q. We could talk a bit more and maybe I could see your wife as well. In addition, I'd like to conduct a physical examination and order some laboratory tests, since some aspects of your history suggest that your erectile troubles may be connected to changes in your body.
A. Your plan sounds fine. I'll ask my wife if she wants to come in.

Having determined the dimensions of the problem faced by the patient, the interviewer then asked a "where do we go from here"—type of question. The possibilities were outlined, at least for the near future, taking into consideration the capabilities of the interviewer to further investigate and possibly manage sexual problems.

The diagnostic interview of the 42-year-old man with an erection complaint tells us the following:

1. His erection troubles were acquired and generalized
2. His erections were partial
3. His sexual interest level and ejaculation were unchanged
4. His wife's experience with her level of sexual desire, lubrication, orgasm, and experience with coital pain were similarly unaltered
5. He was concerned about his erection problems, although his wife was reassuring
6. He wanted to investigate the problem and was prepared to include his wife in the process if she was willing

SUMMARY AND CONCLUSIONS

Health professionals sometimes refrain from asking questions about sexual matters because they do not know what to do with the answers. In pursuing a positive answer to a screening question, one must continue beyond the complaint to the level of a diagnosis. In the history-taking part of establishing a clinical diagnosis, clinicians may need information from some or all of six or seven types of information (see Box 4-1).

Obtaining detailed information about the particular problem (see first item in Box 4-1) entails asking questions relating to six or seven topic areas (depending on whether the problem was uncovered in the process of investigating another concern or whether it was presented as the "chief complaint"; see Box 4-2).

The questions that arise from these six or seven topics can be asked easily within the time frame that many health professionals spend with patients. Answers may provide information about the nature of the problem and suggest a direction in the search for possible contributing factors and the kinds of investigations that may prove necessary. Appendix III provides examples of the use of this seven-question model that could be used for role-plays in an educational setting.

The example of a man with erection difficulties was used as an illustration but it assumed the existence of basic information about his physical and psychiatric health. The conclusion of this diagnostic process was that this 45-year-old married man with diabetes mellitus, a disease known to be associated with sexual dysfunctions,[8] had a two-year history of erectile problems. His erections were consistently partial and unrelated to his wife's sexual response. He and his wife seemed to have substantial concerns about the change in their sexual experiences. The preliminary diagnosis was that of an erectile disorder presumably related to diabetes. Further medical investigations and laboratory studies were warranted (see Chapter 11). Talking with his wife (alone, with her husband, or both) may provide useful diagnostic information and allow for an understanding of her willingness to be involved in a treatment program.

Some primary care clinicians might be satisfied with what has occurred so far and prefer to send the patient to an urologist for further care. This course of action may not be possible. An urologist may not be geographically nearby, and having unburdened himself or herself to one person, the patient may be unwilling to do so again.

Furthermore, the relationship with the patient may be such that there is a preference, and even a request, for the continued therapeutic involvement of the primary care clinician. In other words, circumstances may dictate the actions of the health professional quite apart from his or her personal desire to continue the investigation. If the patient does not want to be referred, the health professional may wish to explore the reasons for the unwillingness. The patient may, for example, have unspoken fears about talking to another health professional.

The health professional may decide to proceed further before referral and can do so by examining the context in which the sexual dysfunction currently appears and has developed. The present and past contexts of sexual problems are the subjects of the next chapter.

REFERENCES

1. Merrill JM, Laux LF, Thornby JI: Why doctors have difficulty with sex histories, *South Med J* 83:613-617, 1990.
2. Segraves KA, Segraves RT, Schoenberg HW: Use of sexual history to differentiate organic from psychogenic impotence, *Arch Sex Behav* 16:125-137, 1987.
3. Kaplan HS: *Disorders of sexual desire*, New York, 1979, Brunner/Mazel, Inc.
4. *Diagnostic and Statistical Manual of Mental Disorders, ed 4, Primary Care Version*, Washington, 1995, American Psychiatric Association.
5. Masters WH, Johnson VE: *Human sexual response*, Boston, 1966, Little, Brown and Company.
6. Kaplan HS: *Sex is Psychosomatic (editorial)*, *J Sex Marital Ther* 1:275-276,1975.
7. Garde K, Lunde I: Female sexual behaviour: a study in a random sample of 40-year old women, *Maturitas* 2:225-240, 1980.
8. Jensen SB: Sexual relationships in couples with a diabetic partner, *J Sex Marital Ther* 11:259-270,1985.

CHAPTER 5

CONTEXT OF SEXUAL DISORDERS: ISSUES AND QUESTIONS IN THE PRESENT AND PAST

Of all the topics we consider, the content of sexual action and interaction has received the least scholarly attention. What people do sexually—alone or with others—and how they think about their sex lives are subjects that have rarely entered the mainstream of social scientific discourse. . .the level of an individual's sexual activity, however indexed over time, is perhaps the most lore ridden (topic) of all.

LAUMANN ET AL, 1994[1]

PROLOGUE

In the process of eliciting information about determinants of sexual dysfunctions, Kaplan incorporated a cross-sectional and a longitudinal view that included all aspects of biological, psychological, and social theorizing[2] (Box 5-2). She specifically described psychosocial contributing factors as "immediate" (Box 5-1) and "remote" (p. 118).

In scrutinizing the foundations of a sexual dysfunction, there is no necessary incompatibility between immediate and remote factors. They can, and often do, coexist. It is not necessary to theorize about an either/or issue. Uncovering immediate contributors requires an analysis of present sexual events. Other than the significant issue of personal comfort of the health professional, primary care clinicians can easily acquire immediate information within the time frame ordinarily spent with patients (although the process may involve more than one visit).

> Other than the significant issue of personal comfort on the part of the health professional, primary care clinicians can easily acquire "immediate" information within the time-frame ordinarily spent with patients (although the process may involve more than one visit).

The process of discovering remote causes is considerably more complex and includes taking a developmental history (the "story" of the person from birth to the onset of present troubles). Acquiring this information involves more time than many primary care clinicians are regularly prepared to allow. In such instances, consulting a mental health professional who is comfortable with the subject of "sex" and skilled in talking to patients about sexual issues might be a reasonable alternative. Nevertheless, the section of this chapter on remote issues may be useful to the primary care health professional for reference purposes on a particular topic or to develop a better understanding of subjects covered if the patient was referred to a specialist.

PRESENT CONTEXT: IMMEDIATE ISSUES AND QUESTIONS

The most illuminating method for uncovering immediate contributors to a sexual dysfunction is through a detailed description of a recent sexual encounter. To be sure, this is not simple for the patient or the health professional. Describing the nature of,

---

Box 5-1

"Immediate" Psychosocial Causes of Sexual Dysfunction

1. Sexual ignorance
2. Fear of failure
3. Excess need to please a partner
4. Spectatoring[2]
5. Failure to communicate sexual preferences
6. Relationship problems

Adapted from Kaplan HS: *The new sex therapy: active treatment of sexual dysfunctions*, New York, 1974, Brunner/Mazel, Inc., pp. 121-136.

Box 5-2

"Remote" Psychosocial Causes of a Sexual Dysfunction

1. Internal conflict over sexual pleasure
2. Restrictive upbringing
3. Developmental sources of sexual conflict
4. Transference
5. Lack of trust
6. Traumatic early sexual experience

Adapted from Kaplan HS: *The new sex therapy: active treatment of sexual dysfunctions*, New York, 1974, Brunner/Mazel, Inc., pp.137-184.

---

for example, an erection problem is very different from telling the story of *"who does what to whom"* in bed (or anywhere else). The facts involved in the static and cross-sectional description of one's current sexual problem seem much easier to talk about than the dynamic and longitudinal view of a sexual encounter involving another person. Patients who spontaneously describe their sexual experiences run the risk of being seen as verbal exhibitionists, and health professionals who ask questions about these events might be viewed as voyeurs. Two factors could prevent either view:

- An attitude of the health professional that sexual function is a proper dimension of health and therefore a legitimate topic for discussion
- The ethical cloak of the health professional, which defines in whose interest questions are being asked (the patient's) and for what purpose (clarification)

Kaplan referred to the process of asking about the minutiae of a sexual encounter as the Sexual Status Examination[4] (pp. 77-84). Because of the great sensitivity involved in revealing specifics, it is best not to ask this at the beginning of an initial visit. Patients should have an opportunity to decide if they feel comfortable disclosing private and personal information to a particular health professional.

Questions can begin with the patient's (or couple, if both are seen together on a first visit) practices in being affectionate with a partner and how this is separated from what is regarded as "sexual."

The following are initial questions that might be asked of a heterosexual man (although they apply equally well to heterosexual women and same-sex partners):

Q. In what ways are you affectionate with your wife (husband, partner)?

Q. Is it possible for this to occur without thinking that some sexual event will automatically occur as a result?

Q. Do you sleep in the same bed together?

Q. What sort of bedclothes do you and your wife (husband, partner) wear?

Q. Do you snuggle together before going to sleep?

Q. Does this involve touching each other?

Q. What are your "geographical" limits to touching?

Q. What are your sexual "signals?"

Q. How do you separate affectionate and sexual signals?

Q. What are you thinking about when something sexual might occur?

Q. What sort of thoughts do you have at that time about the problem that brought you here today?

Much of the questioning revolves around touching, an aspect of human communication that is intimately related to sexual behavior[5] (pp. 204-236). Answers give the interviewer some idea of the level of sexual communication between the partners and also the extent of anticipatory worry about the sexual difficulty. The interviewer often hears that partners used to be affectionate with each other but that, since the onset of sexual troubles, sex and affection have diminished. This is often to the chagrin of both (see "Treatment of HSD" in Chapter 9).

The patient might then be asked to describe the last time that a sexual experience occurred. When a person is obviously uncomfortable with the request, the interviewer should quickly offer to ask specific questions. The focus in particular should be on what occurred just before attempts at intercourse, since the immediate precursors to sexual dysfunctions are often discovered with this kind of inquiry.

> The patient might be asked to describe the last time a sexual experience occurred. When a person is obviously uncomfortable with the request, the interviewer should quickly offer to ask specific questions.

Illustrative questions concerning sexual practices short of vaginal intercourse follow (asked, in this example, of a heterosexual man):

Q. Do you recall the last time a sexual experience occurred with your wife (partner)?

Q. Was the location usual for you?

Q. What occurred before attempt at vaginal entry?

Q. Do you usually touch your wife's (partner's) breasts before intercourse?

Q. As far as you know, how enjoyable is that for her?

Q. How does she let you know?

Q. Does she touch your penis?

Q. What are you thinking about when that happens?

Q. Are you clear with her about how you like your penis touched?

Q. Have you ever ejaculated when she rubbed your penis?

Q. How does she feel about the wetness of your semen?

Q. Do you touch your wife (partner) between her legs?

Q. What are you thinking about when that happens?

Q. How does she react to that?

Q. Are you aware of where her clitoris is?

Q. Do you stimulate her in this area?

Q. Has she told you how she likes to be touched?

Q. Does she come to orgasm when you're touching this area?

Q. Does oral stimulation of your penis take place?

Q. Do you stimulate her genital area orally?

Q. How do each of you feel about that?

Q. What are you thinking about when you're stimulating her orally?

Q. Are there other kinds of sexual experiences that you and your wife (partner) have together before you attempt vaginal entry?

These questions are explicit enough to uncover the following information:

1. Deficits in knowledge about body parts
2. The range of sexual activities engaged in by the patient and partner
3. Attitudes toward different sexual actions
4. The level of sexual communication between patient and partner
5. What occurs in the patient's mind as the experience evolves

These questions will reveal immediate problems such as:

- Sexual ignorance
- Fear of failure
- Excessive need to please the partner
- "Spectatoring"
- Insufficient communication

When these factors exist, they often can be quickly and effectively remedied.

Little objective information existed in the past about common sexual practices of heterosexual, gay, and lesbian couples. The knowledge that HIV/AIDS is usually transmitted sexually and is therefore potentially preventable has resulted in a need for more information about what people do sexually with one another. Laumann and colleagues discussed the occurrence and incidence of various sexual practices (Tables 5-1 and 5-2) used by opposite gender, gay, and lesbian partners[1] (pp. 96-109 and 317-320).

Almost 75% of men and women subjects in the Laumann et al. study reported that fellatio or cunnilingus was performed by an opposite-sex partner at some time in their lives.[1] Rates of experience over the previous year were similar to lifetime experience, yet only about 25% of the respondents experienced fellatio or cunnilingus during their last sexual event. The conclusion of the authors was that oral sex was familiar to many people and that, after experience with this practice, it was at least occasionally incorporated into a person's sexual activity for the remainder of their lives (p. 107). They added, however, that these two sexual activities did not become defining features of sexual activity between women and men—as was the case of vaginal intercourse, or perhaps, kissing (p. 101). Among gay men and lesbians, rates of activity increased as

Table 5-1 Sexual Practices of Men		
	ANY SAME-GENDER PARTNERS IN PAST YEAR (%)	TOTAL POPULATION (%)
Masturbation (1x/wk or > {ly})	69	27
Active oral sex (sp)	89	77
Active oral sex (le)	—	27
Receptive oral sex (sp)	94	79
Receptive oral sex (le)	—	28
Active anal IC (sp)	79	26
Receptive anal IC (sp)	77	—
Anal IC (ly)	—	10
Anal IC (le)	—	2

Adapted from Laumann EO et al: *The social organization of sexuality: sexual practices in the United States,* Chicago, 1994, The University of Chicago Press.
sp, Since puberty; *ly,* last year; *le,* last event;
IC, intercourse.

Table 5-2 Sexual Practices Of Women		
	ANY SAME-GENDER PARTNERS IN PAST YEAR (%)	TOTAL POPULATION (%)
Masturbation (1x/wk or >[1y])	—	8
Active oral sex (sp)	—	68
Active oral sex (le)	—	19
Receptive oral sex (sp)	—	73
Receptive oral sex (le)	—	20
Anal IC (ly)	—	9
Anal IC (le)	—	1

Adapted from Laumann EO et al: *The social organization of sexuality: sexual practices in the United States,* Chicago, 1994, The University of Chicago Press.
sp, Since puberty; *ly,* last year; *le,* last event.
IC, intercourse.

"homosexuality" was defined more narrowly (see below in this chapter for a discussion of homosexuality and problems with the definition).

The interviewer can continue with specific questions about vaginal intercourse (asked, in this example, of a heterosexual woman):

Q. How is a decision made about vaginal entry?
Q. What intercourse position(s) do you usually use?

Q. Is that something that the two of you talk about?

Q. What happens to your excitement level after he enters?

Q. Are you usually wet when he enters?

Q. Does he have any trouble entering because of the stiffness of his penis?

Q. What do you think about when he's inside?

Q. Does he usually tell you before he ejaculates?

Q. Does he usually ejaculate before you're ready?

Q. Do you tell him if you want him to delay ejaculation?

Q. Do you usually come to orgasm when he's inside?

Q. What do the two of you do after he ejaculates?

Q. How do you feel about the wetness of his semen?

Q. What do you think about when you're lying together?

Q. What is your experience with anal intercourse?

Laumann and colleagues had little to say about vaginal intercourse, since the lifetime experience of survey subjects with this sexual practice was virtually universal.[1] Much more was said about anal intercourse, which differed substantially in heterosexual men and women when compared to oral sexual activity (see Tables 5-1 and 5-2). The authors concluded that anal intercourse was "far less likely to become a common or even an occasional sexual practice once it has been experienced" (p. 107). The occurrence of anal intercourse among gay men is of particular interest because of its link to HIV/AIDS transmission. Of interest was the finding that 20% to 25% of the (narrowly defined) homosexual men reported that they have never experienced anal intercourse.

The questions outlined above provide details about the nature of the specific problem and, as well, can reveal information about immediate causes of a sexual dysfunction.

CONTEXT OF THE PAST: REMOTE ISSUES AND QUESTIONS

Some sex therapists say that in the process of assessing someone with a sexual complaint, one does not need to (indeed, *should* not) obtain detailed information about that person's life history unless obstacles arise[6] (p. 416). However, apart from clinical opinion, some research was conducted on the value of linking past and present. Heiman and colleagues studied couples defined as "clinical" (on a waiting list for a sex therapy clinic) and "nonclinical" (obtained from a newspaper ad).[7] She found that issues from "the more distant past" could be important for those with sexual dysfunctions, especially women. Clinical experience supports this point of view. Experience rather than research is the major tool guiding the clinician in clarifying when and under what circumstances detailed exploration of the past should or should not take place.

Circumstances in which an elaborate investigation of the past may *not* be necessary can often be defined in advance. These circumstances represent situations in which, for example, the focus of care is largely educational (as is often the case in lifelong and generalized orgasmic dysfunction in women [see Chapter 12]) or when the patient's status makes it predictable that the mainstay of treatment will be largely "medical" (for example, instances of premature ejaculation in which the focus of care is on the use of medications rather than talk [see Chapter 10]). In the absence of research, two general concepts serve as a clinical rationale for reviewing the patient's past.

The first concept is that it is only *after* the fact that the interviewer knows the items in a patient's past history that may be of potential significance in relation to etiology or treatment. In other words, one does not know if a "smoking gun" is hidden in a particular field until that area is searched.

The second concept is the common sense notion that personality characteristics and facets of a relationship are not left outside the bedroom when people engage in sexual activities. Issues related to personality and the relationship are of as much concern in the bedroom as they are in the kitchen or living room. Elements that went into the formation of both partners need to be explored if one's concept of "sex" is such that the body and mind are inseparable. Only when genital function is the predominant sexual consideration, such as sexual activity between a prostitute and a client, may personality and relationship factors be less meaningful.

> Personality characteristics and facts of a relationship are not left outside the bedroom when people engage in sexual activities. Issues related to personality and the relationship are of as much concern in the bedroom as they are in the kitchen or living room.

SEXUAL-DEVELOPMENTAL HISTORY

As described here, the *sexual-developmental* history is a developmental history with a special focus on the individual's personal sexual evolution. Comprehensive texts on interviewing should be consulted in relation to nonsexual aspects of a developmental history[8] (pp. 65-82). The assumption in this book is that the special aspects of sexual development are "grafted" to the general aspects of a patient's personal and social history. As Gadpaille wrote, "Sexual development does not occur separately from all other aspects of human growth and maturation. To treat it separately is to some degree a distortion"[9] (p. 46).

In a sexual-developmental history, the list of sex-related questions that might be asked is exhaustive to the interviewer and exhausting for the patient. Inevitably, the interviewer is selective and inquires about issues that appear to have relevance to the present problem. The key word is "appear." Different areas appear to be pertinent to different clinicians. To some, all areas of inquiry are relevant. To others, there must be clear and prior justification for particular questions. In either instance, an interviewer should be able to explain the rationale for any question asked.

> To some clinicians, all areas of inquiry are relevant. To others, there must be clear and prior justification for particular questions. Either way, an interviewer should be able to explain the rationale for any question asked.

The psychosocial connections between past and present in relation to sexual problems generally were subjects of speculation and data-oriented research. Intuitive concepts come from analytically oriented psychotherapists and theoreticians, including Freud and his disciples.[10] Data-oriented observations were derived from sources such as:

- Experimental research with primates[11]
- Gender problems in children[12]
- Intersex problems in children[13,14]
- Sex-related surveys[1,15-18]

There is an inclination to consider sexual dysfunctions as a group when, in fact, they are heterogeneous. Lumping them together is, to a large extent, unreasonable (hence the rationale for using the word "dysfunctions" in the plural). If the syndromes are, indeed, heterogeneous, it would not be surprising to find that the etiologies are heterogenous as well. Biopsychosocial issues that relate to girls and women are unlikely to be the same for boys and men. Sexual dysfunctions that are lifelong usually have different bases than those that are acquired. Desire disorders are grouped under the same heading in DSM-IV but their origins may well be different from other sexual dysfunctions.[19] These varied roots result in complex interpretation of information obtained in a sexual-developmental history. The connections between past and present may be obscure, may be a matter of speculation, or may be obvious. Without a diligent search it is not possible to determine which they might be.

> The connections between past and present may be obscure, may be a matter of speculation, or may be obvious. Without a diligent search it is not possible to determine which they might be.

As an interviewer traverses the life span, areas of questioning can be defined for each part, as well as the specific questions to be asked and the rationale for the inquiry.

Childhood

Areas of Inquiry

Areas of inquiry include the following:

1. Family-of-origin practices in the exchange of affection (touching and talking)
2. Gender identity/role issues (feeling of maleness or femaleness as a child, favorite games, gender of friends)
3. Learning about intercourse from a reproductive point of view
4. Learning about body structure in the context of exploratory games ("playing doctor")
5. Reaction of adults to discovering one child investigating another
6. Childhood sexual experience with other children and adults

Suggested Questions

Q. Tell me about where you were born and grew up.
Q. Who was in your family at that time?
Q. Where are they now?
Q. What is the nature of your relationship with them now?
Q. Would family members hug or kiss one another when you were young?
Q. Were you happy with the idea of being a boy (girl) when you were small?
Q. Were your friends in primary school mostly other boys (girls) or mostly girls (boys)?
Q. What were your favorite games in your primary school years?
Q. Were you teased about anything?
Q. What about?
Q. How did you first learn about "how babies are made"?
Q. Did you play "doctor" games?
Q. Were you discovered by adults?
Q. How did they react?

Q. Do you recall having sexual thoughts, feelings, or experiences in your preschool years or before you were a teenager?

Q. Children sometimes have sexual experiences with other children or with adults. Was this part of your experience when you were a child?

Studies of Childhood Sexuality

Systematic research into childhood sexuality is limited, probably because parents and schools are circumspect in allowing children to be subjects of study. In spite of this, there is a substantial amount of accumulated information about childhood sexuality and preadolescent sexual behavior.[9,20-23] Martinson's review of relevant information from fetal life to the preadolescent years provides an understanding of the antecedents to adult sexual thoughts, feelings, and experiences.[22] He reflected on the following manifold developmental experiences of children:

- Sensory responsiveness and maternal attachment of the neonate
- Genital play, questions about sex, sex play among peers, and attitudes of parents toward touch in the young child
- Dating, masturbation, erection, orgasm, and heterosexual sex play in preadolescent years

Preadolescent Sexual Play

Kinsey et al. described the specifics of male preadolescent erotic arousal, sex play, and orgasm[15] (pp. 157-193). Their observations clearly established that the minds and bodies of boys were sexually simmering. They provided similar information in their later volume on females[16] (pp. 101-131) and, as well, commented on the significance of preadolescent sex play (pp. 114-116). They concluded the following:

1. First information about sex and body parts was often obtained in the context of play and was therefore of educational significance.
2. "Some of the preadolescent contacts provided emotional satisfactions that conditioned the female for the acceptance of later sexual activities."
3. Guilt reactions induced by adults discovering a child engaged in sex play in many instances "prevented the female from freely accepting sexual relations in her adult married relationships."
4. Male preadolescent sex activities were more commonly carried over into adolescent years than was preadolescent sex activities for females. This "discontinuity" in girls is more the result of culturally related restraints put on older children than "biological latency."

Cross-cultural studies of sexual behavior demonstrate that in sexually permissive societies, individuals in the middle childhood years are far from sexually disinterested, inactive, or "latent."[24] The concept of latency in these years seems more accurately applied to heterosocial rather than heterosexual relationships.

Touch in Childhood

Many of the studies on which Martinson's review was based were conducted in North America[22] (pp. 57-82). If one considers the variety of attitudes and practices toward sexual development in other cultures, it seems almost impossible to define universal preadolescent developmental norms. Montagu particularly emphasized the significance of touch in early childhood development and its relationship to adult sexual behavior and problems[5] (pp. 204-236). Touching was the subject of experimental investigation when the Harlows deprived primates of a warm and affectionate mother. It was demonstrated that primate offspring were so disturbed in their relational abilities that, among other things, they were unable to mate effectively.[11] While one must be cautious in comparing primates and humans, it is nevertheless interesting to consider the consequences of human childhood deprivation. Not surprisingly, studies of adults who were severely deprived in childhood suggest, among other things, substantial negative repercussions in the areas of relationships and sexual disorders.[25]

Roots of Atypical Sexual Behavior

The meaning of divergence from whatever norms exist in preadolescent years is often unclear in relation to adult sexual problems. These differences are particularly blurred when considering two groups of sexual disorders: sexual dysfunctions and paraphilias. In contrast, the childhood precursors of some atypical forms of adult sexual behavior such as same-sex interest and gender disorders have received a greater degree of attention and seem better defined.[26]

Gender problems in adult life frequently become apparent in childhood and hence it is important to ask about this in a sexual-developmental history. Long-term follow-up of boys with feminine characteristics shows that half or more are sexually atypical as adults.[27] Girls who behave in a boyish fashion (tomboys) usually develop as typical women; a small number emerge with a lesbian orientation (p. 155).

Sex Education

There is a certain ritual to the process of asking about "sex education" in a sexual-developmental history. In practice, the answers tend to be largely uniform. Many people say that sex was not discussed in their parental home and that what was learned as a child came from "the street." One has to distinguish between schooling and education in all matters. The importance of formal sex education courses in schools on adult sexual expression is difficult to assess. In the opinion of Masters, Johnson, and Kolodny[28] (p. 128), more information is learned by the informal process of a child watching his or her parents being affectionate with each other.

Child Sexual Abuse

In the Laumann et al. study, 12% of the men and 17% of the women respondents reported having been touched sexually before puberty or when they were 12 or 13 years old.[1] (Only 'hands-on' experiences [i.e., touching] were asked about to eliminate cases of exhibitionism.) Their data suggest the following:

1. That adult-child sexual contact was not occurring more often than in previous years
2. Girls were most likely to be touched by adult men
3. Boys were most likely to be touched by adolescent women
4. Genital touching was the most common sexual event

5. The most common age of the girls was 7 to 10
6. The common age of the boys was older
7. Experiences were most likely to occur with one adult (although one third had experiences with more than one person)
8. The adult was usually a relative or family friend

An evaluation of the effects of sexually abusive childhood experiences on adult life (a crucial clinical issue) revealed the following:

1. Women respondents answered questions on this topic more often than men
2. More women (70%) than men (48%) reported that the experience affected their lives
3. Nearly all respondents judged the effects to have been negative

The sexual sequelae of adult-child sexual activity include effects on sexual function and sexual practices[29]:

- More sexual partners
- More experience with anal intercourse with an opposite-gender partner
- More oral sexual experience among women
- A greater degree of thinking about sexual issues among men

Significant negative long-term consequences (sexual and nonsexual) to sexual experiences between an adult and female child have previously been reviewed.[30] Given this information about long-term sexual sequelae, there seems little doubt about the need to ask questions about this subject in a sexual-developmental history.

Puberty and Adolescence
Areas of Inquiry

Areas of inquiry include the following:

1. Body changes associated with puberty

   - Age of body growth
   - Pubic hair growth
   - Facial hair growth in boys
   - Breast development and onset of menstrual periods in girls

2. Changes in the size of genital organs
3. Feelings about the above changes in relation to peers
4. Changes in genital function associated with various sexual stimuli, including masturbation

   - Erection and ejaculation in men
   - Vaginal lubrication and orgasm in women

5. Sexual attraction to and sexual experiences with members of the opposite and the same sex
6. Reactions to these experiences
7. Repetitive thoughts about being attracted to same-sex individuals without desire or experience

8. Feelings about important love and sexual experiences through adolescence
9. Appearance of the present sexual problem in early sexual experiences
10. Atypical sexual thoughts, feelings, and experiences
11. Forced sexual experiences
12. Pregnancy
13. Abortion and birth control
14. Sexually transmitted diseases

Suggested Questions

Q. How old were you when you first noticed the development of body changes? (For example, men: becoming taller, voice changing, needing to shave; women: breast development, onset of menstrual periods)

Q. How did the timing of this compare to other kids in your class at school?

Q. How did this affect you?

Q. Did you know what to expect (and if so, how)?

Q. (men) Do you recall having erections before your teens?

Q. (men) Tell me about the first time you remember having an erection.

Q. (men) What do you recall about the first time you ejaculated?

Q. (men) Do you remember having "wet dreams"?

Q. Tell me about your experience with masturbation in your teens.

Q. (women) Did you usually come to orgasm?

Q. How did you feel about stimulating yourself?

Q. What did you think about when you masturbated?

Q. What is your experience with masturbation nowadays?

Q. What do you think about when you're masturbating nowadays?

Q. Boys (girls) often feel a surge of sexual feelings in their teens. What was it like for you in those years?

Q. Sometimes boys (girls) have sexual experiences with other boys (girls) during that time. Was that part of your experience?

Q. What about nowadays? Do you find yourself sexually attracted to other men (women)?

Q. Have you had sexual experiences with other men (women) since puberty?

Q. Boys in their teens who have trouble dating girls sometimes worry about being gay, even though they're not sexually attracted to other boys. Did that happen to you?

Q. Tell me about relationships that were important to you in your high school years?

Q. Was there a sexual component to those relationships apart from intercourse?

Q. What actually took place?

Q. Did intercourse take place?

Q. How did you feel about that?

Q. What were your intercourse experiences like?

Q. How did you feel about having intercourse at that time?

Q. Did the problem that you have now appear at that time?

Q. Did you have sexual thoughts or experiences in those years that you thought were unusual (e.g., being sexually involved with young children)?

Q. Did you have sexual experiences where force was used?

Q. (women) Did you become pregnant in your teens?

Q. (women) Did you ever have an abortion?

Q. Did you ever have a sexually transmitted diseases?

Physical Changes

The timing of the body changes of puberty and the accompanying feelings are usually well remembered. This is typically a time of magnified awareness of physical attributes and self-consciousness about every imperfection. Changes rarely occur in logical fashion. Instead, feet can become larger before legs become longer. Dissatisfaction is virtually universal. When this sense of unattractiveness is added to the surge of sexual feelings that typically occur at puberty, the result is

> When a sense of unattractiveness is added to the surge of sexual feelings that typically occur at puberty, the result is often one of tremendous confusion about romance and "sex."

often one of tremendous confusion about romance and "sex." Memories of this time remain vivid forever, and sometimes they have a major impact on later relationships.

Developmental deviance from age-mates is a potential source of embarrassment and bewilderment. The first girl in a class whose breasts are enlarging may simultaneously be an object of envy from other girls and teasing from boys. Conformity in dress and physical development is high on the list of adolescent aspirations. On an intuitive level, delay in physical development has a negative influence on adolescent sexual experimentation and, because of that, may have a negative effect on adult sexual behavior as well.

Adolescence is a time for relationship experimentation; biology influences when this begins and also its extent. Kinsey et al. found that later onset of puberty in boys (age 15 and over) was associated with a lower level of sexual activity among men in future years. Conversely, early onset of puberty (by age 11) was connected to a higher level of sexual activity throughout a man's life[15] (pp. 302-308).

That the hormonal surge of early adolescence has profound biological consequences is obvious. The onset of menstrual periods in girls can have meanings far beyond the flow of blood. The event presages the beginning of childbearing potential and, in the minds of parents, sexual capacity. Parental pride or dread can be transmitted to the adolescent. Cultural traditions in this area are fascinating. Among some groups in India, a public celebration occurs for an adolescent girl one week after the onset of her first menstrual period. Pride and publicity replaces the shame and secrecy that one sometimes still sees in North America. In more open cultures, the "whole world" knows that a "rite of passage" has taken place.

Erections in a male child occur regularly from infancy onward but awareness is often dated from puberty. Ejaculation must await the pubertal biological clock, although males may report orgasm in response to genital touch for years previously. Spontaneous nocturnal ejaculation (or "wet dreams") occur in over 80% of men at some time in their lives[15] (p. 274) but "are primarily a phenomenon of the teens and the twenties"(p. 243). For those who view nocturnal emissions as entirely a function of biology, it remains a challenge to explain Kinsey et al.'s finding (p. 277) that the frequency was higher for better-educated men. The fact that many women also experience orgasm during sleep is less well known. Over 35% of women contributing to the Kinsey et al. study experienced nocturnal orgasm by the age of 45[16] (p. 196).

Masturbation

The first experience with ejaculation is, for many men, through masturbation. This activity was so common among male adolescents in the Kinsey et al. study (88% for single men between ages 16 and 20) that they stopped asking whether it happened or not and, instead, simply asked at what age it began[15] (p. 238). Masturbation was less usual among females. By age 20, 33% of women had masturbated at least once in their lives to the point of orgasm[16] (p. 173). In a more recent survey, respondents were asked only about their experience in the last year[1] (pp. 80-86). In the age group 18 to 24, 41% of men and 64% of women reported that they didn't masturbate at all; 29% of men and 9% of women reported a frequency of once each week. By age 50, over 50% of the men and 70% of the women did not report masturbating.

Apart from frequency, the authors also studied the relationship between masturbation and *marital status.* In Laumann's opinion, Kinsey's view was that "sexual energy was channeled to autoerotic or coupled sexual outlets in a kind of zero-sum complementarity . . . [and thus] . . . the frequency of masturbation decreases in the context of a stable sexual relationship with an available partner." In a finding that was somewhat different from Kinsey and popular notions, Laumann and his co-authors[1] concluded that the two were disconnected in that:

- Rates of masturbation and coupled sexual activity were *both* high among young cohabiting individuals
- Masturbation had "no set quantitative relation to other partnered sexual activities"

Laumann et al. opinions about masturbation and *sexual drive* were also unconventional and instructive.[1] They described the popular belief that "rates of masturbation rise and fall with the availability of sex partners, suggesting that each individual has a given level of 'sex drive' that needs to be expressed in one way or another." However, in their view, "masturbation is driven primarily by . . . social factors . . . [that] can have complementary, supplementary, or independent status with reference to partnered sex." One implication of this view is that a health professional should exercise caution in interpreting the presence or absence of masturbation activity as an indicator of "sex drive."

The relationship between masturbation in adolescence or later and sexual dysfunctions is clearer in women than men. Kinsey et al. found that among women who masturbated to orgasm before marriage about 85% were described as "responsive" in the first year of marriage[16] (pp. 172-173). Of women who never masturbated before marriage or those who did not come to orgasm with masturbation, about one third did not reach orgasm "in their coitus" in the first year of marriage, and the same situation existed for most by the fifth year (p. 172).

The absence of masturbation experience in men or women in the present means, obviously, the inability to use this information clinically. For example, when asking a man about his present erections under various circumstances, it would be pointless to include a question about masturbation erections if this was not part of his recent sexual experience. Negative attitudes toward self-stimulation can determine whether or not this kind of sexual activity occurs but, in addition, can also influence treatment suggestions. For example, it is ethically unreasonable (and from a practical viewpoint ineffective) to ask a woman who is nonorgasmic to stimulate herself if she regards masturbation as immoral.

Sexual Orientation

The hormonal surge of early adolescence is responsible for body changes and also strongly influences sexual attractions and actions that are typically aimed at the opposite sex, occasionally toward the same sex, and sometimes toward both. The evolution of "love" feelings and sexual experimentation needs to be explored. In a controversial finding, Kinsey et al. found that 37% of men "had at least some overt homosexual experience to the point of orgasm between adolescence and old age"[15] (p. 650). Newer data has resulted in more precise understanding of same-gender feelings and behavior (Table 5-3).

One of the objectives of the study by Laumann and his colleagues was to better understand this area and its relationship to HIV/AIDS transmission and vulnerability.[1] Nine percent of the men and 4% of the women respondents reported at least one sexual experience with a same-gender person since puberty (pp. 294-296). However, a critical distinction was made between same-gender sexual behavior before and after the age of 18. When this separation was made, almost half of the men (42%) who reported sexual experience with another man said that the experience occurred before the age of 18 and did not occur again at any time later in their lives (p. 296). The rates for men who engaged in sexual activity with another man were found to range between 2.7% in the past year and 4.9% with any male partner since age 18 (p. 294).

Any understanding of homosexuality must consider a person's behavior and how that individual thinks and feels. Interviewers in the Laumann et al. study inquired about sexual behavior toward others of the same gender and about how respondents think of themselves.[1] They referred to the latter as "identity" and found that "2.8% of the men and 1.4% of the women reported some level of homosexual (or bisexual) identity"

Table 5-3 Homosexuality: Definitions And Frequencies

	MEN (%)	WOMEN (%)
Sexual experience with SGP in lifetime	9	4
Sexual experience with SGP since age 18	4.9	4.1
Sexual experience with SGP in past 5 years	4.1	2.2
Sexual experience with SGP in last year	2.7	1.3
Self-identification as homosexual or bisexual	2.8	1.4
Desire for SGP without activity or self-identification	5	5

Adapted from Laumann EO et al: *The social organization of sexuality: sexual practices in the United States*, Chicago, 1994, The University of Chicago Press.
SGP, Same gender partner

(p. 293). In addition to behavior and identity, respondents were also asked about same-gender "desire." When all three factors were considered together, the authors found clinically important discrepancies. For example, they found that "about 5% of the men and women in our sample express some same-gender desire but no other indicators of adult activity or self-identification" (p. 301). The authors concluded that their "preliminary analysis provides unambiguous evidence that no single number can be used to provide an accurate characterization of the incidence and prevalence of homosexuality in the population at large" (p. 371).

In the context of a clinical interview with a patient, after the subject of homosexuality is "on the table" in the process of asking about early adolescent sexual behavior, similar questions about adult attractions and experiences with same-sex individuals can be asked easily.

> After the subject of homosexuality is "on the table" in the process of asking about early adolescent sexual behavior, similar questions about adult attractions and experiences with same-sex individuals can be asked easily.

There are many reasons to ask such questions. Problems in adolescence among those emerging with a gay or lesbian identity are legion (see Chapter 7). In addition, worries about homosexuality in boys who are heterosexual but have trouble making contacts with girls are probably common.[31] Obviously, sexual interest in another person of the same sex may profoundly influence a person's sexual interest in, and function with, a heterosexual partner.

Initial Intercourse Experiences

In following the love and sexual experiences of a person throughout their teens and beyond, the interviewer must also be sensitive to what actually occurred and the development of sexual problems at those times. Laumann and colleagues wrote that "first intercourse, especially for women, has traditionally been a landmark event surrounded by a welter of moral strictures and normative concerns about the meaning of virginity, the loss of innocence, the transition to adulthood, and the responsibility for procreation and the next generation"[1] (pp. 322-324). Their opinion was that "much of the research on age at first intercourse during the mid- to late 1980s was motivated by an interest on contraceptive use and AIDS awareness among teenagers" and that several surveys (including their own) "overwhelmingly suggest that there has been a significant change in the early heterosexual life of young women in the United States." In their study, 19% of female respondents had vaginal intercourse by age 15, and 90% of males had intercourse by age 20 to 24 (pp. 326-327). The authors concluded the following from their own studies on first intercourse, as well as those of others:

1. First vaginal intercourse is occurring at younger ages
2. More people are engaging in premarital sexual activity with a partner earlier in their lives
3. Gender differences are evident in that "men start earlier, have more partners and are motivated by curiosity and self interest; women begin later, have sex with spouses or more serious lovers, and use birth control more than men"

Thompson provided a different perspective on first intercourse in young women.[32] On the basis of direct interviews of teenage girls, she detailed the elements determining the outcome of this experience. Girls with negative feelings and opinions described:

- An absence of former sexual awareness (including lack of preparatory experiences with petting, masturbation, sexual fantasy, desire, or contraception)
- Lack of control
- Vaginal pain
- Boredom
- Sexual pessimism

In contrast, girls with positive feelings and opinions:

- Approached intercourse with a sense of sexual desire, control, and knowledge
- Were contraceptively prepared
- Described mothers who were "open" about their own bodies, intimacies, and relationships

The positive group anticipated pleasurable intercourse within a mental and physical life-context that included sexual fantasy, masturbation, and petting. These were sexually optimistic young women who knew their own minds and bodies.

A study of "clinical" (on a waiting list for a "sex" clinic) and "nonclinical" (obtained through a newspaper ad) couples found that "sexual and emotional" responses to the first coitus appeared to be far more significant for women than for men.[7]

Sexual Function Difficulties

A study of over 1800 English teenagers concerning sexual issues (including problems), as well as a follow-up study of the same population when they were in their mid-20s, revealed that about one fourth "had a sex problem which they had never discussed with anyone."[33] These difficulties included anxiety over "performance," guilt feelings, change in sexual interest, and concern about masturbation. The extent to which concerns were carried over from adolescence to adulthood was not stated but the likelihood is that there were many.

Atypical Experiences

There is surprisingly little information about the epidemiology and childhood precursors of adolescent or adult paraphilias (previously known as perversions or sexual deviations (see "Nonparaphilic and Paraphilic Compulsive Sexual Behaviors: Sexual Issues and Questions" in Chapter 8). An exception to this lack of information is the finding that those who have been sexually active with children were sometimes themselves the target of the same kind of sexual behavior when they were children.[34] When looking retrospectively, paraphilic behavior often begins in adolescence.[35] In one study, "over 50% of the various categories of paraphilias had developed their deviant sexual arousal pattern prior to age 18."[35] However, the extent to which paraphilic behavior can be an occasional and "benign" aspect of adolescent sexual development is unknown. Gender identity disorders are said to crystallize in this same period also.[36]

> In one study, "over 50% of the various categories of paraphilias developed their deviant sexual arousal pattern before age 18."[35]

Sexual Assault

Laumann and his colleagues[1] (p. 333) asked respondents about "forced sex" rather than "rape" for two reasons:

- Rape was considered a legal rather than a descriptive term
- They wanted to "cast a wider net for coerced sexual events, recognizing that meeting the legal standards for rape does not exhaust the category of women being coerced to have sex"

A small number of men (1%) and a large number of women (22%) reported being sexually forced by a man (p. 335). In other words, "more than one in five women has experienced what she considers to be an incident in which she was forced to do something sexual that she did not want to do"(p. 335). The experience of women in this survey was described as being consistent with other surveys of sexual assault. The fact that forced sexual experiences can have profound effects on sexual function in women and men is well documented.[1,37,38] Diminished sexual desire appears to be one of the main consequences.

Pregnancy and Abortion

The effect of pregnancy and abortion on later sexual function depends on the circumstances. The results of various birth control approaches on sexual function have been reviewed[39] (pp. 404-410). The sexual impact of birth control pills in particular is subtle, in that sexual desire may be lessened in some individuals.[40]

Sexually Transmitted Diseases

The differentiation between Sexually Transmitted Infections and Sexually Transmitted Diseases (STIs and STDs) is explained by the fact that not everyone with an infection is symptomatic and therefore may not know they have a disease. Such disorders are not, of course, limited to puberty and adolescence; however, bacterial and viral infections occur most commonly in the 18 to 24 year old age group.[1] The frequency is thought to be related to a greater number of sexual partners, which "is the most succinct measure of the extent of exposure to infection" (pp. 385-386).

An interviewer may have to extrapolate the effect of sexually transmitted diseases on sexual function, since there is little information on this subject in the medical literature. One related exception is the modification of sexual practices in homosexual men in response to the AIDS epidemic. For example, changes are described in the use of condoms and the exclusion of anal intercourse in sexual activities[1] (pp.432-437).[41]

Adulthood
Areas of Inquiry

Areas of inquiry include the following:

1. Romantic relationships from quantitative and qualitative viewpoints
2. Sexual aspects of romantic relationships
3. Marriages and their sexual components
4. Reasons for the ending of important premarital and marital connections and the extent to which sexual problems were significant

5. Changes in sexual experiences before and after marriage
6. Covert or overt sexual experiences with other partners during marriage or committed relationships
7. The nature of a person's sexual response with (other) current and previous sexual partners
8. Reproductive issues

Suggested Questions

Q. Tell me about previous relationships that meant a lot to you.

Q. What were your sexual experiences like in those relationships?

Q. Why did those relationships end?

Q. Did you ever have the same kind of sexual problem that you have now?

Q. How long did you and your wife (husband, partner) know each other before living together?

Q. What was your sexual relationship like in those days?

Q. What were your living arrangements during that time?

Q. When your living circumstances changed, what effect did that have on your sexual relationship?

Q. Sometimes people who have a close relationship also have sexual experiences with other partners for various reasons; one reason is to test themselves to see if a particular sexual problem appears with someone else. Have sexual relationships with others for this or any other reason been part of your experience?

Q. How did you manage sexually on those occasions?

Q. To what extent is your wife (husband, partner) aware of those experiences?

Q. What was her (his) reaction?

Q. (If patient has children) Tell me about your sexual experiences when you were (your wife was) pregnant.

Q. (If patient has no children) Have you decided against having children or have you had some fertility difficulty?

RATIONALE FOR QUESTIONS

Relationships before marriage are interpersonal and sexual testing opportunities. Problem patterns may become evident as an interviewer explores the reasons for developing links with others and why they become disrupted, for example:

- Changes in living arrangements may imply alterations in expectations that, in turn, may have profound effects on a couple's sexual experiences
- Marriage may result in changes in a couple's sexual experiences
- Another area is the possible presence of other sexual partners

Kinsey et al. found that about 50% of married men reported having sexual intercourse with women other than their wives at some time in their married lives[15] (p. 585). Among women, about one fourth had similar experiences by age 40[16] (p. 416). Information on this subject provided in the Laumann et al. study was markedly different[1] (pp. 212-216). "Over 90 percent of the women and over 75 percent of the men in every cohort, report fidelity within their marriage, over its entirety" (p. 214).

Whatever the motivation for other relationships, it is useful to know whether or not the particular sexual problem that presently exists was present during those other occasions. When planning treatment, the health professional must also know if another current relationship is transient or committed. A productive treatment outcome could be difficult in the presence of an unseen third person with whom the patient has a substantial relationship.

Issues relating to reproduction can have profound effects on sexual experiences. Opposing ideas on the topic of having children can disrupt an otherwise harmonious couple. The process of trying to "make a baby" because of infertility problems results in sexual experiences that are structured, devoid of passion, and empty of feelings. It is hardly astonishing that problems might develop in such circumstances.

Most observers describe a constantly diminishing level of sexual interest in women through the period of pregnancy.[42] In contrast, Masters and Johnson described an increasing degree of sexual interest in pregnant women in the second trimester[43] (pp. 158-159).

The Older Years

Areas of Inquiry

Areas of inquiry include the following:

1. The nature of current relationships
2. How the past and present compare sexually
3. The frequency of sexual activities
4. The range of sexual experiences
5. The extent of understanding and expectation of alterations in sexual function in the aging process
6. Changes in sexual response

   - Extent and speed of vaginal lubrication (women)
   - Effective stimuli for erections, the rapidity and stiffness of erections, the length of time to obtain another erection after ejaculation, and the length of time required to come to orgasm (men)

7. Experience with the use of postmenopausal hormones (women)
8. Connections between health and sex

Suggested Questions

Q. What has your sexual relationship with your wife (husband, partner) in general been like in recent years?

Q. What were your sexual experiences as a couple like before the development of the problem you mentioned?

Q. How often does sexual activity occur now?

Q. What takes place now sexually when you and your wife (husband, partner) are together?

Q. What sort of sexual changes were you expecting as you became older?

Q. (women) Many women experience changes in the amount or speed of vaginal lubrication with menopause. What is your experience?

Q. (women) What is your experience with estrogens or other hormones after your menopause?

Q. (men) Have you noticed any change in the speed with which you get an erection compared to, say, five years ago?

Q. (men) Is there any change in the stiffness of your erections now compared to, say, five years ago?

Q. (men) Is there any change in how long it takes you to have another erection after you've ejaculated once compared to, say, five years ago?

Q. (men) Is there any change in how long it takes you to ejaculate or come to orgasm now compared to, say, five years ago?

Q. Have health problems influenced your sexual experiences?

Studies of Sexuality and Aging

The Kinsey surveys included very few older people and as a result others researched this gap in sex-related information.[15,16] Pfeiffer and his colleagues studied an elderly group at the Duke University Center for the Study of Aging and Human Development.[44] Their findings include the following:

- Sex has an important role in the lives of many elderly persons
- There is a tendency toward declining sexual activity with age

Of major consequence is the fact that they also saw exceptions in the form of patterns of stable, and even increasing, sexual activity.

In an effort to supplement the available information about sex and aging, Consumers Union (CU) undertook a survey of older readers of the magazine, *Consumer Reports*.[45] The result was the book, *"Love, Sex and Aging,"* based on written responses to a questionnaire completed by 4246 people over age 50 (of which 2456 were over the age of 60). The survey was obviously biased in that the sample:

- Was self-selected
- Consisted of people of higher than average income and education and better than average health and who had greater interest in the topic

However, the results are nevertheless significant because they describe what is sexually positive and possible in men and women as aging occurs.

The CU survey related 15 nonsexual factors (e.g., age, income, and the "empty-nest syndrome") to marital happiness. Only one was found to be "closely associated"—the quality of communication. When the quality was low, sexual activity suffered. This conclusion may have diagnostic implications and therapeutic ramifications. Clinicians need to gauge the overall quality of the relationship in the assessment of sexual difficulties. The nature of sexual activities a couple enjoys may represent vital information, depending on the problem presented.

> Clinicians need to guage the overall quality of the relationship in the assessment of sexual difficulties.

In reading through Kinsey's surveys, it was also clearly evident that the acceptability of various sexual activities depended at least partly on the era in which a person was raised. For example, many older couples living in the 90s grew up in a time when it was considered improper for a woman to touch or stimulate a man's penis. Given this culture-based attitude, Masters and Johnson's observation, for example, of the older man's need for tactile stimulation to develop or maintain an erection may result in major sexual difficulties.[43]

Sexuality of Aging Men (Box 5-3)

In relation to men specifically, Kinsey et al. declared that of eleven factors that "are of primary importance in determining the frequency and sources of human sexual outlet," none seems more important than age.[15] "Having reached a peak in adolescence, sexual activity in the male drops steadily from then into old age." While this finding of diminished sexual activity in aging men has been confirmed by others, studies[46] also show the following:

1. A wide variation in individual rates of decline
2. Decreased sexual desire (although to a lesser extent than sexual activity)
3. Increased prevalence of erectile dysfunction
4. A general decrease in genital and extragenital reactions to sexual stimulation

The Duke University study also examined the determinants of sexual behavior in middle age and old age and found that, among men, many factors influenced the extent of sexual behavior,[44] including:

- Past sexual experience
- Age
- Subjective and objective health
- Social class

In the CU Survey, four specific questions were asked of men about their erections.[45] Of the 2402 male respondents the following observations were noted:

- Their refractory period (the time it takes to have another erection after orgasm) was longer (65%)
- It took longer to get an erection (50%)

Box 5-3

Summary of Sexual Function Changes in Aging Men[45-47]

- Quality of communication closely associated with marital happiness
- Sexual satisfaction—no difference
- Sexual desire generally decreased but wide variation
- Sexual activity generally decreased but wide variation
- Erection—some required longer time to become erect
- Erectile dysfunction—increased prevalence
- Erection following orgasm—some required increased time
- NPT testing—many aspects decreased
- Bio-available testosterone—decreased
- Luteinizing hormone—increased
- Ejaculation—often longer time from vaginal entry to orgasm

NPT, Nocturnal penile tumescence.

- Their penis was less stiff when fully erect (44%)
- They more frequently lost their erection during sexual activity (32%)

Ejaculation and orgasm changes in men were also described in the same survey. Ejaculation usually (not always) slowed so that there was a longer time from vaginal entry to orgasm. In addition, orgasms did not occur with every sexual experience.

More recent observations on male physiology have added important information to our knowledge about sexual changes in aging men. These changes seem to be mediated by hormonal, neural, and vascular mechanisms. Schiavi and his colleagues took physiological studies beyond others by examining the sexual function of *healthy* aging men.[46] Schiavi summarized from this study[47] as follows:

1. No reported difference in sexual or marital satisfaction in spite of age-related changes in the sexual desire and sexual activity of study subjects
2. A wide variation in levels of sexual desire, response, and activity among even the oldest of the subjects
3. A marked decrease on many aspects of Nocturnal Penile Tumescence (NPT) testing
4. A highly significant decrease in the amount of bio-available testosterone and an increase in circulating luteinizing hormone (confirming previous reports of an age-related decline in gonadal function, but he also noted that "the magnitude and extent of the hormonal–behavioral correlations observed . . . does not support the notion that hormonal factors are important determinants of individual differences")

In examining possible causes of changes in erection function specifically, another study looked at 39 healthy and sexually functional men ranging in age from 21 to 82 and related the observation of decreasing erectile capacity in aging men to decreasing sensory/neural and autonomic function rather than hormones.[48]

Schiavi concluded about sexuality in men that: "aging is associated with a decrease in sexual desire, arousal and activity even when the effects of illness, medication and psychopathology are minimized or eliminated . . . [and that] . . . a proportion of subjects in the oldest age group . . . remained sexually active and had regular intercourse in the presence of a marked decrement in erectile capacity . . . It would appear that in these individuals, the value that sexuality had in their lives, the frequency and range of their past sexual behaviors, their motivation and ability to experiment and develop compensatory sexual strategies and the supportive attitude of their partners were instrumental in their continuing sexual activity, their sexual satisfaction and the self-perception of not being sexually dysfunctional."[47]

Sexuality of Aging Women

The Duke University study also drew conclusions that were specific to women.[44] The authors believe that the level of activity in women reflected "the availability of a socially sanctioned, sexually capable partner." Relatively few factors (compared to men) were determined to influence the level of sexual activity:

- Marital status
- Age
- Extent of enjoyment derived from sexual experiences in earlier years

In a general population survey of sexual desire in midlife, Hallstrom and Samuelsson interviewed 497 women living with a spouse, on two occasions, six years apart.[49] Ages of the women were 38, 46, 50, and 54 at the time of the first interview. The research strategy allowed the authors to study age and cohort effects. Their conclusions were that sexual desire showed considerable stability over time but that a substantial proportion of their subjects (27%) experienced a major change in sexual desire, mostly a decrease. Ten percent of their subjects demonstrated an increase. Decreased sexual desire was predicted by:

1. High sexual desire at the first interview
2. Lack of a confiding relationship
3. Insufficient support from a spouse
4. Alcoholism in a spouse
5. Major depression

Increased sexual desire was predicted by:

1. A low level of desire in the first interview
2. Negative marital relations before the first interview
3. Mental disorder at the time of the first interview

The CU Survey (Table 5-4) included responses from 1844 women who were 50 years, or more, old[45] (pp. 311-346).

Brecher, the author of the CU report, commented on the apparent inconsistency between the decline in frequencies of sexual activities in men and women and the positive qualitative comments that accompanied the returned survey questionnaires.[45] "The

Table 5-4 Sexual Function In Aging Women

	AGE		
	50s (%)	60s (%)	70s (%)
Sexually active	91	91	79
Frequency/wk in married women	1.3	1.0	0.7
Vaginal lubrication, "right amount"	48	35	23
Orgasm frequency, almost every time	←——— 45 - 53 ———→		
Interest in sex—strong or moderate	75	67	59
Sexual relationship very or moderately important	83	73	63

Adapted from Brecher EM: *Love, sex and aging*, Boston, 1984, Little, Brown and Company.

enjoyment of sex can and sometimes does increase with age even as the frequency may decrease . . . [and in addition] . . . respondents . . . have found techniques for maintaining . . . their enjoyment of sex despite physiological changes . . . " (p. 346).

IMPACT OF HORMONAL CHANGES ON SEXUALITY IN AGING WOMEN

To understand the effects of aging on sexuality in women, some attention was given to the hormonal variations that occur in the peri- and postmenopausal years and the effects of those changes. Sherwin explained that there is a virtual cessation in the production of estradiol (the principal estrogen) by the ovary at the time of menopause (before menopause, 95% is derived from this source).[50] In addition, testosterone production from the ovary (a source of about 25% of testosterone in premenopausal years) becomes negligible at the same time in about 50% of women. Both hormones were described as having effects on the brain, as well as on peripheral tissues.

In the absence of estrogen, the vaginal epithelium becomes attenuated and pale due to diminished vascularity. The consequences of this can be atrophic changes, which in turn, can lead to inflammation or ulceration. All of this can result in diminished vaginal lubrication, which, in turn, might intuitively be expected to cause discomfort or pain with intercourse. Vaginal lubrication and pain with intercourse were investigated in the Laumann et al. study.[1] When women age 50 to 59 were asked if "trouble lubricating" had been a problem within the past year, 46% said "yes." However, a much smaller number (16%) of women respondents in this same age group reported "pain during sex." Clinically, postmenopausal women who use oral estrogens or estrogen vaginal cream generally find enhanced lubrication and the elimination of dyspareunia. It appears then that postmenopausal vaginal atrophy and diminished elimination of discomfort or pain with intercourse are not necessarily followed by dyspareunia but when postmenopausal dyspareunia does occur it is frequently accompanied by diminished vaginal lubrication.

While vaginal atrophy is a consistent finding in postmenopausal women, this is less so in women who regularly engage in intercourse. This observation may be even more prominent for those whose sexual activity involves masturbation.[51] The relationship between the thickness of the vaginal mucosa and vaginal lubrication is not entirely clear. Although the two often are thought to be closely related, Masters and Johnson described three women who responded with considerable vaginal lubrication in spite of a thin and atrophic mucosa[43] (p. 234).

Studies of the absence of testosterone in women (which occurs suddenly when both ovaries are surgically removed) and its therapeutic use confirm that testosterone is associated with an enhancement of sexual desire, interest, and enjoyment of sex in some postmenopausal women.[52] Sherwin concluded elsewhere that "in women as well as in men, testosterone has its major effect on the cognitive, motivational, or libidinal aspects of sexual behavior such as desire and fantasies and not on physiological responses . . . [and that] . . . the likelihood . . . [is that] . . . the mechanisms impact directly on the brain."[50] From a therapeutic viewpoint, she also suggested treatment with testosterone in instances of surgically induced menopause, as well as in instances of natural menopause that is accompanied by a change (decrease) in sexual desire (see Chapter 9 for a more detailed discussion of the use of testosterone to treat sexual desire disorders in postmenopausal women).

SUMMARY

Investigation of a sexual problem begins with a description. However, understanding possible origins may entail the following:

- Detailed history-taking
- Physical examination (possibly)
- Laboratory studies (possibly)

Considering the etiology of a problem requires awareness of the context in which it exists. The interviewer needs a structure for obtaining this contextual information.

Kaplan's system for arranging explanatory information was to separate immediate and remote factors that might further understanding of the reasons for a sexual dysfunction.[2]

Immediate issues are best discovered during a patient's description of details of a sexual encounter as it takes place in the present. Describing the process of "who does what to whom" is considerably more disconcerting to health professional and patient than simply stating the fact that a problem exists and outlining what it is. Nevertheless, in the absence of objective measures, this process is a necessity, since the health professional depends entirely on the patient's words in attempting to understand the nature of a sexual dysfunction. However difficult talking about sexual details may appear, practice by the health professional makes this progressively easier.

Remote factors become apparent when reviewing a person's developmental history, particularly when the focus is on the evolution of his or her sexual development (hence the term *sexual-developmental history*). Although this process may not always seem necessary, the importance of past experiences may not be apparent until *after* the fact.

Primary care health professionals are able to acquire information about immediate factors within the time frame that they usually spend with patients (although the process may involve more than one visit). However, detailed inquiry into remote factors is more complex and time consuming and, as a result, may be more realistically undertaken by a health professional who has a special interest in sexual issues.

The sexual life cycle closely follows the unfolding of the individual. Through childhood, puberty and adolescence, adulthood and the older years, the interviewer traces the sexual thoughts, feelings, dreams, and events in the patient's life, all the while searching for anything that might help explain the reasons for a dysfunction in the present and for ways to correct it. Areas of inquiry arise for each period of time, as do questions. The rationale for the questions asked derive from the data: what is known about positive and negative happenings during each period.

When talking to an adult about "sex" during their childhood, the health professional is partly operating in a vacuum, since only a limited amount of knowledge is available. This lack of knowledge, for example, about sexual norms, probably results from the reluctance of parents and schools to allow children to be subjects of study. In contrast, much is known about adolescence—the multicolored picture of this period is a time of enormous sexual ferment, physically as well as in thought and behavior. Much can be learned about an adult by carefully detailing what took place in their mind and in their actions during their teenage years. Ways of thinking and behavior seem to crystallize at this time. The consolidation of adulthood often provides information about the appearance of sexual problems in, for example, the context of previous relationships.

Changes in the older years, including sexual alterations, are often a source of confusion. The virtual conspiracy of silence surrounding sexuality and aging relates partly to the great difficulty that many health professionals (especially students) find in talking about this subject to older patients and partly to the self-restraint displayed by those same patients.

When sexual dysfunctions occur, regardless of age, the health professional needs a structure within which to organize an assessment. This topic will be discussed in the next chapter.

REFERENCES

1. Laumann EO et al: *The social organization of sexuality: sexual practices in the United States*, Chicago, 1994, The University of Chicago Press.
2. Kaplan HS: *The new sex therapy: active treatment of sexual dysfunctions*, New York, 1974 Brunner/Mazel, Inc.
3. Masters WH, Johnson VE: *Human sexual inadequacy*, Boston, 1970, Little, Brown and Company.
4. Kaplan HS: *The evaluation of sexual disorders: psychological and medical aspects*, New York, 1983, Brunner/Mazel, Inc.
5. Montagu A: *Touching*, ed 3, New York, 1986, Harper & Row, Publishers, Inc.
6. Bancroft J: *Human sexuality and its problems*, ed 2, U.K., 1989, Churchill Livingstone.
7. Heiman JR et al: Historical and current factors discriminating sexually functional from sexually dysfunctional married couples, *J Marital Fam Ther* 12:163-174, 1986.
8. Morrison J: *The first interview: revised for DSM-IV*, New York, 1995, The Guilford Press.
9. Gadpaille WJ: *The cycles of sex*, New York, 1975, Charles Scribner's Sons.
10. Freud S: The transformations of puberty: [3] the libido theory. In Freud S: *On sexuality: three essays on the theory of sexuality and other works*, Middlesex, 1905/1977, Penguin Books, pp 138-140.
11. Harlow HF, Harlow MK: The affectional systems. In Schrier AM, Harlow HF, Stollitz F (editors): *Behavior of non-human primates*, Vol II, New York, 1965, Academic Press.
12. Green R: *The "sissy boy syndrome" and the development of homosexuality*, New Haven and London, 1987, Yale University Press.
13. Money J, Ehrhardt AA: *Man and woman, boy and girl*, Baltimore, 1972, The Johns Hopkins University Press.
14. Diamond M, Sigmundson K: Sex reassignment at birth: a long term review and clinical implications, *Arch Pediatr Adolesc Med* 151:298-304, 1997.
15. Kinsey AC, Pomeroy WB, Martin CE: *Sexual behavior in the human male*, Philadelphia and London, 1949, W.B. Saunders.
16. Kinsey AC et al: *Sexual behavior in the human female*, Philadelphia and London, 1953, W.B. Saunders.
17. Spira A, Bajos N, and the ACSF group: *Sexual behavior and AIDS*, Brookfield, 1994, Ashgate Publishing Company.
18. Johnson AM et al: *Sexual attitudes and lifestyles*, Oxford, 1994, Blackwell Scientific Publications.
19. *Diagnostic and statistical manual of mental disorders*, ed 4, Washington, 1994, American Psychiatric Association.
20. Rutter M: Psychosexual development. In Rutter M: *Scientific foundations of developmental psychiatry*, London, 1980, William Heinemann Medical Books Limited.
21. Money J: *Gay, straight, and in-between: the sexology of erotic orientation*, New York, 1988, Oxford University Press.
22. Martinson FM: Normal sexual development in infancy and early childhood. In Ryan F, Lane S (editors): *Juvenile sex offending: causes, consequences, and correction*, Boston, 1991, Lexington Books.
23. Frayser SG: Defining normal childhood sexuality: an anthropological approach. *Annual Review of Sex Research* 5:173-217, 1994.

24. Ford CS, Beach FA: *Patterns of sexual behavior*, New York, 1951, Harper & Row.

25. Robins LN: *Deviant children grown up*, Baltimore, 1966, Williams and Wilkins.

26. Zucker K, Bradley S: *Gender identity disorder and psychosexual problems in children and adolescents*, New York, 1995, The Guilford Press.

27. Green R: Children called "sissy" and "tomboy," adolescents who cross-dress, and adults who want to change sex. In Green R (editor): *Human sexuality: a health practitioner's text*, ed 2, Baltimore/London, 1979, The Williams and Wilkins Company, pp 151-162.

28. Masters WH, Johnson VE, Kolodny RC: *Sex and human loving*, Boston, 1986, Little, Brown and Company.

29. Wyatt G: Child sexual abuse and its effects on sexual functioning, *Annual Review of Sex Research* 2:249-266, 1991.

30. Browne A, Finkelhor D: Impact of child sexual abuse: a review of the research, *Psychol Bull* 99:66-77, 1986.

31. Ovesey L, Woods SM: Pseudohomosexuality and homosexuality: psychodynamics as a guide to treatment. In Marmor J (editor): *Homosexual behavior*, New York, 1980, Basic Books, Inc.

32. Thompson S: Putting a big thing into a little hole: teenage girls' accounts of sexual initiation, *J Sex Res* 27:341-361, 1990.

33. Schofield M: *The sexual behaviour of young people*, Boston, 1965, Little, Brown and Company.

34. Freund K, Kuban M: The basis of the abused-abuser theory of pedophilia: a further elaboration on an earlier study, *Arch Sex Behav* 23:553-563, 1994.

35. Abel GG, Rouleau JL, Cunningham-Rathner J: Sexually aggressive behavior. In Curran WJ, McGarry AL, Shah SA (editors): *Forensic psychiatry and psychology: Perspectives and standards for interdisciplinary practice*, Philadelphia, 1986, F.A. Davis Company.

36. Newman LE: Treatment for the parents of feminine boys, *Am J Psychiatry* 133:683-687, 1976.

37. Feldman-Summers S, Gordon PE, Meagher JR: The impact of rape on sexual satisfaction, *J Abnorm Psychol* 88(1):101-105, 1979.

38. Masters WH: Sexual dysfunction as an aftermath of sexual assault of men by women, *J Sex Marital Ther* 12(1):35-45, 1986.

39. Kolodny RC, Masters WH, Johnson VE: *Textbook of sexual medicine*, Boston, 1979, Little, Brown and Company.

40. Marcotte DB et al: Physiologic changes accompanying oral contraceptive use, *Br J Psychiatry* 116:165-167, 1970.

41. Schechter MT et al: Patterns of sexual behavior and condom use in a cohort of homosexual men, *Am J Public Health* 78:1535-1538, 1988.

42. Reamy K, Whyte SE: Sexuality in pregnancy and the puerperium: a review, *Obstet Gynecol Surv*, 40(1):1-13, 1985.

43. Masters WH, Johnson VE: *Human sexual response*, Boston, 1966, Little, Brown and Company.

44. Pfeiffer E, Davis GC: Determinents of sexual behavior in middle and old age, *J Am Geriatr Soc* 20:151-158, 1972.

45. Brecher EM: *Love, sex and aging*, Boston, 1984, Little, Brown and Company.

46. Schiavi RC et al: Healthy aging and male sexual function, *Am J Psychiatry* 147:766-771, 1990.

47. Schiavi R: Sexuality and aging in men, *Annual Review of Sex Research* 1:227-249, 1990.

48. Rowland DL et al: Aging and sexual function in men, *Arch Sex Behav* 22:545-557, 1993.

49. Hallstrom T, Samuelsson S: Changes in women's sexual desire in middle life: the longitudinal study of women in Gottenburg, *Arch Sex Behav* 19:259-268, 1990.

50. Sherwin BB: Menopause and sexuality, *Can J Obstet/Gynecol Women's Health Care* 4:254-260, 1992.

51. Leiblum S: Vaginal atrophy in the postmenopausal woman, *JAMA* 294:2195-2198, 1983.

52. Sherwin BB, Gelfand MM, Brender W: Androgen enhances sexual motivation in females: a prospective, crossover study of sex steroid administration in the surgical menopause, *Psychosom Med* 47:339-351, 1985.

CHAPTER 6

ASSESSING SEXUAL DYSFUNCTIONS AND DIFFICULTIES: THE PROCESS

In an age when scientific disciplines are becoming increasingly specialized, it is more and more difficult to bring together new knowledge in a manner that helps us comprehensively to understand the human condition. Sexuality is a prime example of the growing need for such a synthesis . . . for the medical profession, sex provides as good a model of psychosomatic relationships as one can find . . . a proper understanding of human sexuality demands a truly psychosomatic approach.

BANCROFT, 1989[1]

Not all clinicians who specialize in the care of people with sexual disorders agree on the necessity of the entire process described in this chapter and for the length of time it involves. For example, Kaplan[2] (pp. 91-92) states that:

- About 60% of her assessments take place in a single 40 minute session with a couple or a symptomatic patient alone
- A second session is necessary in about 20% of cases
- More time is required when a situation is especially complex

> Kaplan states that about 60% of her assessments take place in a single 40 minute session with a couple or a symptomatic patient alone, that a second session is necessary in about 20%, and that more time is required when a situation is especially complex

A single history-taking session, while considerably less thorough than the process described in this and the previous chapter, is particularly applicable to a primary care setting. If nothing else, it indicates that much can be accomplished with many patients within a limited period of time.

WINDOW OF OPPORTUNITY

Patients often arrive alone when initially visiting a health professional and it is in this context that a sexual problem typically surfaces—frequently during a discussion of some other topic. What happens subsequently can develop in one of two ways:

- The focus immediately shifts to the area of "sex"
- A plan is developed with the patient to talk about this new topic at another time

The extent to which a patient feels a sense of urgency, the amount of professional time available, and the clinical skills of the professional dictate which path is taken. There are benefits to each approach. Talking about a sexual problem when the subject is broached is appealing, since it allows an interviewer to take advantage of this "window of opportunity." However, the idea of talking at a later time is attractive

> Talking about a sexual problem when the subject is broached is appealing, since it allows an interviewer to take advantage of this "window of opportunity." However, the idea of talking at a later time is attractive because it allows for unhurried conversation. Time may be needed for the gradual unfolding of a painful story that may never have been told

because it allows for (presumably) unhurried conversation. Time may be needed to allow for the gradual unfolding of a painful story that may never have been told.

Some health professionals (especially nonpsychiatric physicians and health professionals who have a limited amount of time) prefer not to hear a lengthy account of a sexual difficulty, conduct only a brief assessment, then refer the patient. Part II considers when referral is reasonable and, conversely, when a sexual problem can be assessed more elaborately and managed on a primary care level. When undertaking a more comprehensive assessment, health professionals may want greater structure (outlined later in this chapter).

THE PATIENT'S PARTNER

Although patients may be unaccompanied when first seen, another person may be present in spirit, that is, the patient's sexual partner. Learning about the existence of this other person allows for the possibility of their inclusion on a subsequent visit. The partner may be initially absent for several reasons, including:

1. Involvement of a sexual partner on a first visit is unusual (unless the visit is structured this way)
2. People tend to blame themselves for sexual problems and therefore may not understand the necessity of including a partner
3. A patient may be embarrassed to talk explicitly when a partner is present and thus not want the other person to be present

If the professional thinks it is important to include the partner in discussions of the problem, this should be explained to the patient.

The rationale for including a partner is twofold:

- Diagnostic
- Therapeutic

While considerable diagnostic (past-oriented) information can be obtained from one person alone, a partner may have a different point of view. This was demonstrated by a study that compared separately obtained interview data from men with erectile difficulties and their wives.[3] Frequent discrepancies were found in the information obtained such that, for example, in 18% of the cases the diagnosis was changed. The authors provided several examples, one of which follows:

A 59-year-old salesman: "Patient reports that impotence began within the last year, after years of infrequent sex. He said that in this, his second marriage, he feels desire but suffers fear of failure with his wife. He reports no erections with masturbation and partial morning erections. Pertinent medical history is a history of cocaine and heroin abuse, ending in 1961, and prostatitis. The patient's wife indicated that this was his third marriage, and that the potency difficulty began at least three years ago but that sex had been so infrequent (occurring only at her insistence) that she felt any erectile difficulties were less important than the low desire."[3]

Apart from the issue of diagnosis, the other person often needs to be involved when trying to effect change (future-oriented). The authors again provided an example:

A 58-year-old accountant: "Patient reported no sexual problems in his first marriage, which ended with his wife's sudden death in 1982. He was unable to achieve intercourse with his new fiancee, despite a close and desiring relationship during the last 18 months. He has had diabetes for 10 years, and the NPT workup showed serious erectile abnormalities warranting prosthesis recommendation. Interview with patient's fiancee revealed that she was not at all dissatisfied with the status quo and may have chosen Mr. C in part because of lack of sexual intercourse in the relationship. Pre-operative conjoint counseling was recommended to explore issues of mutual motivation for surgery."[3]

The above examples demonstrates that, from diagnostic and treatment perspectives, what can be accomplished might be quite limited if discussions are held with only one partner.

When the connections between two people are substantial (planning to marry and living apart; single and living together; married), one should be skeptical when hearing that the other person does not want to be involved, since the statement may not be accurate. An invitation extended to the other person may, in fact, never have been delivered and, if it was, consideration must be given to *how* it was delivered. Often it becomes evident that the *patient* is the one who is reticent, saying that the problem is one's own and does not and should not involve the partner.

INTERVIEWING A SOLO PATIENT

The phrase "solo patient" describes someone who sees a health professional alone. The term reflects any of the following:

1. Absence of a current sexual partner
2. Marital status (unmarried)
3. Living arrangements (living alone)
4. Unwillingness of a partner to be involved

Solo patients referred to a sex-specialty clinic or professional are often men who have problems with erections or premature ejaculation. These difficulties are frequently cited as the major reason for the disintegration of a recent relationship. With the other person absent, this interpretation is one-sided and limited in scope. The tenacity with which a patient presents a problem needs to be judged. If the patient is equivocal, this might provide the health professional an opportunity to assist in reexamining the contribution of sexual problems to the fracture in the relationship. If the patient is inflexible, a confrontation only may increase the distance between the patient and his clinician.

Solo patients referred to a sex-speciality clinic or professional are often men who have problems with erections or premature ejaculation. These difficulties are frequently cited as the major reason for the disintegration of a recent relationship. With the other person absent, an interpretation is one-sided and limited in scope

A 25-year-old man was referred after the breakup of a two-year relationship with a woman with whom he had been living. When sexually stimulated, he was unable to develop a full erection. The same situation existed when he occasionally masturbated or when he woke up in the morning. The last occasion he recalled having a full erection under any circumstance was four years before. He was an intensely introverted man and one of few words. He said that erection problems were usual for him but worse now because he was depressed over the disruption of a relationship that he had hoped would end in marriage. He attributed the breakup to his sexual "performance" and was sure that nothing else (such as his inability to communicate or excessive drinking) could have contributed. His family doctor chose not to contradict directly and instead initially discussed the patient's sexual function in greater detail, as well as his depressed mood. As the patient's mood lifted, other issues were brought into the discussion without difficulty.

Despite being evaluated alone, the initial assessment of a solo man can be quite useful. He receives the powerful information that he is not alone in having whatever the problem is and that some of the possible origins can be investigated. In some instances (e.g., a primarily medical or psychiatric etiology of erection problems), one can also be therapeutically helpful. However, in some situations, the health professional may have to insist that for treatment purposes the patient must have a sexual partner. All too frequently, the patient's reply is that the very presence of this problem prevents him from establishing such a relationship, since women "expect" him to "perform" within a few dates. This dilemma may seem to be a *"Catch 22"* situation (except that some men seem to have no difficulty finding sexual partners in spite of their troubles). The interviewer might then reasonably conclude that personality issues and "social skills" are included in addition to "performance" problems. In such instances, the focus of treatment may shift to include these factors as well.

A smaller percentage of solo patients are women who describe trouble reaching orgasm or having pain with intercourse. They, too, worry about the impact of this on their relationship. The timing of a request for help is different from men in that solo women usually ask for assistance in anticipation of the dissolution of a partnership, rather than after. Their thinking is, typically, that if they are unable to fulfill the sexual needs of a man, he will leave.

A 22-year-old woman was referred because of vaginal pain that had been evident since she began to include intercourse in her sexual activities three years before. She had a regular sexual partner for the previous two years. In that relationship, her level of sexual desire had not diminished, she lubricated easily, and had no difficulty coming to orgasm on the rare occasions that intercourse occurred. Avoidance of coital pain had been high on her list of sexual priorities. She and her boyfriend were sexually active with one another (not including intercourse) several times each week but she had become certain that he would not remain in the relationship much longer if intercourse was not included in their sexual experiences. Although the boyfriend appeared satisfied with the arrangement, her concept of the sexual requirements of men was that the absence of intercourse, however temporary, was unacceptable. She was not reassured by his protestations to the contrary. She was referred to a gynecologist and was found to have endometriosis after an examination for laparoscopy. Surgery resolved her dyspareunia; however, when the relationship ended, she had little choice but to consider nonsexual factors.

INTERVIEWING A COUPLE

The word "couple" obviously includes those who are married but it also includes individuals who are single (in terms of marital status) but living together, whether in a heterosexual or homosexual relationship.

Given a choice, many health professionals prefer to begin by talking with a couple together rather than with each person separately, recognizing benefits and limitations to both arrangements. The advantages of interviewing a couple together seem to far outweigh the disadvantages.

First, in an initial conjoint visit, the "therapist" is clearly established as responsible to both parties and therefore aligned with neither. When an individual is first seen alone, there is always the danger that the person not initially seen will feel:

> In an initial conjoint visit, the "therapist" clearly establishes a responsibility to both people and therefore aligns with neither. When an individual is first seen alone, there is always the danger that the person not initially seen will feel:
> - Left out
> - That an alliance has been formed between the other two
> - That the reason for the inclusion is primarily as a target for blame

- Left out
- That an alliance has been formed between the other two
- That the reason for including the partner is primarily as a target for blame

Second, an initial visit together presents the clinician with the opportunity to:

- Evaluate the quality of the relationship between partners
- Consider the extent to which conflicts contribute to the genesis of the sexual problem
- Think about how discord might interfere with resolution of the problem

Affectionate gestures, sitting arrangements, and facial expressions may reveal clues about love or its absence.

Third, sexual problems are often complicated by an absence of the two partners candidly talking together. This reticence may have always been present or may have become a more recent casualty of their troubles. It is truly remarkable to observe two people sitting in the same room trying jointly to explain to a third person (a stranger) what happens sexually between them when they have not talked previously to one another about these very same events. Although technically part of

> It is truly remarkable to observe two people sitting in the same room trying jointly to explain to a third person what happens sexually between them when they have not talked previously to one another about these very same events

---

Box 6-1

Areas to Avoid When Talking to a Couple in an Initial Assessment

1. Other recent or current sexual partners
2. Past sexual partners
3. Masturbation
4. Sexual fantasies
5. Past STDs
6. Atypical sexual practices

---

an "assessment," this process is almost invariably therapeutic. In other words, treatment often begins with the first visit.

Limitations of an initial conjoint visit extend to six areas and are self-imposed by the health professional because the information may be damaging to the couple or ruin the relationship between the interviewer and one of the two partners (Box 6-1). To be sure, information in all six areas can and should be gained when each person is seen individually (Box 6-1).

First, one should avoid asking about other recent or current partners, even if discussed by the couple before the visit. When previously revealed to the other person, often only the skimpiest of information was given. One is likely to hear about a third person in the context of an attack by one partner against the other. It is preferable not to worsen matters by increasing the high level of tension that may already exist. More information can be acquired harmlessly simply by asking the other partner (not the one who was active outside the relationship) what they understand about what had occurred.

A couple in their 20s and married eight years were referred because of two problems:

- The man's rapid ejaculation
- The woman's sexual disinterest

Before the first visit, the woman phoned to ask if she could be seen alone initially and requested that her phone call not be revealed in any subsequent visits when she and her husband were seen as a couple. It was explained to her that when an individual in a long-term relationship was referred, both people were ordinarily seen together initially and then separately. She agreed to the process and they were seen together on the first visit. (In retrospect it might have been wiser to reverse the order.) The husband's ejaculation difficulty seemed lifelong, and the wife's sexual disinterest appeared acquired in that it had existed for about two years. She stated that about two years before, she had been briefly interested in another man who was also married. When the husband was asked what he understood about this relationship, he indicated that:

• The man had been a friend of his
• His friend and his wife had kissed a few times
• The romance lasted a few weeks
• His wife and the other man had not seen one another in over a year

When interviewed alone, the wife told a different story, namely:

• She had been in love with this other man for many years
• The relationship was continuing
• Sexual activities occurred regularly with him
• She was far from sexually disinterested in this other relationship

The wife continued to explain that because of attachments to their children neither she nor the other man wanted to break up their marriages. She asked if there was some way her husband's rapid ejaculation could be controlled and her sexual interest in her husband regenerated. As a result of the visit, she understood that the problem with her husband was only partly sexual, that the problem was mostly one that involved other aspects of their relationship, such as trust and commitment. She was unsure about what to do and accepted referral to a psychotherapist for continued exploration of her options.

Second, it is best to avoid asking about past sexual partners. Previous relationships are generally known to current partners but there is an almost unspoken agreement between couples not to discuss details, particularly sexual minutiae. Such information only invites uncomplimentary comparisons (such as penis size or a different way of coming to orgasm).

Third, the health professional should be very cautious about introducing the subject of masturbation. For many, this topic is very private, as well as embarrassing. If one partner introduces the subject, discussions can continue on an abstract level. One can also discover just how much this has been discussed between the two people. Individual experiences are best left to individual visits. The health professional should avoid forcing one partner into a revelation about masturbatory experiences in the presence of the other. At another time and when talking in confidence, one partner might be encouraged to reveal aspects of this activity to the other.

Fourth, questions about sexual fantasies should be omitted during an initial conjoint visit. Masturbation is a private act; what occurs in thought is even more so. Sexual fantasies often involve a person other than the usual sexual partner and therefore may be misinterpreted as meaning a lack of sexual desire or love.[4]

Fifth, although acquiring a history of past STDs is essential it is best to do so when the patient is seen alone to avoid potentially damaging a current relationship. When an interviewer asks about past STDs in the presence of a partner, the question may also entail coercing that person into talking about a past relationship that may have been private.

Sixth, it is not advisable to ask about atypical sexual practices when both partners are present. For example, when interviewing a couple, one would not ask a man if he dresses in women's clothing. A truthful answer is unlikely and could be damaging if it were revealed (see "The Second Visit" below in this chapter for further discussion of "secrets").

FIRST VISIT   (see illustrations provided in Appendices I and II)

Explanation of the Assessment Process

Whenever meeting with a patient in response to a specific sexual complaint, one should first explain some aspects of what is about to occur. Patients have immediate questions: Who is this person we are about to talk to? What kind of professional experience do they have? What should I expect today? What is the matter with me? Can it be fixed? What will it take to do so? Why am I so nervous? How much will it cost? (As much related to humiliation and embarrassment as money.)

Some of these questions can be answered immediately (introductions, duration of visits, purpose of visits, the use of audio-visual equipment such as tape recorders) but others represent the very rationale for an elaborate inquiry-assessment and therefore must await the end of the process. Even then, a clear accounting may not be easily given.

Before discussing the sexual problem that resulted in the visit, the interviewer should:

1. Describe what is about to occur, since patients do not know what to expect in spite of any previous explanation
2. Be sensitive to the fact that in such circumstances repetition may be necessary, since people tend to absorb only a small amount of what is initially said
3. Be aware that talking about sexual matters is usually embarrassing and foreign
4. Be aware that discussing sexual matters with a stranger may be even more embarrassing and foreign, since the reaction of the stranger is an unknown factor

Introduction to the First Visit

The introduction to the first visit can begin with the declaration that, while its purpose is clearly to talk about sexual troubles, the interviewer wants to initially learn more about the background of the patients. Being explicit about the rationale for background questions is necessary; otherwise, people may wonder about the reasons for questions that might seem irrelevant.

The interviewer could then clarify:

- Ages
- Occupations
- Duration of the relationship
- Living arrangements
- Children
- Health (including psychological health)
- Medications
- Use of alcohol, drugs, and tobacco
- Previous efforts at resolving the sexual dilemma(s)

The purpose in asking about past therapeutic efforts of health professionals is not to denigrate colleagues but to know in a practical sense what has not worked previously, so that the same ineffective approaches are not repeated.

In asking about occupation, the interviewer should be aware that some people are involuntarily unemployed and feel guilty about this, an attitude one would like to avoid enhancing. One way to approach this subject is to not actually ask directly about occupation but rather to ask how one "spends their days."

Likewise, since some couples choose not to marry or have children (and the interviewer is best seen as nonjudgmental), direct questions about marriage and children can be avoided in favor of equally revealing questions about how long the couple has known each other and who else lives with them. If necessary, more direct questions can be asked at a later time. A nonjudgmental way to inquire about the absence of children is to simply ask if this is a result of infertility or a deliberate decision.

> A nonjudgmental way to inquire about the absence of children is to ask if this is a result of infertility or a deliberate decision.

The Chief Complaint

The chief complaint (CC) is a brief and pointed statement of the patients' main concern. When, during the conversation, it is reasonable to turn to the specific sexual trouble, the interviewer may ask about it in (at least) one of two ways:

- Directly—by inquiring of each partner separately what, from their point of view, is the main reason(s) for the visit
- Indirectly—by asking the patient(s) to retrace the steps that resulted in the current visit

The latter seems less precipitous and thus somewhat softer. The indirect approach involves the patient(s) explaining, for example, whose decision it was to talk to a health professional, what was actually said, what the response was, and, if the partner was not involved, what feelings he or she had about the outcome. Since each partner may have a somewhat different perspective, both should be encouraged to state the chief complaint separately and from their personal point of view.

History of the Present Illness

The history of the present illness (HPI) refers to clarification of the chief complaint. Given the limitations of a first couple interview described above in this chapter (see "Interviewing A Couple"), this means the HPI of *this* relationship. Most of the first visit is occupied with the HPI and includes four areas of inquiry:

1. Definition of the problem using the outline described in Chapter 4
2. Elaboration of sexual activities that do not include intercourse (using the outline described in the portion of Chapter 5 titled "Present Context: Immediate Issues and Questions")
3. Extent of exchanges of affection between the two partners
4. Quality of the relationship

If the "patient" is a couple, the interviewer should ask frequently if what was just said by one also represents the opinion of the other.

SECOND VISIT

The portion of Chapter 5 titled "The Context of the Past: Remote Issues and Questions" is the focus of the second visit, when each of the partners are seen alone. However, it is usually best to *begin* by asking the person what their impressions were of the *first* visit. It is sometimes revealing to also ask whether sexual activities occurred since the last visit, and, if so, whether there was any change. Sometimes, talking on one occasion is sufficiently therapeutic to resolve the troubles. Dramatic change resulting from one visit is more likely to occur when there is a reformulation of the problem (e.g., the "problem" becomes a nonissue) rather than any actual change.

A 35-year-old woman was seen because of a concern that she did not have orgasms with intercourse. She was easily orgasmic in other sexual experiences with her husband. They lived together in another city but she was taking a refresher course elsewhere for six weeks and was determined to resolve their sexual difficulties during that time. It became clear during the first visit that the concerns about orgasm with intercourse were more her husband's concern. She was sexually content. Reassurance about the normality of her sexual response was gratefully received. When seen one week later, she related that her husband visited her on the weekend, and in talking together they decided that their sexual concerns had evaporated. As a result, they had mutually satisfying sexual experiences, including intercourse. The second visit was also the last visit and did not include a sexual-developmental history, since the problem had "disappeared."

Before beginning the sexual-developmental history, the interviewer might also ask if the patient deliberately omitted anything from the first interview because of not wanting to hurt their partner's feelings. This question provides an early opportunity for the emergence of secrets that may be significant in understanding the sexual problems. Secrets can include:

- The existence of other partners
- Desire for a form of sexual activity thought to be unacceptable to the partner
- Thoughts such as sexual fantasies
- Masturbation

Hidden information may be diagnostically important, since it may tell an interviewer whether, for example, a problem is situational (see introduction to PART II). Likewise, secret information may be therapeutically important in that it may influence the decision of the health professional to treat both partners together or recommend that they be seen separately. The interviewer cannot be neutral when in possession of a significant secret "belonging" to only one of the partners.

The second (and solo) visit also permits the interviewer to ask questions related to the six areas avoided on the first visit (see "Interviewing A Couple," discussed earlier in this chapter). The interviewer can explain the reasons for previously omitting these questions and the rationale for addressing these issues in the absence of the partner. An alternative approach is to integrate these questions (so they could be asked in context) into a sexual-developmental history (see Chapter 5).

THIRD (OR FOURTH) VISIT

Meeting with a couple again after each partner is seen separately can accomplish several objectives.

1. It is always instructive to *listen* to the results of previous interviews. Treatment is not separate from other aspects of the whole process and actually *begins when patients are initially* seen. In other words, the assessment itself can be therapeutic. Communication difficulties and the couple's limitations in solving *any* problem together become apparent when previous visits *have not* promoted substantive discussion between the partners. For example, previous discussion may have resulted in:

> Treatment is not separate from other aspects of the whole process and actually begins when patients are initially seen, that is, the assessment itself can be therapeutic

   - Reformulation of a problem so that the initial sexual complaint is now seen as subsidiary to another problem that requires more immediate attention (e.g., intense relationship discord)
   - The decision that the presence of a third person (e.g., the health professional) in the endeavor is undesirable
   - Making the *etiology* of the sexual difficulty and therefore what is *therapeutically* required more evident than it might have been previously (e.g., the effect of a sexual assault in a patient's past)
   - Confirmation that the focus on a particular sexual complaint is, indeed, correct

2. Focus on the couple's sexual activity. Their description of any changes that occurred may also reveal reasons for the shift and provide information about interfering factors

3. The interviewer is provided with the opportunity to:
   - Review the main elements of the history
   - Consider the possibility of using other forms of investigation
   - Discuss therapeutic options (including the provision of reading materials), logistics of continued visits, or aspects of referral

Hawton suggested that a "formulation" be presented to the couple at this time in which predisposing, precipitating, and perpetuating factors are outlined[5] (pp. 118-122). He described the four reasons for doing so, as follows. A formulation:

   - Provides the partners with further understanding of their difficulties
   - Encourages a sense of optimism about the outcome
   - Provides a rational basis for treatment
   - Enables the therapist to check that the information obtained has been correctly understood

While providing a formulation is a desirable objective, it is not always easy to structure information in this way.

A 25-year-old woman was seen with her husband. They were married for two years and were seen because of her concerns about not reaching orgasm during sexual activity with her husband. She was regularly orgasmic when masturbating alone, a fact of which he was unaware until after the first visit. Both were shy and talked little together about sexual, and nonsexual, issues.

Information gained from meeting separately with the woman follows:

1. She was concerned about her husband leaving her because of her "inadequate" sexual response
2. She revealed a lifelong self-deprecatory opinion of herself
3. She had brief episodes of depression
4. She sometimes injured herself as punishment
5. She wondered what her husband saw in her
6. Her mother was a harshly critical person who implied that she (the patient) could not complete tasks productively
7. She talked fondly of her mother and worried only about her husband
8. She hoped that becoming orgasmic with her husband would result in him being more sexually content

Information gained from meeting with the husband alone follows:

1. He said that his biggest concern was his wife's (seemingly) unalterable negative view of herself
2. He hoped she would be more sexually active, if not orgasmic
3. Despite his many attempts at reassurance, she would not accept his protestations that he was sexually content

During the third visit, sexual and nonsexual issues were discussed, as well as the possible relationship between the two: her sexual self-depreciation being one more area of her life in which her mood disorder impaired her ability to function. Two treatment suggestions were made: (1) the Masters and Johnson format of sex therapy[6] as an approach to some of their sexual concerns with the objective being the wife becoming orgasmic with her husband and (2) that the wife's apparent mood disorder be given separate attention by a psychiatrist. The couple accepted both recommendations.

PHYSICAL EXAMINATION

The main theme of Part I of this book is talk and thus the specifics of a physical examination are not reviewed here. This information can be found elsewhere.[1,5] ([5]pp. 111-117)[7] While there is disagreement among sex specialists about the need for a physical examination in all cases of patients appearing with sexual problems in a specialized setting,[1] there is no difference of opinion about the wisdom of such an examination by a *physician in primary care.* The objective of this examination can be one or a combination of the following:

- Reassurance
- Diagnosis
- Education

An examination can be reassuring, if only to inform a patient that no obvious disease is present. In addition, the primary care *physician* is the only health professional that can provide (initially and before any specialists are involved) diagnostic information based on a physical examination. Given the frequency with which there is contact between physicians and the general population, the primary care physician is also in an excellent position to provide educational input[8,9] (see introduction to PART II).

Bancroft reviewed the specific indications for a physical examination in the context of a specialized setting providing care for those with sexual difficulties[1] (p. 417). These also represent circumstances in which the primary care physician might be particularly vigilant. In women, the specific indications include the following:

1. Pain or discomfort during sex activity
2. Recent history of ill health or physical symptoms apart from the sexual problem
3. Recent onset of loss of sexual desire with no apparent cause
4. Any woman in the peri- or postmenopausal age group with a sexual problem
5. History of marked menstrual irregularity or infertility
6. History of abnormal puberty or other endocrine disorder
7. When the patient believes that a physical cause is most likely or suspects that there is something abnormal about her genitalia

In men (p. 424), specific indications are similar except for the additional suggestion of an examination for *all men* over the age of 50 with a sexual problem.

It is apparent that talking during a physical examination can provide a dimension of understanding that is not easily obtained otherwise. Outside of an examination room, the following dialogue between a sex-specialist and a woman patient is not unusual:

Q. Do you think that your genital anatomy is in any way abnormal?
A. I'm not sure.
Q. Well, have you ever asked your family doctor about it during a pelvic examination?
A. Not really. I figured I'd be told if there was anything wrong.
Q. Well, if nothing is said, a person might worry anyway that something isn't right.
A. That's true. Now that you mention it, there is something I wanted to ask someone about. . . .

A complete or partial physical examination should, under some circumstances, be included in the evaluation of a sexual complaint (see introduction to PART II).

> Sex specialists disagree about the need for a physical examination in all cases of patients appearing with sexual problems in a specialized setting. However, there is no disagreement about the wisdom of an examination by a physician in primary care. The objective of this examination can be one or a combination of the following:
>
> - Reassurance
> - Diagnosis
> - Education

> In evaluating negative structural findings, one must recognize that people are examined in a sexually "resting" state and that the opposite is true of sexual troubles, namely, that they represent difficulties with function that often becomes apparent only in the "active" state. The two situations may not result in the same physical findings

However, some humility is required in interpreting negative physical findings. A patient may conclude that "nothing was found" and therefore depart the examination room with the thought that "it's all in my head." In evaluating negative structural findings, one must recognize that people are examined in a sexually "resting" state and that the opposite is true of sexual troubles, namely, that they represent difficulties with function that often becomes apparent only in the "active" state. The two situations may not result in the same physical findings. This should be explained to patients *before* a physical examination so that the limitations of such an examination are understood, particularly if (as is often the case) no structural abnormality is, in fact, detected. The examiner could also explain before the examination that, if there is an obvious problem, it probably would have been discovered before the referral. This is said in an effort to diminish unrealistic expectations.

Some sexual dysfunctions such as a lifelong inexperience with orgasm in a woman and premature ejaculation in a man are rarely a result of disorders of the genitalia or other body organs and thus do not ordinarily require a physical examination as part of an assessment. However, in relation to some other sexual complaints, an understanding of the body's structural status must be an integral part of an assessment. Two examples are:

- Erectile dysfunction that is not clearly situational (see Chapter 11)
- Pain or discomfort associated with vaginal entry (see Chapter 13)

When including a physical examination in an assessment, the purpose should be explained as diagnostic and educational. In relation to the educational "agenda," the examiner might also suggest the possible inclusion of the person's sexual partner (with the explicit acceptance of both) in the examination room. There may be some hesitation in responding to this idea because it is, obviously, unconventional and the patient may be embarrassed as well. After the rationale is explained, the suggestion is often accepted, since in a harmonious relationship, the partner is an ally rather than an obstacle. The idea of having a partner present during the physical examination was first suggested by Masters and Johnson and was discussed by them particularly in relation to the assessment of vaginismus[6] (pp. 262-263). Their explanation of the purpose was that the partner would then have a clear demonstration of muscular constriction at the vaginal opening.

In conducting a woman's pelvic examination, a useful approach is for her to be lying (at about a 45 degree angle) on an examination table in such a way that she can observe the examination with the aid of a handheld mirror. The patient is invited to ask questions (as is her partner) while receiving a brief explanation of the structure and function of the genitalia. One patient was known to voice her appreciation of this method by comparing it to the usual alternative where she "would lie on (my) back and count the flies in the light fixture." Since this method encourages talk, it is particularly useful in the problem of intercourse-related vaginal pain in that the patient can describe exactly what hurts and where.

"Entry dyspareunia" inevitably results in the anticipation of discomfort when anything is inserted into the woman's vagina. Understandably, the expectation of pain is disconcerting to the patient during a physician's vaginal examination and in sexual activity with a partner. In an attempt to diminish the fear of anticipated discomfort, the examiner can explicitly transfer control to the patient by telling her:

You are the "boss" when it comes to your body. I won't put my finger into your vagina. You hold my wrist and gently and slowly insert my finger. I don't want to do anything that will cause you pain. During a vaginal examination, my intention is to get a clearer idea of the location of your discomfort and see if I can discover any particular reason for it.

With the "you are the boss" theme, the examiner presents a model of communication that usually contrasts starkly with what occurs at home with the patient's partner and in the examination room with other physicians. In the past, the woman in this situation typically felt an absence of influence over what occurred sexually and "shut down" entirely to avoid the inevitable pain. In becoming "the boss" in the examination room, she exerts control over the amount of vaginal discomfort she feels and the conditions under which it occurs. After this occurs successfully in the examination room, the couple can adapt to her being the "boss" (at least over her vagina) in sexual situations at home.

The response of women patients to this suggestion is usually spectacular. A powerful rationale for the inclusion of the partner in the examination therefore may be as much in the area of couple communication as a demonstration of the control that the woman could exercise. This aspect of the physical examination is an example of a diagnostic procedure that is also therapeutic.

There are at least two problem areas in the genital examination of men:

- Compared to women there is much less organized teaching in medical schools about practical aspects of examining male genitalia. The pelvic examination of women is often taught with the assistance of women volunteers who provide "feedback" during the examination. For reasons that are unclear, only the occasional medical school provides a program for teaching genital examinations of men—to the detriment of women and men physicians and all of their male patients.

  > The pelvic examination of women is often taught with the assistance of women volunteers who provide "feedback" during the examination. Only a few medical schools provide a program for teaching the genital examination of men—to the detriment of women and men physicians and all of their male patients

  One might have legitimate concerns about the diagnostic capabilities of young physicians in relation to male genitalia. Other than sexual dysfunctions, cancers of the male genital system represent one fourth of newly diagnosed cancers in American males.[10] Testicular cancer in particular, although unusual, is the most common malignancy in men 15 to 44 years of age.[11]

- Examination of the genitalia and anus is one of the reasons patients give for a preference for a physician of a particular sex (usually for the same sex—in contrast to "strictly medical areas" in which there was no preference).[12] Even for genitalia and anus examinations, the reasons why patients want a same-sex physician are not entirely clear. One of men's fears might be that of developing an erection during the examination. Some physicians seem apprehensive about this as well, not knowing what to do or say in such circumstances. Health professionals who work with men with spinal injuries know that simply touching a patient's penis might result in a reflex erection. Although erections in such men are often well received in spite of the presence of a health professional, the same can not be said of able-bodied men. However, something can be learned from the process of examining men with spinal injuries that might be of more general value. Professionals who care for these patients have learned to talk to them beforehand about the possible occurrence of an erection. With able-bodied men, talking about the possible development of an erection during an initial examination probably lessens the chance of it happening and certainly diminishes any potential embarrassment or self-consciousness if it does. One might say to an able-bodied patient:

Sometimes a man's penis gets bigger or erects in nonsexual situations such as during an examination. This is entirely normal and matches our knowledge that direct touch is an important way in which erections develop.

SUMMARY AND CONCLUSIONS

Although *assessment* is usually differentiated from *treatment*, the treatment of a sexual problem often begins immediately when the patient is first seen. In view of the secrecy that so often accompanies sexual problems, open discussion becomes therapeutic. The assessment of a sexual dysfunction is influenced by, among other things, whether the "patient" is an individual or couple. If a substantial relationship exists, both partners should be seen (otherwise, the clinician may encounter considerable therapeutic limitations). Ideally, the first assessment visit involves seeing both partners together. This is advantageous for the following reasons:

1. Both partners are "defined" as patients
2. The health professional is equally committed to both partners
3. The situation encourages partner discussion
4. The clinician can directly observe some facets of the relationship

Limitations of a first conjoint visit include avoidance of six topics:

1. Other recent current sexual partners
2. Past sexual partners
3. Masturbation
4. Sexual fantasies
5. Past STDs
6. Atypical sexual practices

Information about these issues should be obtained when an individual is seen alone.

The content of the first visit concentrates on the "chief complaint" and the "history of the present illness." This entails obtaining information about the problem using the structure outlined in Chapter 4 and in the part of Chapter 5 titled "Present Context: Immediate Issues and Questions," asking about non-intercourse sexual activities, affection, and quality of the relationship. During the second visit, each person is seen alone, and information obtained relates to another part of Chapter 5, titled "Context of the Past: Remote issues and Questions." In the third visit, both partners are brought together again and the focus of the content is on summarizing information from the previous two visits, formulating explanations for the difficulties, and discussing treatment options and approaches. A physical examination is included when this has not previously taken place or when there is a special need to clarify information obtained by history-taking.

REFERENCES

1. Bancroft J: *Human sexuality and its problems*, ed 2, U.K., 1989, Churchill Livingstone.
2. Kaplan HS: *The sexual desire disorders*, New York, 1995, Brunner/Mazel, Inc.
3. Tiefer L, Melman A: Interview of wives: a necessary adjunct in the evaluation of impotence, *Sexuality Disabil* 6:167-175, 1983.
4. Hessellund H: Masturbation and sexual fantasies in married couples, *Arch Sex Behav* 5:133-147, 1976.
5. Hawton K: *Sex therapy: a practical guide*. New York, 1985, Oxford University Press.
6. Masters WH, Johnson VE: *Human sexual inadequacy*, Boston, 1970, Little, Brown and Company.
7. Kaplan HS: *The evaluation of sexual disorders: psychological and medical aspects*, New York, 1983, Brunner/Mazel, Inc.
8. Ferguson KJ, Stapleton JT, Helms CM: Physicians' effectiveness in assessing risk for human immunodeficiency virus infection, *Arch Intern Med* 151:561-564, 1991.
9. Daicar T: The role of the educational pelvic examination, *J Soc Obstet Gynecol Can* 13:31-35, 1991.
10. Gilliland FD, Key CR: Male genital cancers, *Cancer* 75(1 Suppl):295-315, 1995.
11. Forman D, Moller H: Testicular cancer, *Cancer Surv* 19-20:323-341, 1994.
12. Fennema K, Meyer DL, Owen N: Sex of physician: patients' preferences and stereotypes, *J Fam Prac* 30:441-446, 1990.

CHAPTER 7

TALKING ABOUT SEXUAL ISSUES: GENDER AND SEXUAL ORIENTATION

Intuitively, there might seem to be good reasons to try to match the gender of the interviewer to the gender of the respondent . . . potential respondents were offered the choice of a male or female interviewer if there appeared to be any hesitation about agreeing to give the interview . . . the majority had no clear preference . . .

JOHNSON ET AL, 1994[1]

The effectiveness of any interviewing technique is, in the last analysis, to be determined by the quality of the data that are obtained.

KINSEY ET AL, 1949[2]

GENDER: ISSUES AND QUESTIONS

When Talking About Sexual Issues, do Health Professional and Patient Genders Matter?

When talking about sexual issues with a patient, does it make any difference if the health professional is a man and the patient is a woman (or vice versa)? What if both are women or both are men? The answer to the question of whether gender matters is, "yes."

A 24-year-old woman medical student joined a 45-year-old psychiatrist/sex therapist in a consultation regarding erection difficulty in a heterosexual couple. The medical student stated privately beforehand that she was apprehensive about talking to patients about sexual issues, since this was not encouraged during her previous training and she hadn't done so before.

This visit was the first for the couple. The senior clinician began the interview by asking both partners about themselves. When the woman partner answered her part of the question, she was looking at the woman medical student much of the time. When the details of the couple's sexual encounters were discussed, this was even more evident. The medical student completed her Sexual Medicine clinical experience within the same time as the assessment. The senior clinician continued to follow the couple in treatment by himself without difficulty for the next three months.

Gender is probably always an influence when people are talking about sexual issues. Gender makes a difference because two people of the same gender talk the same language to each other. There is an immediate and implicit assumption of communality of development and experience—probably the principal reason that many women patients seem to preferentially choose women physicians. When talking to one another about sexual issues, men are more comfortable talking with other men (other things being equal such as the absence of homophobia), since both understand what it means to have an erection and to ejaculate. The same can be said of women and, for example, the sexual significance of menstrual periods and breastfeeding.

> Gender makes a difference because two people of the same gender talk the same language to each other. There is an immediate and implicit assumption of communality of development and experience.

Does the importance of gender mean that male health professionals are unable to comprehend the sexual experiences of women and vice versa? Of course not. One thing it *does* mean is that when health science students are *beginning* to talk with patients about sexual issues, it is far easier for women students to talk with women patients and for male students to talk with male patients. As confidence develops, the student advances into the less familiar territory of the thoughts and experiences of the other group. Ultimately, patients want help with problems, and, as important as gender might be to some, *competence* is the crucial factor.

> Ultimately, patients want help with problems, and, as important as gender might be to some, competence is the crucial factor.

A 45-year-old woman was referred to a (male) sex-specialist by her (female) family physician because of lack of sexual activity in her relationship with her husband. The patient was sexually assaulted five years before by a (male) psychiatrist. She reported that, despite the referral, her current family physician had difficulty understanding her problems. The patient said that her family physician told her that her vagina was "tight as a drum, like that of a 16 year old." The family physician was also reported as having said that she, herself, was envious and was sure that the patient's husband was quite pleased with the state of his wife's vagina. In fact, the patient had not had any sexual experiences with her husband (or anyone else) for the five years since her sexual assault. Furthermore, the patient felt that her family doctor was unsympathetic, and she was obviously unhappy over the way her situation was handled. Unfortunately, she was unable to talk with her family physician about what she felt to be the latter's insensitive approach.

In extrapolating from their studies on sexual physiology, Masters and Johnson concluded that therapist gender was a matter of consequence in the treatment of dysfunctional couples[3] (p. 4). They believed that the presence of a man and a woman was essential to their research on sexual physiology since ". . . no man will ever fully understand a woman's sexual function or dysfunction . . . [and] . . . the exact converse applies to any woman." Hence they developed the concept of the "dual-sex therapy team" in sex therapy in which each partner has a "friend in court" and an "interpreter."

Two considerations balance the logic and sensitivity of the dual-sex therapy team approach:

1. The issue of competence is ignored when one thinks *only* about the primacy of gender
2. Practicality (insufficient numbers of trained personnel and limited health care financial resources) usually dictate that treatment be provided by one person rather than two

When a single therapist versus a dual sex-therapy team approach was examined from a research perspective, it did not seem to result in any difference in outcome.[4] Sixty-five sexually dysfunctional couples were randomly assigned to treatment by (1) a male or (2) female professional working alone or (3) a dual-sex cotherapy team. The treatment results were the same in all three circumstances. Moreover, it made no difference to the outcome if the therapist who was working alone was a man or woman and the patient was of the same or opposite sex.

A woman was referred to a "sex clinic" by her family physician because of a diminution in her feelings of sexual desire. The referral specified that she be seen by a woman therapist. Although the clinic usually accommodated such requests, it was not possible to do so in this circumstance. The referring physician was told this situation and was also told that one of the male therapists could see the patient within a short time. The referring physician discussed this with the patient and the referral proceeded. The issue of gender difference and its possible impact on history-taking and treatment was explicitly raised by the therapist at the beginning of the first visit and the patient was encouraged to indicate if and when she thought this might be an impediment to anything taking place in the consulting room. Furthermore, the therapist told her that if their gender difference proved to be a problem, he would help her find a woman therapist with whom she might be more comfortable. By the middle of the first visit, and in response to a question by the therapist, the patient said that her discomfort in talking with a man about sexual concerns was much less problematical than she anticipated. The issue of gender did not arise again in the subsequent six months of care.

Suggested Question to Ask Early in the Interview When Patient and Interviewer are Opposite Genders: "HOW DO YOU FEEL ABOUT TALKING TO A MAN (WOMAN) ABOUT SEXUAL MATTERS?"

Does Talking About Sexual Issues Evoke Sexual Feelings in the Patient Toward the Health Professional, and is There a Connection Between Talk, Feelings, and Professional Sexual Misconduct?

The answer to the above question is, "maybe." However, the real question should be: are such connections the norm? The answer is unequivocally, "no." If the answer was positive, it is logical to expect that sex therapists (who spend much of their professional time talking to people about sexual issues) would have to constantly contend with their own, and their patient's, sexual feelings toward each another, as well as the consequences of those feelings. Most professionals working in the area of Sexual Medicine would declare that these are baseless worries.

Nevertheless, the questions are important, since sexual misconduct concerns are prevalent in all health professions. When talking about sexual issues with patients, health professionals exercise a greater degree of caution now than in previous years—a result of social sensitivity to the problem of sexual abuse by individuals in positions of authority (e.g., teachers, clergy, and health professionals). When explaining the reasons for avoiding discussions of "sex" with patients, some health professionals anecdotally include worries that any inquiry about sexual issues may provoke such an accusation.

It is instructive to consider what science demonstrates about the issues of talking to patients about sexual issues, sexual feelings in the health professional toward patients (and vice versa), and professional sexual misconduct. While not all the questions have answers, information exists for some. For example, connections between sexual feeling of the psychologists and sexual misconduct have been examined.[5] In this study, 95% of men and 76% of women report sexual attraction to a client at some time in their careers, although only 9.4% of men and 2.5% of women acted on those feelings. The authors conclude that the two phenomena were (mostly) different— "therapist-client sexual intimacy must be clearly differentiated from the experience of sexual attraction to clients." Despite the fact that the attraction to clients was the norm for men and women psychologists, two thirds of respondents to the survey felt "guilty, anxious or confused" about having such feelings. Although information is not yet available concerning other health professionals, there is little reason to expect different results.

> "therapist-client sexual intimacy must be clearly differentiated from the experience of sexual attraction to clients."[5]

A second study of psychologists by the same group confirmed the finding about sexual attraction from the previous study.[6] The authors also report the following data:

1. Almost 60% of respondents reported feeling sexually aroused in the presence of a client
2. Over 50% reported hugs, flirting, and statements of sexual attraction from the client toward the psychologist
3. Client disrobing was "exceptionally rare"
4. Over one third "reported both male and female client (apparent) sexual arousal during sessions"
5. Ten percent of therapists had a complaint filed against them
6. This happened to men three times more often than women
7. Therapists who had some sexual involvement with clients were four times more likely to have had a previous complaint lodged against them (malpractice, ethics or licensing) than those who did not experience such involvement

Concerns of Canadian physicians regarding the connections between sexual talk, feelings, and misconduct became complex as a result of the involvement of the Canadian Medical Protective Association (CMPA; the defense union formed by physicians against malpractice suits). In the early 1990s, the topic of professional sexual misconduct received an almost frenzied degree of public and professional attention in

Canada. In the midst of this upheaval the CMPA issued a bulletin that included the following definition of patient sexual abuse: (patient sexual abuse can be construed during the process of) "Requesting details of sexual history or sexual preferences when not clinically indicated for the type of consultation or presenting problem."[7]

The CMPA warning to physicians served only to underline the inhibitions many already felt when faced with talking about "sex" with their patients. For Canadian professionals having clinical, teaching, and research responsibilities concerning sexual problems, the CMPA bulletin was not a welcome statement since it provoked more questions than it answered:

1. Was there a concern that questions about sexual matters might be misinterpreted by the patient as a sexual invitation by the physician?
2. Was there a worry that including "sex" in the context of a routine medical consultation was, *ipso facto*, an imposition on a patient?
3. Did the definition of sexual abuse represent the attitude of organized medicine or of malpractice insurance companies (a lawyer wrote the CMPA article)?
4. To what extent was the statement part of a larger social concern about sexual abuse?
5. Was there a worry that including "sex" in a medical history might uncover or provoke sexual feelings in the patient toward the physician?
6. (Most importantly), what was the evidence on which the recommendations in the bulletin concerning sex history-taking were based?

The CMPA bulletin failed to take into account the complexity of professional sexual misconduct and the fact that the precursors involve much more than talking about sexual matters. Precursors usually entail problems over "boundaries." The concept of boundaries has gained much attention, particularly within the medical disciplines of Psychiatry and Family Practice. The word *boundary* refers to the unseen line between health professional and patient, and the present focus is on what constitutes crossing over that line for both parties.

A distinction is made between *boundary crossings* and *boundary violations*.[8] "Boundary crossings" are not necessarily harmful (e.g., attending the funeral of a patient who died). A "boundary violation" is a "crossing" that is harmful (e.g., sexual misconduct). The CMPA might view *questions* about sexual issues to represent a "crossing" or even constitute a "violation" unless ". . . clinically indicated for the type of consultation or presenting problem."[7]

Use of the "permission" technique described in Chapters 2 and 3 might substantially lessen the possibility that questions about sexual matters may be interpreted as a "crossing" or a "violation." However, permission is not the equivalent of license. Permission is given to talk about a subject. It is not assent to a question that has not yet been asked. The manner in which questions are posed, or the language used, might, for example, represent a boundary crossing or violation.

Does Disclosure of the Health Professional's Sexual Experiences Help the Patient?

When a health professional has a patient who has sexual difficulties, one might legitimately wonder about the value of disclosing one's own sexual thoughts and experiences. After all, most woman (including women health professionals) have, for example, had at least an occasional time when intercourse caused vaginal discomfort. Likewise, most men have, at some time, probably experienced rapid ejaculation in intercourse. (Neither of these are the same as a sexual dysfunction, which, among other things, is persistent). Logic indicates that this might be useful information to have for a patient with a similar problem. It might even allow a patient to be more optimistic about the result of a treatment program if it was explained that this also happened to oneself. Intuition provides more guidance to professionals on what to do or say in this situation than science.

As logical as self-disclosure might seem, the small amount of research on this subject does not support a great benefit to sharing one's sexual thoughts and experiences with a patient. A survey of 63 male psychologists found that sexual experiences were the least common of the types of disclosure made.[9] From a clinical viewpoint, there are strong opposing opinions to the notion of professional self-disclosure in this area.

First, the crucial question to be answered is: would it help to make the patient better, which, after all, is the "job" of the health professional (or to use more recent jargon, the "objective")? While patients often find it reassuring to know that others have also experienced sexual problems, the mechanism of self-disclosure by a health professional is not the best method. Information is often available from, for example, self-help books and the Internet. Patients want something *different* from a health professional than what they can easily get elsewhere. Patients want specific help in finding a solution to their *own* sexual predicament and are less interested in the personal difficulties of the health care provider.

Second, it may be difficult to separate discussion of professional self-disclosure on sexual matters from the issues of professional sexual misconduct and boundaries. Self-disclosure may be seen, at least, if not more, as a "boundary crossing." Health professionals should be aware that there may be an inclination by "fact finders" (for example, licensing organizations) to consider the presence of boundary violations (or even boundary crossings) to be "presumptive evidence of allegations of sexual misconduct."[8]

Self-disclosure, in particular, was one of the issues examined by a Massachusetts task force that was established for the purpose of developing guidelines on maintenance of boundaries in psychotherapy.[10] While specific to psychotherapists, the ideas generated are unquestionably serious issues for other health care professionals as well. The guidelines acknowledge that in some areas, self-disclosure is accepted. One area is in the treatment of substance abuse. Another is in the selection of a health professional with the same sexual orientation (gay or lesbian). However, the guidelines also categorically state that, "It is never appropriate for physicians practicing psychotherapy . . . to disclose details of their sexual lives."

Suggested Statement in Response to a Patient Asking About a Health Professional's Sexual Experiences: **"YOU CAME TO SEE ME TO DISCOVER THE EXPLANATION FOR YOUR OWN TROUBLES AND TO FIND HELP TO DO SOMETHING ABOUT THEM. I DON'T BELIEVE THAT TALKING ABOUT MY SEXUAL EXPERIENCES ASSISTS YOU IN DOING THAT."**

In a corollary to the issue of "boundary violation," some think that "excessive distance" from a patient (rather than excessive involvement) might constitute another example of a violation.[11] In this view, an act of "omission is at least as dangerous as (one of) commission." If one accepts this, *avoiding* the subject of "sex" in a history might be seen as an act of omission constituting a "boundary violation."

SEXUAL ORIENTATION: ISSUES AND QUESTIONS

". . . homosexuality . . . [should] . . . not be defined by behavior but by the predominant erotic attraction to others of the same sex . . . One need not engage in sexual activity to be homosexual, any more than one need engage in sexual activity to be considered heterosexual."

RICHARD ISAY, 1969[12]

All of the issues and questions related to the subject of sexual orientation can not possibly be reviewed in this chapter. The focus in this section is on matters that are problematic in primary health care. Developmental and frequency aspects of homosexuality are included in Chapter 5 (see "Puberty and Adolescence—Sexual Orientation").

Terminology

The word "homosexual" is often used in the community and among health professionals to define people who have sexual connections with same-sex partners. However, some prefer use of the words "gay" and "lesbian" and find the word "homosexual" uncomfortable and even offensive. One disadvantage to the use of the word "gay" to describe both groups is that it tends to render individuals apart from gay men as somewhat invisible.[13]

A second objection to the word "homosexuality" is that it leaves out the subject of "heterosexuality" as something that is an equally interesting subject to study (Tiefer L, personal communication, 1997). (The origins of both are only beginning to become unraveled).

> A problem with the word *homosexuality* is the emphasis on the sexual part of the relationship rather than the caring that might exist between two people.

A third problem with the word "homosexuality" is the emphasis on the sexual part of the relationship rather than the caring that might exist between the two people.

The word "homosexuality" implies a meaning that is clear and specific but in fact the opposite is true. For example, does "homosexuality" refer to *sexual behavior* only, without considering what is in a person's *mind*? Or could it refer to the exact opposite, considering only what is in one's mind without reference to sexual behavior? Could someone be homosexual but sexually inactive just like a person who is heterosexual and sexually inactive? If the interviewer *is* considering mind-issues apart from behavior, does that include only sexual images such as fantasies, or feelings of love for a partner as well?

In fact, there are at least three ways to define sexual orientation:

- Behavior
- Fantasy
- Self-identification

(See "Sexual Orientation" in Chapter 5 and Table 5-3 for more discussion on the definition of "homosexuality" and the variety of meanings of the word).

Why is it Necessary for a Health Care Professional to Know the Sexual Orientation of a Patient?

Interest in the health and happiness of the patient is one of the principal reasons for knowing about a patient's sexuality, including their sexual orientation (see "Why Discussion Should Occur" in Chapter 1; see also Box 1-2). (Before homosexuality was deleted from the system of psychiatric diagnoses, the principal rationale for asking about sexual orientation was diagnostic).[14]

Gay men and lesbians may have an increased vulnerability to some medical and emotional disorders. Examples of such medical disorders in men[15] include the following:

- HIV/AIDS in those who engage in anal intercourse with other men
- Other STDs
- Hepatitis
- Anal cancer
- Urethritis

Examples of a possible increased risk of medical disorders in lesbians include the following:

- Ovarian cancer as a result of loss of the protective effect of pregnancy[16] (although an increasing number of lesbians are choosing to have children) and the use of oral contraceptives[17]
- Breast cancer because of increased risk among women who have not given birth
- Cervical cancer based partly on the "false assumption that lesbians do not engage in risk behaviors for cervical cancer . . . [when in fact] the majority of respondents to surveys . . . report a history of heterosexual activity, often involving multiple partners"[18]
- STDs (including HIV/AIDS) among bisexual women[15]

Gay men and lesbians may also have an increased vulnerability to problems affecting mental health[13,15]:

- Acceptance
- Ostracism
- Discrimination
- Personal losses
- Stigmatization
- Depression
- Violence (anti-gay and battering)
- Substance abuse

Risk of suicide has been reported as a particular issue among gay adolescents.[19] A population-based study of over 36,000 US junior and senior high school students indicated that bisexuality/homosexuality was a substantial risk factor for attempted suicide in male (but not female) adolescents.[20] A large proportion (27%) of men with eating disorders are reported to be primarily gay or bisexual.[21] The National Lesbian Health Care Survey provides more specific information about lesbians and reported on information gained from 1925 respondents (a 42% response rate).[22] The survey found that 30% of respondents used alcohol more than once weekly and 6% used it daily, about 75% "had received counseling at some time, and half had done so for reasons of sadness and depression."[22]

In addition to medical and mental health issues, there is evidence that sexual concerns among gay men are not identical to those in heterosexual men.[23] In one study, homosexual men cited that the following occurred at least once in their lifetime:

- Painful receptive anal intercourse
- Concerns about the "normality" of their thoughts, feelings, or fantasies
- Harassment for being gay/homosexual/bisexual

(In a comparative group of heterosexual men, premature ejaculation and low sexual desire were most common).

What is the Relevance of Past Homosexual Behavior to a Current Sexual Dysfunction?

In the course of asking someone about sexual orientation issues, the health professional might discover, for example, that the patient has had same-sex sexual experiences in the past or same-sex sexual fantasies in the present. What does this mean? In some instances sexual orientation may be a peripheral factor; in others, it may be central.

A 30-year-old woman with her husband of four years was referred by her family physician to a "sex clinic" with her husband of four years because of her diminished sexual desire. The couple were initially seen together, but when she was subsequently seen alone, it became apparent that her sexual interest was far from absent and that her sexual fantasies included both men and women. Unknown to her husband, and apart from her relationships with men in her teens and beyond, she lived with another woman in a romantic and sexual relationship for about three years in her early 20s. She regarded herself as bisexual and said that her sexual desire had never been a problem in the past with women or men (*including* her husband). She was deeply in love with her husband and concerned about their present sexual difficulties, which, she thought, more likely involved his erection problems than her sexual orientation. With an ultimately successful treatment focus on his situational erectile disorder, the sexual desire issue disappeared.

A 19-year-old student was referred by his family physician because of an inability to ejaculate. He had not previously disclosed to other health professionals that he could ejaculate when alone and when with a male partner. His principal sexual concern was the inability to have the same experience when having intercourse with a woman. In that circumstance, ejaculation could occur only if he simultaneously fantasized about having a sexual encounter with a man. He was distressed about being able to ejaculate only in this way and was concerned that this might indicate that he was gay. He described his fantasies during masturbation as involving only men since he began at the age of 13 and added that men were included when he thought about his most pleasurable sexual experiences with a partner. His apparent reluctance to accept his homosexuality led him to attempts at intercourse with four different women, which resulted in an inability to ejaculate without fantasizing about men on all four occasions.

Suggested Question Directed Toward a Man and Asked in the Context of a Discussion About a Sexual Dysfunction: "**WHAT IS YOUR OPINION ABOUT THE CONNECTION BETWEEN THE PROBLEM OF ____ (E.G., ERECTIONS) AND YOUR SEXUAL EXPERIENCES WITH OTHER MEN (WOMEN)?**"

Disclosure of Sexual Orientation to Health Professionals

Primary care health professionals learn about the sexual orientation of their patients in two ways:

- The information is spontaneously revealed
- The patient waits for the health professional to ask specific questions

Of these two possibilities, survey data indicate that many gay men and lesbians choose the latter. These surveys leave unclear the answer to the question of the impact of HIV/AIDS on the extent of disclosure.

Interviews were conducted with 623 gay men in the United Kingdom who were registered with a general practitioner.[24] Forty-four percent of the men had not revealed their sexual orientation to their family doctor. This was true as well for 44% of the 77 men who were HIV positive (in most instances, they were tested in a specialized clinic).

One part of another study of 105 bisexual men assessed the degree to which male subjects revealed their sexual attraction to other men to various people in their network.[25] Only 23% "fully disclosed" this information to a "doctor or clinic" and, even more surprisingly, only 53% disclosed this information to a "counselor or psychologist."

A group of 424 bisexual and lesbian respondents to another survey indicated that over one third (37.5%) "believed that disclosure of sexual orientation to their physician would adversely affect their health care."[26] In addition, over one third of the respondents "said that they would like to disclose their sexual orientation to the physician providing their gynecologic care, yet they hesitated to do so."[26] Moreover, 60% indicated that they would be willing to discuss their sexual orientation *if the information was not put in the medical record*. In the experience of respondents (apart from opinions and desires), only 41% disclosed their sexual orientation.

Primary care health professionals learn about the sexual orientation of their patients in two ways:

- The information is spontaneously revealed
- The health professional asks specific questions

Of these two possibilities, survey data indicate that many gay men and lesbians choose the latter.

Suggestions for physicians regarding sexual orientation:

1. Offer to not record sexual orientation information in the medical record
2. Allow a friend or partner to be present during the examination
3. Include the friend or partner in treatment discussions
4. Ask questions in a manner that does not presume heterosexuality

The authors of this study concluded with some concrete suggestions for physicians:

1. Offer to not record sexual orientation information in the medical record
2. Allow a friend or partner to be present during the examination
3. Include the friend or partner in treatment discussions
4. Ask questions in a manner that does not presume heterosexuality

Of 622 men and women subscribers to a gay newspaper who responded to a questionnaire survey, 49% of the respondents explicitly revealed to their primary health professional that they were homosexual.[27] However, an additional 34% said they would provide this information to their health professional if they "thought it was important." This finding suggests that many gay patients may be willing to reveal their sexual orientation if asked and if the rationale for the question is made clear.

"Homophobia" (defined as "the irrational fear, distrust, and/or hatred of lesbian/gay people") seems to be the main deterrent to disclosure of one's status as gay or lesbian to health care professionals.[13] Some regard an attitude of "Heterosexism" (defined as a "world-view value system that prizes heterosexuality") with homophobia. Heterosexism assumes that heterosexuality is the only appropriate manifestation of love and sexuality and devalues homosexuality and all that is not heterosexual.[13] In one of the surveys described above, 89% of respondents who rated their primary health professional's attitude as very supportive candidly discussed their sexual orientation with that person, compared to 48% of those who judged their health professional to be hostile.[27] As a result of homophobic attitudes among health professionals, many lesbians reportedly turned to "complementary health care providers. . . . [and are therefore] . . . . unlikely to receive any of the standard medical screening tests. . . . The effects of this alienation. . . . *may result in a significant increase in morbidity and mortality*".[28]

What Questions Does One Ask?

Given that there *is* reason to ask about sexual orientation in a health setting and that the majority of patients do not reveal this information spontaneously, what question(s) does one ask? How does one determine sexual orientation anyway? By self-identification? By the fantasies of a person? By the sex of sexual partners? By some combination of these elements?

> "orientational identity and sexual behavior are not synonymous and require separate and specific inquiry."[28]

Questions that help establish sexual orientation are theoretical and have a serious practical application as well. For example, in one survey, 78% to 80% of lesbians reported sexual activity with a man in the previous one to five years. The author concluded from this report that "orientational identity and sexual behavior are not synonymous and require separate and specific inquiry".[28] Such information might, for example, be helpful in learning about the origin of a patient's STD.

In asking for "identifying information" from a new patient, one usual question relates to clarification of the person's living circumstances. If the patient is living with someone, the interviewer can simply ask if the relationship is one that is also romantic (apart from sharing the cost of the accommodations). If the gender of the other person has not already been identified (unusual), this question too can easily be asked.

Another approach to clarifying the sexual orientation of a patient is to use the screening outline provided in Chapter 3. However, one of the problems with this approach is having to wait until the subject of "sex" arises in the "Review of Systems." If one *does* delay until this point, the specific question(s) asked by a health professional become influenced by their purpose(s). For example, one reason is to simply clarify the sexual orientation of a new patient while learning about the person in the first few visits. Another intention might be to consider an STD in the differential diagnosis of a patient with a particular medical complaint. A third purpose might be to clarify the nature of the relationship between a patient who is depressed and a friend who just died.

The Chapter 3 screening method (with suggested questions) is easily applied to sexual orientation questions involving a new patient. The four-question model (see Figure 3-4) entails asking:

1. A preamble/permission question
2. A question that addresses the issue of whether the person is sexually active
3. Whether the partner(s) was(were) a man, a woman, or both
4. If the patient has any sexual concerns (see Figure 3-4)

A question about the gender of the partner immediately (but implicitly) tells the patient that the interviewer is not assuming that person to be heterosexual. "Simply *having* a nonjudgmental, non homophobic attitude is not enough. The responsible practitioner needs to *convey* his or her nonjudgmental attitude to all patients."[28] On the basis of clinical impression, questioning the possibility of same-sex sexual experiences by a health professional is easily accepted by most patients and does not elicit the same response from people as in a social situation.

> Questions from a health professional regarding same-sex sexual experiences are easily accepted by most patients and do not elicit the same response from people as in a social situation.

Initial use of the undifferentiated word "partner" (rather than spouse, husband, wife, boyfriend, or girlfriend) also conveys to the patient that the interviewer is not making any assumption regarding sexual orientation. Furthermore, this approach is beneficial in talking to heterosexual patients, since it also implicitly dispels any supposition of particular linkages with sexual activity (such as marriage).

With gay and heterosexual patients, use of the word "partner" conveys an attitude of acceptance. The health care professional must attend to such issues during an interview, in the use of patient forms, and in waiting room information pamphlets.

Last, clinicians should be clear about the sexual orientation of the patient *before* questions about birth control are asked. To do otherwise risks alienating the patient. (The comment refers to the order of questions not the relevancy. The health professional should not assume that questions about birth control are immaterial because someone is a lesbian. What determines the relevancy is the patient's behavior).

Confidentiality

When a gay or lesbian patient is in a partnership, the health care professional should inquire about the involvement of the partner in appointments and the extent to which the partner's influence is desired in any future medical emergency involving the patient. O'Hanlan suggests that couples be encouraged to consider preparing a medical power of attorney, particularly before elective surgery or obstetric delivery.[28]

Fearing repercussions, many gay and lesbian patients are unwilling to reveal their sexual orientation unless this information is not recorded in their medical record. One suggested possibility under such circumstances is a coded entry in the chart.[29]

What Does the Heterosexual Health Professional Know About Homosexuality and the Sexual Practices of Gay Men and Lesbians?

When a heterosexual health professional talks about sexual issues with a patient who is gay or lesbian, it should not be any different than talking to a heterosexual person, but it often is. The heterosexual health professional should consider their personal attitudes and knowledge about homosexuality. Gays and lesbians are often quite tolerant of professional knowledge-deficits, providing it is acknowledged and does not extend beyond the "garden variety" lack of information.

A gay male couple in their 40s was referred to a professionally experienced (heterosexual) sex therapist for assessment of an erectile concern of one partner. One of the two men was himself a health care professional and explicitly stated on the first visit that he had "checked out" the therapist before proceeding with the appointment. (The patient never said what facets of the therapist made him acceptable but the implication was that it was connected to his professional attitude). The therapist agreed to continue seeing the couple in treatment but made it understood that, since the majority of his patients were heterosexual, he would need to be taught some aspects of the sexual practices of gay men. They were completely at ease with the professional's request for more information.

Suggested Statement and Question to a Gay Man or Lesbian in the context of an HPI: **Man or Lesbian in the Context of an HPI: "I KNOW VERY LITTLE ABOUT THE ACTIVITIES OF GAY MEN (OR LESBIANS) WHEN THEY ARE BEING SEXUAL WITH ONE ANOTHER. IS IT OKAY IF I IF I ASK YOU ABOUT THEM?"**

Additional Question if the Answer is, `yes': **"TELL ME WHAT YOU AND YOUR PARTNER USUALLY DO TOGETHER."**

The principal driving force behind the recent large-scale "sex" surveys has been presence of the HIV/AIDS epidemic together with the absence of reliable information about community sexual practices (see Table 1-1 in Chapter 1). As a result of these surveys, more is known concerning gay and lesbian sexual activities. For example, in the French survey, gay and bisexual men described the following most common sexual activities during their last intercourse:

- Stroking each other tenderly (96%)
- Reciprocal masturbation (77% to 82%)
- Fellatio—active or passive (72% to 76%)
- Anal penetration—active or passive (28% to 36%)

Anal penetration occurred without a condom in 12% to 15%. Inserting a fist in the anus was unusual (6%)[30] (p. 131). (See also Tables 5-1 and 5-3 in Chapter 5).

What Information Can a Health Professional Provide to Patients about Sexual Orientation and Sex-related Issues?

PFLAG (Parents, Families and Friends of Lesbians and Gays) is an international organization that is devoted to support, education, and advocacy. PFLAG circulates a list of recommended readings (most in paperback) on various sexual orientation issues. Some readings are directed toward parents, spouses, and children of gays and lesbians; others focus on particular subjects such as religion and spirituality, history and civil rights, and HIV/AIDS.

Most large cities in North America have speciality bookstores devoted to gay, lesbian, and bisexual themes. Health professionals could direct patients to such locations. Several recent publications seem particularly useful (for patients and for health professionals):

- *Becoming gay: the journey to self-acceptance*, Isay R (author): a sensitive and readable book on self-acceptance and the development of homosexuality in the individual. It is written from the perspective of a practicing gay psychoanalyst[12]
- *A natural history of homosexuality*, Mondimore FM (author): an informative review of all aspects of the topic of homosexuality from its history to recently published research into genetics and the brain[31]
- *The complete guide to safer sex*, McIlvenna T (author): in addition to sexual orientation issues, this material (available in paperback) offers a thorough review of all aspects of safe sex behavior[32]

Last, the Internet is a significant resource on gay, lesbian and bisexual issues and includes a large amount of information (see Appendix IV).[33]

SUMMARY

The gender of the participants in a health care interview that includes sexual issues and the sexual orientation of the patient are pervasive factors regardless of the setting, be it medical or mental health. These two issues always must be considered.

Usually, the fact that the health professional is a man or woman does not interfere with talking about "sex," regardless of the gender of the patient. However, for some, the gender of the professional is important (e.g., some women patients have a sense of satisfaction and safety only when talking with other women). The expectation of comfort seems mostly related to a communality of life experience.

Some health professionals might be concerned that they or their patient will become sexually stimulated by a discussion of the topic. Sexual feelings may, in fact, appear, but when they occur, they are often results of factors that are not necessarily related to any specific discussion about sexual issues. Whatever the reason for the patient or professional developing sexual feelings, only infrequently does the other person know, and less common still is the possibility that either may act on those feelings. "Boundary violations" that result from sexual feelings, including professional sexual misconduct, interfere with the entire relationship between health professional and patient. Professional self-disclosure in relation to sexual issues (other than sexual orientation) may do the same. At very least, self-disclosure is unconventional, if not unproductive.

In contrast to the gender of the participants in the interview (obvious to all) their sexual orientation is often hidden. Primary care professionals must have this information because of its direct relationship to a patient's health and happiness. Gay men and lesbians seem particularly vulnerable to some disorders, and importantly the expectation of a homophobic reception interferes with many undergoing regular screening procedures.

There are two ways that a health professional discovers the sexual orientation of a patient:

- The patient spontaneously reveals the information
- Specific questions are asked

Studies show that the former happens in only a minority of situations. An interviewer might ask about whom the patient lives with and whether the relationship is one that is also romantic or involves sexual experiences. Somewhat later in the interview, within a Review of Systems (ROS), the screening outline presented in Chapter 3 suggests a single straightforward question that asks the patient if their sexual partner is a man or woman or both. Using the word "partner" and not making assumptions about the gender of the other person conveys an attitude of acceptance. Questions about birth control without first clarifying a patient's sexual orientation risks alienating that person. Clinicians would also do well to discuss issues related to confidentiality: whether and how information about sexual orientation should be recorded in the medical record, and the extent to which a partner is involved in the patient's medical care.

To better understand their patients, heterosexual health professionals should learn more about the nature of gay and lesbian relationships, and specifically, about the sexual practices that their patients experience.

Some of this information is acquired by talk; some is acquired by reading. Patients should also be encouraged to make use of the self-help literature and information on the Internet.

REFERENCES

1. Johnson AM et al: *Sexual attitudes and lifestyles*, Oxford, 1994, Blackwell Scientific Publications.
2. Kinsey AC, Pomeroy WB, Martin CE: *Sexual behavior in the human male*, Philadelphia and London, 1949, W.B. Saunders.
3. Masters WH, Johnson VE: *Human sexual inadequacy*, Boston, 1970, Little, Brown & Company.
4. LoPiccolo J et al: Effectiveness of single therapists versus cotherapy teams in sex therapy, *J Consult Clin Psychol* 53:287-294, 1985.
5. Pope KS, Keith-Speigel P, Tabachnick BG: Sexual attraction to clients: the human therapist and the (sometimes) inhuman training system, *Am Psychol* 41:147-158, 1986.
6. Pope KS, Tabachnick BG: Therapists' anger, hate, fear, and sexual feelings: national survey of therapist responses, client characteristics, critical events, formal complaints, and training, *Profess Psychol: Res Pract* 24:142-152, 1993.

7. *Information letter*: The Canadian Medical Protective Association 7:2, 1992.

8. Gutheil TG, Gabbard GO: The concept of boundaries in clinical practice: theoretical and risk-management dimensions, *Am J Psychiatry* 150:188-196, 1993.

9. Berg-Cross L: Therapist self-disclosure to clients in psychotherapy, *Psychother Private Prac* 2:57-64, 1984.

10. Hundert EM, Applebaum PS: Boundaries in psychotherapy: model guidelines, *Psychiatry: Interpersonal and Biol Processes* 58:345-356, 1995.

11. Lewin RA: The concept of boundaries in clinical practice: theoretical and risk-management dimensions: comment, *Am J Psychiatry* 151:294, 1994.

12. Isay R: *Becoming gay: the journey to self-acceptance*, New York, 1996, Pantheon Books.

13. Harrison AE: Primary care of lesbian and gay patients: educating ourselves and our students, *Fam Med* 28:10-23, 1996.

14. Marmor J: Epilogue: homosexuality and the issue of mental illness. In Marmor J (editor): *Homosexual behavior: a reappraisal*, New York, 1980, Basic Books, Inc.

15. Council on Scientific Affairs, American Medical Association: Health care needs of gay men and lesbian women in the United States, *JAMA* 275:1354-1359, 1996.

16. Cramer DW et al. Determinents of ovarian cancer risk. 1. Reproductive experiences and family history. *J Nat Cancer Inst* 71:711-716, 1983.

17. Lee NC et al: The reduction in risk of ovarian cancer associated with oral-contraceptive use, *N Eng J Med* 316:650-655, 1987.

18. Rankow EJ: Breast and cervical cancer amongst lesbians, *Womens Health Issues* 5:123-129, 1995.

19. Kournay RFC: Suicide among homosexual adolescents, *J Homosexuality* 13:111-117, 1987.

20. Remafedi G et al: The relationship between suicide risk and sexual orientation: results of a population-based study, *Am J Public Health* 88:57-60, 1998.

21. Carlat et al: Eating disorders in males: a report on 135 patients, *Am J Psychiatry* 154:1127-1132, 1997.

22. Bradford J, Ryan C, Rothblum ED: National lesbian health care survey: implications for mental health, *J Consult Clin Psychol* 62:228-242, 1994.

23. Rosser BRS et al: Sexual difficulties, concerns, and satisfaction in homosexual men: an empirical study with implications for HIV prevention, *J Sex Marital Ther* 23:61-73, 1997.

24. Fitzpatrick R et al: Perceptions of general practice among homosexual men, *Br J Gen Prac* 44:80-82, 1994.

25. Stokes JP, McKirnan DJ, Burzette RG: Sexual behavior, condom use, disclosure of sexuality, and stability of sexual orientation in bisexual men, *J Sex Res* 30:202-213, 1993.

26. Smith et al: Health care attitudes and experiences during gynecologic care among lesbians and bisexuals, *Am J Public Health* 75:1085-1087, 1985.

27. Dardick L, Grady KE: Openness between gay persons and health professionals, *Ann Intern Med* 93:115-119, 1980.

28. O'Hanlan AK: Lesbian health and homophobia: perspectives for the treating obstetrician/gynecologist, *Current Problems in Obstetrics, Gynecology and Fertility* 18: 97-133, 1995

29. White J, Levinson W: Primary care of lesbian patients, *J Gen Intern Med* 8:41-47, 1993.

30. Spira A, Bajos N, and the ACSF group: *Sexual behavior and AIDS*, Brookfield, 1994, Ashgate Publishing Company.

31. Mondimore FM: *A natural history of homosexuality*, Baltimore and London, 1996, The Johns Hopkins University Press.

32. McIlvenna T (editor): *The complete guide to safer sex*, Fort Lee, 1992, Barricade Books Inc.

33. Weinrich JD: Strange bedfellows: homosexuality, gay liberation, and the Internet, *J Sex Ed Ther* 22:58-66, 1997.

TALKING ABOUT SEXUAL ISSUES: MEDICAL, PSYCHIATRIC, AND SEXUAL DISORDERS (Apart From Dysfunctions)

The nature of [a patient's response to the presence of a sexual difficulty] is influenced by cultural background, personality characteristics, the individual's prior experiences, and the dynamics of [the] marital relationship . . . . It seems important to use a multi-factorial model . . . that integrates psychological variables with biological processes in order to better understand the effect of . . . medical illness on human sexuality.

SCHIAVI, 1990[1]

MEDICAL DISORDERS

Physical Illnesses and Disability in Adults: Sexual Issues and Questions

> Avoidance of sexual issues that partly results from the gloomy attitude of some health professionals is contraindicated by clinical experience and research findings that emphasize the benefit that patients can derive when intervention is offered.[3]

While a wide variety of sexual problems exist in those with a chronic medical illness, a "pessimistic stereotype" on the part of a health care provider about the sexual potential of patients can result in professional inactivity.[2] From a biological point of view, the appearance of sexual problems is hardly surprising when body systems that contribute to sexual function (hormonal, gynecological, urological, neurological, and cardiovascular) are affected. Yet the avoidance of sexual issues, which partly results from the gloomy attitude of some health professionals, is contraindicated by clinical experience and research findings that emphasize the benefit patients can derive when intervention is offered.[3]

Sexual dysfunctions that occur in the desire and arousal phases of the sex response cycle (see Chapter 3) seem more common than others in the context of chronic medical disorders.[4] The orgasm phase appears less vulnerable to disruption by illness (apart from neurological disorders and side effects of some medications—see Appendix V). Observations about the vulnerability of different parts of the sex response cycle seem equally valid in men and women. A common finding in various studies is the appearance of multiple sexual problems, rather than any one in particular.

> Over 70% of 384 patients referred to a sexual rehabilitation service were seen only once or twice, but 50% of the patients who were followed up had a positive view of the consultation and their present sexual status.

"Numerous studies have documented that patients with disabilities related to diabetes, myocardial infarctions, or strokes . . . want information about sexual function from their primary-care team but rarely solicit or receive sex education relevant to their medical problems"[4] (p. 320). Findings from one study of cancer patients state the same conclusions and are revealing from a primary care perspective.[5] Over 70% of 384 patients referred to a sexual rehabilitation service were seen only once or twice, but almost 50% of the patients who were followed-up had a positive view of the consultation and their present sexual status. "Patients . . . who are distressed enough about sexual issues to ask for help usually want *education* and *crisis intervention* rather than conventional sex therapy."[5] In a needs study of cancer patients, over 50% indicated they would feel most comfortable discussing sexual and social concerns with their physician.[6] In response to the sexual and fertility needs of patients with cancer, Schover has written an informative and sensitive self-help book.[7]

The focus of attention in this section of the book is on adults with acquired illnesses and disability, but one must remember that individuals with congenital disorders grow into adulthood with sexual consequences to their disorders that are, in some respects, quite different from those that develop later in life. Overprotective behavior by parents, personal devaluation, desexualization by others, deficits in knowledge about sexual anatomy and physiology, lack of knowledge of sexual practices, lack of experience in relationships, and social isolation are only some of the elements identified as being influential factors in such a child[8] (p. 244).

In addition to the issues and questions outlined in previous chapters and in the section on Psychiatric Disorders below in this Chapter, some particular issues and questions

Table 8-1 Sexual Issues in a Medical and Psychiatric Examination

EXAMINATION SECTION	SEXUAL ISSUES
Identifying information (II)	• Relationship status • Sexual orientation (possibly)
History of present illness (HPI)	Sexual symptom(s) of disorder
Personal and social history (P and SHx)	• Childhood sexual experiences with adults • Sexual orientation • Past romantic and sexual experiences
Review of systems (ROS)	Sexual Disorders • Sexual dysfunctions • Paraphilias • Gender identity

Past medical history (PMHx)	• STDs (past and present)
	• Reproduction
	    Birth control
	    Effect of pregnancy on illness
	    Effect of illness on pregnancy and
	    child care
	    Abortion
	• Bowel and bladder problems
	• Motor difficulties

Physical Examination (Px)	Signs of disease affecting sexual function
Mental status (MS)	Thoughts of sexual violence
Treatment (Rx)	Sexual side effects of drugs

arise around the topic of sexuality associated with medical illness and disability in adults with acquired disorders. Table 8-1 outlines one approach to considering sexual issues in a conventional medical and psychiatric history. In this structure, the interviewer asks about sexual and sex-related issues that might be relevant to each stage of the history. As an alternative, the health professional might also consider specific areas of inquiry. Szasz outlined seven such areas in patients with a severe physical disability[9] as follows:

1. Sexual response
2. Fertility
3. Motor functions
4. Urinary/bowel/gas control
5. Partnership
6. Sexual self-view
7. Sexual interest.

Some of these areas are discussed elsewhere in this book (e.g., symptoms of sexual dysfunction in Chapter 4 and Part II); others are addressed below.

ISSUE #1: What was the Sexual Status of the Patient *Before* the Onset of the Illness or Disability?

When sexual function is apparently disrupted at the time of the onset of an illness or disability, the assumption is often made that the latter was the cause of the sexual problem. This is not always so. Only a thorough history reveals the accuracy of this supposition.

A 44-year-old man was referred because of erectile difficulties. One year before, he was diagnosed with diabetes mellitus. Since erectile problems are well known to be a symptom of diabetes, the referring physician assumed that the two were related and suggested that the patient receive intracavernosal injections as the then preferred form of treatment.[10]

The patient and his wife wanted to explore other forms of treatment, hence the referral. History revealed that the patient, indeed, had erectile difficulties with his wife but had full and prolonged erections with masturbation (which took place about once per month) and in the morning upon awakening. Furthermore, when questioned about his previous sexual function, it became apparent that he had experienced erectile problems from time-to-time since he married 18 years ago at the age of 26. The diagnosis of a situational erectile disorder (see Chapter 11) was made and he was reassured about the lack of connection between his erection function and his diabetes. The suggestion of intracavernosal injections was not accepted and a talk-oriented form of treatment was initiated with the patient and his wife. While the patient continued to have erectile difficulties after treatment, they occurred far less frequently and the wife and the husband were more satisfied with their sexual relationship.

Suggested Question to be Asked in the Context of the History of the Present Illness (HPI) or Review of Systems (ROS): "TELL ME ABOUT YOUR SEXUAL RELATIONSHIP WITH YOUR WIFE (HUSBAND, PARTNER) BEFORE YOU DEVELOPED (FOR EXAMPLE) DIABETES."

ISSUE #2: What is the Patient's *Mood* and How Does it Influence His or Her *Attitude* Toward Sexual Activity With a Partner?

Physical illness or disability can result in someone feeling undesirable and undesired as a partner generally and a sexual partner specifically. Other professionals use the terms *devaluation* and *desexualization* to refer to these phenomena[8] (p. 243). (These attitudes should be distinguished from an acute depressive disorder when a person may feel self-deprecatory). Family members, friends, and the community may reinforce thoughts of "devaluation" and "desexualization." The question may be heard: "Why can't people see me as someone who has a handicap rather than someone who *is* handicapped?"[11]

A 37-year-old woman was diagnosed with multiple sclerosis four years before referral. She worked full-time as a secretary and her symptoms were, so far, invisible. She was married for ten years but left her husband because of his involvement with another woman. In her past sexual experiences (alone and with a partner), she came to orgasm easily and regularly but this ceased altogether about two years before.

To her surprise, men asked her out on dates, and some continued to be interested in her "even" after they discovered her illness. She was fearful about resuming a sexual relationship with a man because she viewed herself as undesirable. When she did resume a sexual relationship, her (current) male partner wondered why she did not come to orgasm and whether he was somehow at fault. She wondered if there was some way that her problem with orgasm could be reversed. Knowing that the "stimulus" intensity provided by a vibrator would be much greater when compared to her usual sexual experiences and being aware through history-taking that she had never used one in the past, her family doctor suggested this approach to her. With her persistence in the length of time she used the vibrator (over one half hour) and in the number of times she tried (many), she eventually came to orgasm again—initially when alone and then with her partner.

Suggested Questions to be Asked in the Context of the History of the Present Illness (HPI) or Review of Systems (ROS): "HOW HAS (FOR EXAMPLE) MULTIPLE SCLEROSIS INFLUENCED THE WAY YOU FEEL ABOUT YOURSELF GENERALLY AND HAS IT INFLUENCED OTHERS ROMANTICALLY INTERESTED IN YOU?"

Additional Question: "HOW HAS (FOR EXAMPLE) MULTIPLE SCLEROSIS INFLUENCED THE WAY YOU FEEL ABOUT YOURSELF SEXUALLY?"

ISSUE #3: Does the Patient have any *Symptoms* (e.g., Pain or Motor Problems) that would Interfere with being Affectionate or with Sexual Experiences?

> Intimacy does not require sexual inter-course. Virtually no disability precludes some form, of physical closeness in bed.[9]

Some kinds of illnesses (e.g., rheumatoid arthritis) might significantly interfere with being affectionate and with sexual activities. The same might be said of disabilities that result in the need for a wheelchair. Movements that entail hugging or holding may be a problem, quite apart from more complex actions which involve, for example, transfer from a wheelchair to a bed or undressing. However, "intimacy does not require sexual intercourse. Virtually no disability precludes some form of physical closeness in bed."[9]

A 45-year-old married woman developed rheumatoid arthritis 20 years before. It now affects joints, including her hands, hips, knees, and ankles. She walks with a cane and, much of the time, uses a motorscooter. She and her husband were always very affectionate with one another and although less sexually interested compared to the early part of her marriage, she felt that a sexual relationship was important to a couple and that every effort should be made for it to continue. Among other problems, intercourse became progressively difficult because she could not easily spread her legs. As a result, she and her husband gradually focused their sexual/genital experiences on him stimulating her clitoris with his fingers and she stimulating him orally. These sexual practices were familiar to them since before their marriage and remained greatly satisfying to both.

Suggested Question to be Asked in the Context of the History of the Present Illness (HPI) or Review of Systems (ROS): "HOW HAVE YOUR PROBLEMS (FOR EXAMPLE) WITH YOUR JOINTS AFFECTED YOUR SEXUAL EXPERIENCES OR LOVEMAKING?"

ISSUE #4: Has the Patient's Sexual Function been Affected by *Treatment for the* Disorder?

Medications (see Appendix V) and surgical procedures, especially those affecting body systems described at the beginning of this chapter, can have profound and direct effects on sexual function.

The 35-year-old wife of a 55-year-old man phoned for an appointment because of her husband's relative sexual inactivity. They were married for four years, she for the first time and he for the second. Their sexual activity was satisfying to both until his prostate surgery (TURP) two years before. Since then, his erections were partial:

- During sexual activity with his wife
- On awakening in the morning
- During masturbation

Moreover, his ejaculation was retrograde (which to him, was like not ejaculating at all) and his orgasm was much less intense.

He was angry about not having been alerted before surgery that these phenomena might occur and said that, had he known, he would have at least obtained a second opinion. His wife was chagrined at his apparent loss of sexual desire. Because of his great difficulty in adjusting to this new situation, they were referred to a sex-specialist, who was also a mental health professional. After a period in which the husband was seen alone in psychotherapy, his anger diminished and his sexual desire returned, much to the pleasure of his wife. Sildenafil (viagra) was successfully used to treat his generalized erectile dysfunction. However, much to their disappointment, attempts at becoming pregnant were unsuccessful.

Suggested Question to be Asked in the Context of Reviewing the Patient's Treatment Course: **HAVE THERE BEEN ANY SEXUAL SIDE EFFECTS FROM THE MEDICATIONS THAT YOU'RE TAKING (OR SURGERY THAT OCCURRED)?"**

Additional Question if the Answer is, "yes": **"WHAT KIND OF CHANGES HAVE YOU NOTICED?"**

ISSUE #5: Are there *Reproductive Consequences* to the Patient's Illness or Disability?

When considering reproductive consequences, illnesses and disabilities that most affect people in their childbearing and childrearing years are of greatest concern. Included are, for example, spinal-cord injuries and autoimmune diseases such as multiple sclerosis and rheumatoid arthritis. Reproductive consequences involve the ability to conceive and include factors such as genetics, prenatal care, childbirth and postnatal childcare.

A 23-year-old man fractured several vertebrae in a motorcycle accident. His spinal cord was severely injured at the mid-thoracic level. As a result, he was unable to walk and required a wheelchair. His girlfriend with whom he had been living for six months (and intended to marry) could not continue to live with someone who was paraplegic and, as a result, they separated. He seemed depressed but was unwilling to talk with a health professional about his reaction to the disrupted relationship.

In the course of his rehabilitation program, he was informed that if he wished, someone was available for him to talk with about sexual issues. Approximately two years later, he was interested in seeing a health professional after he became romantically involved with another woman. At that time, he also stated his great desire to father a child. His genital function was such that he was able to have reflex erections but could not ejaculate. However, he knew from other men in similar situations that intercourse was possible and that obtaining semen to impregnate a woman might also be possible through the process of electroejaculation or vibratory stimulation.[12] He was referred to a urologist who specialized in this form of care to obtain more information.

Question to be Asked in the Context of Rehabilitation: "**WHAT IS YOUR OPINION ABOUT SOMEONE IN YOUR SITUATION HAVING CHILDREN?**"

Addition Question: "**IS THIS SOMETHING YOU WANT SOME MEDICAL ASSISTANCE WITH NOW OR POSSIBLY SOMETIME IN THE FUTURE?**"

PSYCHIATRIC DISORDERS

In 1972, Pinderhughes, Grace, and Reyna, surveyed 18 psychiatrists in a Boston Veterans Administration Hospital. Not only did physicians believe that the great majority of psychiatric disorders could be caused by sexual anxiety, but two thirds agreed that sexual activity could slow recovery from an acute episode of psychiatric illness. In the same hospital, however, only 40% of patients surveyed recalled discussing sexual issues with their psychiatrists.

SCHOVER AND JENSEN, 1988[13]

Psychiatric Disorders: Sexual Issues and Questions

Some health professionals (particularly nonpsychiatric physicians) and many people in the community believe that psychiatrists and others who work in the mental health field are especially knowledgeable about sexual issues (if not inordinately interested in this area). In truth in talking to patients about sexual problems, psychiatrists, for example, seem no more and no less knowledgeable and skilled than other physicians.[14]

As indicated above, Table 8-1 outlines one approach to considering sexual issues in a conventional medical and psychiatric history. In this structure, the interviewer asks about sexual and sex-related issues that might be relevant to *each* stage of the history.

Alternatively, the interviewer could focus on specific sexual and sex-related issues. There are at least seven topics that should be addressed in the course of a conventional psychiatric history. While it may not be appropriate to ask about all of these issues during the first visit, they should be included sometime during the first few meetings with the patient. The seven areas are described below, with brief case histories and suggested questions.

ISSUE #1: Does the Patient have a Sexual *Symptom of a Psychiatric Disorder?*

Psychiatric disorders are generally so pervasive that they interfere with all aspects of a patient's day-to-day function, so much so that it is difficult to conceive of "sex" not being affected in some way or other. In other words, "sex" is almost always disrupted when a psychiatric illness develops and therefore is almost always evident as a symptom. In treating people with psychiatric disorders, one is reminded of Freud's appeal to other clinicians to think about love and work when considering the impact of a mental disorder on a patient.

When thinking about sexual symptoms of a psychiatric disorder, depression is a handy example, partly because it is so common. While DSM-IV outlines The Diagnostic Criteria for a Major Depressive Episode, disrupted sexual function is not specifically included.[15] Yet it seems to be conventional wisdom that sexual interest or desire is diminished when a person is depressed. Paradoxically, at the same time that diminished sexual desire in depression is assumed, a question about this may not even be asked.

A 29-year-old woman with a bipolar disorder was admitted to hospital because of depression. Her chief worry was difficulty in finding a boyfriend. Questions asked included those related to sleep, energy, appetite for food, present mood, and thoughts of suicide. No sex-related questions were included in her history despite the fact that in a previous episode of mania and unlike her usual behavior she was sexually indiscriminate, had five different sexual partners in a two-week period, and, as a result, became pregnant and subsequently had a therapeutic abortion.

When seen as an outpatient some months later, the psychiatrist to whom she was referred included questions about her present sexual status in his initial interview. She felt that her sexual desire changed radically in that there was a complete absence of interest. She attributed this change to her medications. Her psychiatrist thought that medication side effects could be an explanation but also wondered whether her persistent depression was the principal cause. His belief was confirmed when the patient's sexual desire level again increased during an episode of elevated mood three months later. However, since the connection between her mood and sexual behavior was discussed in recent visits, the patient became amenable to continuing the birth control measures she had recently begun.

Suggested Question to be Asked in the Context of the History of the Present Illness (HPI): "**SOME PEOPLE FIND THAT WHEN THEY ARE DEPRESSED, SEXUAL THOUGHTS OR EXPERIENCES CHANGE. HAS THIS HAPPENED TO YOU?**"

Alternative Question: "**HAVE YOU NOTICED ANY CHANGE IN YOURSELF SEXUALLY?**"

ISSUE #2: Is there any Sex-related Facet of the Patient's *Personal and Social (developmental) History* that Might Help Explain the Present Episode of Psychiatric Illness?

In the assessment of a psychiatric disorder, the interviewer considers the symptoms of the disease and the patient's life history in an attempt to understand (1) why the patient is ill and (2) why the patient is ill at this time. Since love and sex are part of individual development, it becomes important to understand how these two issues evolved over the lifetime of a patient. The interviewer particularly wants to know about significant negative events, including possible sexual assault as a child or as an adult. On a psychiatry inpatient service, over 80% of patients describe a history of sexual or physical assault as a child or an adult.[16]

A 44-year-old woman was in hospital because of depression. Early in the initial interview and in the course of a developmental history, she talked about her father having been sexually involved with her when she was a child. The interviewer inquired sensitively into some of the details. In response to specific questions, she talked about the following:

- Having been raped repeatedly from about the age of six to eleven
- Not having discussed this with anyone prior to the current admission
- The impact of these events on her relationships with others (she found trusting others to be difficult)
- The impact on her personal development (she blamed herself).

In subsequent months, she began to come to terms with her childhood sexual experiences, and her periods of depression seemed to diminish in frequency and intensity. While sexual activity with a partner was not always pleasurable in the present, the "flashbacks" that had regularly been associated with such experience in the past occurred appreciably less often and represented considerable less interference.

Suggested Question to be Asked in the Context of a Personal and Social (developmental) History: "WHEN YOU WERE A CHILD, DID YOU HAVE ANY SEXUAL EXPERIENCE WITH AN ADULT?

Additional Question: "AS AN ADULT, HAS ANYONE EVER FORCED YOU INTO A SEXUAL EXPERIENCE?"

ISSUE #3: Are There *Reproductive* Consequences to Women Patients that are Apparent in the Review of Systems?

A serious mental illness in a woman can have enormous repercussions from a reproductive viewpoint, including:

1. The effect of pregnancy and child care on the course of the illness
2. The effect of the illness on the developing fetus
3. Postnatal care of the child
4. Genetic considerations

Despite the importance of reproductive issues, questions about the topic seem infrequent in mental health histories. A survey of 94 psychotic women (ages 18-45) found that 75% of the patients never talked about family planning with a professional.[17]

A 25-year-old pregnant woman with schizophrenia was seen in the emergency room of a general hospital because of a recent worsening of symptoms, including auditory hallucinations and the thought that her fetus was actually the devil. She was seen previously in the same emergency room on four occasions over the same number of years and was hospitalized once. Her background history disclosed that:

1. She was presently in the second trimester of pregnancy
2. Did not have a family physician
3. Was not on any antipsychotic medication
4. Had been living on the street
5. Had not been using any form of contraception

She was seen every few months by a community psychiatric outreach service. That clinic was unaware that she was pregnant and had no information concerning her sexual or reproductive history. Also, no related information was included in the recorded history from her previous hospital admission. With antipsychotic medication, careful communication with the community psychiatric service, and regular care by a family physician attached to the clinic, she gave birth some months later to an apparently healthy baby. At that time, and with her consent, a tubal ligation was performed.

Suggested Questions to be Asked of Women in the Context of a Review of Systems (ROS):

"HAVE YOU EVER BEEN PREGNANT?"
"WHAT HAPPENED TO THE PREGNANCY?"
"WHAT HAPPENED TO YOUR (FOR EXAMPLE) DEPRESSION WHEN YOU WERE PREGNANT BEFORE?
"ARE YOU HAVING INTERCOURSE WITH OTHER PEOPLE?"
"ARE YOU USING ANY KIND OF BIRTH CONTROL?"
"IS THIS SOMETHING YOU WOULD LIKE TO DO?"

ISSUE #4: Are there *STD-related* Consequences to the Patient's Illness that are also Apparent in the Review of Systems?

Individuals with chronic mental illness were, in the past, often thought to be sexually stagnant, and therefore concerns about the consequences of sexual experiences were relatively few. While restrictive policies of mental hospitals allowed little sexual activity to occur, the process of "deinstitutionalization" has provided patients with opportunity for greater sexual spontaneity. The result of this freedom is the recognition that many patients with a chronic mental illness are far from sexually inactive. However, such patients "are likely to exhibit problem-solving, planning, and judgmental deficits that increase vulnerability to casual, transient, coercive, or exploitative sexual relationships".[18] In one study, 44% patients with the diagnosis of schizophrenia who were sexually active in the preceding six months infrequently used condoms on a consistent basis in spite of substantial risk of HIV transmission.[19] It seems evident that those with chronic mental illness represent a high-risk population for HIV/AIDS infection.

A 23-year-old man was brought to an emergency room by police because he threatened others as a result of believing that his thoughts were being electronically monitored. He had been living on the street for over one year and was occasionally followed by a community mental health team because of his schizophrenia. His symptoms diminished over several days and it became apparent that part of his present symptoms resulted from his use of intravenous amphetamines on many occasions in the previous several months. Needles were usually reused and obtained from others.

In addition, he engaged in intercourse with three different women (also on the street) in the past month, and never used a condom. He tested negative for HIV but positive for Hepatitis C. The mental health service had not known previously about his use of IV drugs (and therefore, sharing needles) and assumed him to be sexually inactive. Both issues became an immediate focus of his care. He agreed to participate in a needle exchange program but thought that condoms were unnecessary because of his low level of sexual desire. He was, however, willing to continue talk about condom use.

Suggested Question to be Asked the Initial History, or ROS: "HOW MANY MEN OR WOMEN HAVE YOU BEEN SEXUALLY ACTIVE WITH IN THE PAST SEVERAL MONTHS?"

Additional Question: "DID YOUR SEXUAL EXPERIENCES INCLUDE HAVING INTERCOURSE?"

Additional Question: "WHEN YOU HAD INTERCOURSE (ANAL OR VAGINAL), WERE THERE TIMES WHEN YOU DIDN'T USE A CONDOM?"

ISSUE #5: Is there any Other Sex-related Aspect of the Patient's Review of Systems (such as a sexual disorder in addition to the current psychiatric disorder)?

DSM-IV contains a category of illness titled: "Sexual and Gender Identity Disorders"[15] One of these disorders might coexist with the psychiatric illness being considered.

A 19-year-old single male was admitted to hospital because of depression. He was interviewed by a resident who could talk easily with patients about sexual problems because of a recent and special educational experience in a clinic that focused on patients with sexual disorders. The patient identified problems in a relationship with a woman as an important reason for his present mood state. He was asked specifically about the sexual part of that relationship and answered that it was "not quite satisfactory." He was then asked specifically about having desire, erection, or ejaculation difficulties before the current episode of illness. He said none of these problems occurred but that what was sexually "unsatisfactory" was her disinterest and their virtual absence of sexual experiences together. In asking him about other sexual issues, the patient described the following:

- Unknown to his partner he would wear women's clothes approximately once each week when alone
- Cross-dressing was part of his sexual life since he was 14
- He became sexually excited when cross-dressed and would masturbate

He also indicated that he often had such fantasies when with his girlfriend and (contrary to what he had previously reported) that they would interfere with his erections when he attempted to engage in sexual intercourse. He was referred to a sex-specialist for consultation while in hospital who saw him in continuing care after discharge.

Suggested Question to be Asked in the Context of a Review of Systems (ROS) or Personal and Social (developmental) History: "**DO YOU HAVE ANY SEXUAL CONCERNS (PROBLEMS OR DIFFICULTIES) THAT EXISTED BEFORE THE DEVELOPMENT OF THIS CURRENT PROBLEM AND THAT WE HAVEN'T YET TALKED ABOUT?**"

Alternatively, One Might Ask Specific Questions:
- About Sexual Dysfunctions): "**DO YOU HAVE SEXUAL DIFFICULTIES WHEN YOU ARE ACTIVE (OR INVOLVED) WITH A PARTNER (OR ALONE)?**"
- (About Gender Disorders) see below in this Chapter
- (About Paraphilias) see below in this Chapter

ISSUE #6: Is there any Sex-related Facet of the Patient's Mental Status (such as thoughts of sexual *aggression or violence*)?

Residents in Psychiatry are usually taught to ask questions of patients concerning thoughts of homicide. Yet, judging by newspaper reports, acts (and presumably thoughts) of sexual violence seem far more common. Given the propensity of men to act aggressively or even violently when disinhibited and the fact that acts of sexual violence by women are much less usual, a question on this subject should be directed toward male patients.

A 26-year-old man was admitted to hospital with the diagnosis of schizophrenia. When asked, he admitted to thoughts about injuring himself and others with a knife in response to voices telling him to do this. He felt he had the potential to act violently, although he had never done so in the past. He spontaneously described himself as "gay." No questions were asked about any sexual matters (including his sexual orientation), or about any possible connection between sexual thoughts or hallucinations and violence.

He responded quickly to antipsychotic medication and was discharged from hospital. When asked about the content of his hallucinations some months later as an outpatient, he described his previous thoughts of sexual violence and said that they had almost disappeared. He was sure that other people currently considered him to be "gay." Questions about his sexual fantasies and experiences with other men revealed that he was exclusively heterosexual. Thoughts of sexual violence returned when he stopped his medication. He was quickly rehospitalized and carefully supervised until the safety of others could be assured.

Suggested Question to be Asked in the Context of a Mental Status Examination of a Man: "**HAVE YOU EVER HAD THOUGHTS ABOUT BEING SEXUALLY AGGRESSIVE OR VIOLENT TOWARD A WOMAN OR ANOTHER MAN? (OR YOURSELF)?**"

Issue #7: Is The Patient Receiving Any Form Of Treatment That Might Interfere With Sexual Function?

Since symptoms of psychiatric disorders are so widespread in their manifestations, any form of treatment that is successful will likely be sexually beneficial. In fact, asking about current sexual and interpersonal function may be one way of gauging therapeutic progress. However, some kinds of treatment (especially psychotropic drugs) are notorious for having a negative effect on sexual function (see Appendix V).[20,21] Men may have problems with erection or ejaculation. Women may have problems related to orgasm. Both may find that sexual desire has changed. Infrequently, patients complain about sexual side-effects of drugs spontaneously. More likely, they will not talk about this unless specifically asked.

A 36-year-old divorced man was admitted to hospital because of depression. In his opinion, his divorce was the precipitating factor in this current episode of illness. Questions included the following topics:

- Sleep
- Energy
- Suicide thoughts
- Weight change
- Interests

No questions about "sex" were asked throughout the hospitalization in spite of his concerns about his past relationship with his former wife. His treatment had involved various drugs, including

- Fluoxetine
- Desyrel
- Pimozide

No questions were ever asked about any sexual side-effects of these substances despite, for example, the frequent reports of sexual side-effects with the use of SSRIs. When seen some months later as an outpatient, his depression had markedly improved. Sex-related questions were asked at that time and he revealed that he was distressed about not ejaculating. A "drug holiday" (see Chapter 10) was suggested and ejaculation was successfully accomplished on the following weekend.

Suggested Question to be Asked in the Context of an Inquiry into Previous or Current Treatment(s): "HAVE YOU NOTICED ANY SEXUAL SIDE-EFFECTS OF THE MEDICATION(S) YOU ARE USING?"

A More Specific Alternative Question is: "HAVE YOU NOTICED ANY EFFECT OF THE MEDICATION YOU ARE USING ON YOUR SEXUAL DESIRE, ERECTIONS, OR EJACULATION (IN MEN) OR SEXUAL DESIRE, VAGINAL LUBRICATION, COMING TO ORGASM, OR INTERCOURSE PAIN (IN WOMEN)?"

SEXUAL DISORDERS (APART FROM SEXUAL DYSFUNCTIONS)
Sexual Sequelae of Child Sexual Abuse in Adults: Sexual Issues and Questions
Epidemiology of Child Sexual Abuse

Childhood sexual experiences with adults seem to be extraordinarily common. Prevalence rates vary according to the following parameters:

1. Definition used, which, in turn, reflects such factors as the sample studied (college students, clinical, or community populations—each progressively higher in prevalence)
2. Types of sexual incidents ('hands-on' or 'hands-off')
3. Age limit of "childhood"
4. Interviewing methods

Rates of child sexual abuse range from 6% to 62% for women and 3% to 31% for men.[22] Wyatt's definition used in her research as it related to the issues of age and consent seems particularly sensible: "incidents involving a victim 12 years or younger are included as sexually abusive, regardless of the victim's consent, because children cannot understand sex-related incidents in which they are being asked to participate. Incidents occurring with victims ages 13 to 17 that were nonconsensual and involved coercion, regardless of the age of the perpetrator were also included. . .".[22]

Long-term Sexual Consequences of Child Sexual Abuse

While the general outcome of child sexual abuse on adults is well reviewed, a relatively small amount of attention seems to have been specifically given to long-term sexual sequelae.[23] Many observations on the sexual impact are from uncontrolled studies. Reported effects on adult women include the following phenomena[22]:

1. Avoidance of the sexual act that was forced on the person as a child
2. Extremes in sexual activity (lack of interest or a compulsive desire)
3. A high number of sexual partners
4. Less use of birth control, with more unplanned pregnancies, more abortions, and increased risk of acquiring a sexually transmitted disease
5. Specific sexual dysfunctions (anorgasmia, dyspareunia, vaginismus)

Reported effects on adult men include the following[24]:

1. Low sexual interest
2. Erectile difficulties
3. Increased homosexual practices
4. Sexual identity confusion
5. Fear and guilt about sexual pleasure
6. Sexually victimizing others

Child Sexual Abuse and History-taking in the Adult Patient in Primary Care

The clinical identification of child sexual abuse in a primary care setting requires asking a screening question that is descriptive, has no implication of judgment and does not include an opinion about consent. The term *sexual abuse* in a screening question does *not* fulfill any of these criteria, in contrast to the question suggested in Chapter 5 and repeated here.

> The majority of sexually abusive experiences in childhood are remembered in adult life so that the primary care clinician does not need to contend with the issue of whether the events are "repressed" or whether they are, in fact, "recovered memories."[25]

> Acquiring details of a childhood sexual experience with an adult is important to understanding the personal meaning of child sexual abuse but women and men both attest to the infrequency of such questions from health professionals.

Suggested Question to be Asked in the Context of a Review of Systems (ROS) or Developmental History: "CHILDREN SOMETIMES HAVE SEXUAL EXPERIENCES WITH OTHER CHILDREN OR WITH ADULTS. WAS THIS PART OF YOUR EXPERIENCE WHEN YOU WERE A CHILD?"

The majority of sexually abusive experiences in childhood are remembered in adult life so that the primary care clinician need not contend with the issue of whether the events are "repressed" or whether they are, in fact, "recovered memories."[25] That is, primary care health professionals should consider as "sexually abused," patients who recall the childhood sexual experiences. The concepts of "recovered memories" and the False Memory Syndrome provokes immensely strong feelings and tremendous antagonism.[26] Sorting out conflicts over memory as it pertains to any particular patient should be left to specialists in the field of child sexual abuse.

Acquiring the details of the childhood sexual experience(s) with an adult is important to understanding the personal meaning of child sexual abuse but women and men both often attest to the infrequency of such questions from health professionals.

A 27-year-old nurse was referred to a sex specialist from a psychiatrist. She described a history of child sexual abuse with the deep and repellent concern that she could become sexually aroused only when she had fantasies of being sexually assaulted by a man. As a child from age five to eleven, she was repeatedly stimulated orally by her uncle and several of his friends and was also regularly coerced into stimulating them orally to the point of them ejaculating in her mouth. Intercourse never took place. Typically, she was threatened with the disruption of the family if the secret was revealed.

The details of these sexual events were discussed with her after some initial reluctance. She acknowledged that the process of describing her childhood sexual experiences was painful and that she had never described them before. She said with gratitude that it was a relief to put the memories into words and added that, as a result, she was convinced that the interviewer was the first health professional who truly understood what she experienced as a child. As she was able to reveal these events, her fantasies of being assaulted diminished in frequency and intensity.

A 24-year-old law student was referred with his wife because of his inability to consummate his marriage of two years. During sexual activity alone or with his wife, he had no difficulty obtaining and maintaining full erections. However, whenever vaginal intercourse was attempted, he continually experienced erectile loss. This same sequence of sexual events occurred regularly in his few previous relationships and, as a result, he had never experienced intercourse. His wife experienced no vaginal pain during pelvic examinations and described no fear of intercourse. In fact, she was distressed at the absence of intercourse because she wanted to become pregnant. When seen alone and during the course of obtaining a sexual-developmental history, the husband revealed having been anally raped by a male cousin on several occasions when he (the patient) was about eleven years old. The patient did not see a connection between the past and present sexual events and, as a consequence, had never raised this issue before with a health professional, including the psychiatrist he had seen because of repeated episodes of depression.

The treatment plan was to initially see him alone in individual psychotherapy, after which both partners would be seen together in sex therapy. At the beginning, the husband questioned whether his sexual inclinations were toward men, since he had never had intercourse with a woman. In fact, his sexual fantasies involved men and women, a fact that he revealed with a sense of shame. He gradually became more accepting of having bisexual fantasies but was adamant about not wanting sexual experiences with other men.

> When he and his wife were seen together, he revealed his childhood experiences to her and, much to his surprise, she remained quite supportive and loving. While continuing to be apprehensive about losing his erections, they completed a sex therapy program together and several months later were regularly including intercourse in their sexual experiences.

A health professional should not be satisfied with simply knowing that "child sexual abuse" had occurred and repeating this phrase to other professionals as if its meaning was self-evident. The rationale for obtaining details extends to the following:

> **Questioning about details should avoid anything that may appear as a repetition of the sexual assault.**

1. Not conveying the idea that what took place is so horrible that it is, in fact, unspeakable
2. Understanding the context in which the events occurred (where, with whom, ages of the participants, the relationship with the other person)
3. Becoming aware of the possible connections between past and present (the nature of sexual activities, and response both then and now)

Questioning about details should avoid anything that may appear as a repetition of the sexual assault. Asking about details should not be done precipitously but rather with a signal to the patient that, if OK from their point of view, this aspect of their experience will be discussed on another occasion in the near future. Wyatt provided a list of detailed and explicit questions.[22]

Child Sexual Abuse and Primary Care Intervention

When primary care clinicians encounter a patient who had sexual experiences in childhood with an adult, several initial approaches are possible. The extent of care often depends on what the patient wants at that time. For example, some patients feel that the experience is far behind them and has little or no relevance to present concerns. However, the fact that the childhood sexual experiences are inquired about and discussed (even briefly) in the present indicates to the patient that he or she can return at some time in the future to discuss this topic again if so desired. Other patients may want to consider their childhood sexual experiences further in a preliminary way before embarking on any serious examination with a health professional. In this circumstance, informative reading materials can be helpful, particularly first-person accounts—some of which are especially powerful.[27] When the patient wants in-depth dissection, referral to a mental health professional is warranted, especially a mental health professional who has clinical experience in this area.

Sometimes treatment for nonsexual issues relating to child sexual abuse simply ends without any attention to sexual concerns. "It's almost as though we don't see the word *sex* in sexual abuse. But sexual abuse does cause *sexual* harm" (italics added).[28] Some patients who are reluctant to focus on these sexual issues might benefit by reading a self-help book that highlights this area.[28] When more extensive care is necessary, referral to a sex therapist may be required.

Nonparaphilic and Paraphilic Compulsive Sexual Behaviors: Sexual Issues and Questions

Compulsive sexual behaviors (CSBs) include nonparaphilic and paraphilic actions.

Definition of Nonparaphilic Compulsive Sexual Behaviors

In a review of CSBs, Travin, defined nonparaphilic compulsive sexual behaviors "as normative behavior carried to extremes".[29] Examples include:

- Compulsive use of erotic videos, magazines and computer programs
- Uncontrolled masturbation
- Unrestrained use of prostitutes
- Numerous, brief, and emotionally superficial sexual liaisons (previously referred to as Satyriasis in men and Nymphomania in women)

Nonparaphilic sexual behaviors usually involve repetitive actions over many years, the expenditure of large amounts of time and money, and interference with personal and family responsibilities. The uncontrolled nature of the activity robs the person of pleasure. Nonparaphilic behaviors usually involve men but include women as well. Judging by referrals to sex-specialty clinics, nonparaphilic CSBs are common.

Terminology and Nonparaphilic Compulsive Sexual Behaviors

Phrases used to describe CSBs that are nonparaphilic include *sexual addictions*[30] and *obsessive-compulsive disorder.*[31] Both terms elicit objections: "addiction" because no substance is ingested and there are no physiological consequences to the behavior or its cessation, and "obsessive-compulsive disorder" because obsessions and compulsions are usually considered by patients to be intrusive, senseless, and distressing, whereas CSBs are regarded by patients (at least initially) as pleasurable.[32]

Definition of Paraphilias

Paraphilias are defined in DSM-IV as "recurrent, intense sexual urges, fantasies, or behaviors that involve unusual objects, activities, or situations and cause clinically significant distress or impairment in social, occupational or other important areas of functioning"[15] (p. 493). The DSM-III-R definition of paraphilias was slightly different: "response to sexual objects or situations that are not part of normative arousal-activity patterns and that in varying degrees may interfere with the capacity for reciprocal affectionate activity"[33] (p. 279). The most visible and dramatic paraphilic actions are illegal in most jurisdictions and range in severity from sexual behavior that affects other people indirectly (e.g., exhibitionism: displaying one's genitalia in public) to those that are direct and violent (e.g., sexual sadism: becoming sexually aroused by causing pain to others). Not surprisingly, individuals who display illegal sexual behavior often first come to the attention of others after being arrested by the police.

Terminology and Epidemiology of Paraphilias

The word "paraphilia" replaces the older word "perversion" and the more recent phrase, "sexual deviation." The frequency of paraphilic behavior in the community is not known, partly because individuals with paraphilias are extremely secretive about their sexual activities. DSM-IV, however, deduces that paraphilias are far from rare, given the "large commercial market in paraphilic pornography and paraphernalia"[15] (p. 524). An additional reason for the mystery about the prevalence of paraphilias is because researchers tend to omit questions about such practices in sexology[34-36] or psychiatric[37,38] surveys.

In a clinical context (and, perhaps, in a research context as well), most people with paraphilias will not spontaneously reveal this aspect of their behavior. Because of the illegality of many paraphilic actions and the great impact of these (and nonparaphilic behavior) on close relationships, people may not even admit to such actions when questioned. The majority of individuals who demonstrate paraphilias are men, for reasons that are a matter of debate. The degree to which paraphilic and nonparaphilic behavior are separate or on a continuum is unclear, as is the extent of overlap.

Compulsive Sexual Behaviors: Initial Evaluation

> Some paraphilic and most nonparaphilic behaviors do not result in legal problems. Thus primary care clinicians are becoming increasingly involved with such patients

Primary care clinicians generally have little to do therapeutically with sexual offenders, since they are quickly diverted to the legal system and thence to the mental health system. However, given the fact that some paraphilic and most nonparaphilic behaviors do not ordinarily result in legal problems, primary care clinicians are becoming increasingly involved with such patients, at least in their identification, if not their care. Health professionals may be asked to talk with such patients by a distraught partner who may have just discovered what is occurring. Although there may be a strong professional temptation to immediately refer the patient to a psychiatrist or psychologist, a thorough assessment should be conducted first. Individuals reporting CSBs have been described as representing a heterogeneous group[32], as follows:

1. Typically a man in his late 20s who has had the CSB for almost nine years
2. Impairment that was psychological (subjective distress), relationship (marital discord), or occupational
3. Comorbidity with several psychiatric disorders, including:

   - Substance abuse (64%)
   - Major depression or dysthymia (39%)
   - Phobic disorder (42%)

Suggested Screening-type of Question Concerning Nonparaphilic CSBs to be Asked in the Context of a Review of Systems (ROS): "**DO YOU EVER FEEL THAT YOUR USUAL SEXUAL EXPERIENCES ARE OUT OF CONTROL?**"

Suggested Screening-type of Question Concerning Paraphilic CSBs to be Asked in the Context of a Rreview of Systems (ROS): "**WHEN YOU WANT TO BE SEXUAL, DO YOU ENGAGE IN SEXUAL ACTIVITIES THAT OTHER PEOPLE FIND UNUSUAL?**"

> Maintaining a nonjudgmental attitude becomes particularly important for the health professional if the relationship with the patient is to survive. The interviewer must remain dispassionate. Doing so may be difficult, since many CSBs represent sexual behavior that is foreign (and sometimes repellent) to many health professionals.

Creating a screening question about paraphilic CSBs without sounding judgmental is difficult. There is less likelihood that the word "unusual" would be interpreted as judgmental if the question is phrased so that any judgment is attributed to others rather than the interviewer. Maintaining a nonjudgemental attitude becomes particularly important for the health professional if the relationship with the patient is to survive. For that to happen, the interviewer must remain dispassionate. Doing so may be difficult since many CSBs represent sexual behavior that is quite foreign (and sometimes repellent) to many health professionals.

When talking to a patient about CSBs, and for reasons discussed in Chapter 6 (see "Interviewing a Couple"), it is best to meet with that person alone rather than with a partner, since the information revealed may be damaging to the couple relationship. In addition, patients will likely be much more candid when seen alone. Given the embarrassment and sense of shame that usually accompanies atypical sexual behavior, the patient is not likely to have previously discussed this subject with anyone.

Confidentiality (see "Privacy, Confidentiality, and Security" in Chapter 2) are usually serious issues in the evaluation of CSBs. Laws regarding confidentiality are determined by individual states and provinces in North America, so that the possibility of making generalized recommendations to health professionals on a country-wide basis is limited. Thus, health professionals working in a specific jurisdiction must be aware of the legal contexts in which their practice takes place in order to provide optimal care to their patients and to protect themselves. Health professionals are usually not lawyers and therefore are unschooled in legal interpretations involved in reporting. State and provincial health professional organizations should provide guidance to their members.

> Health professionals working in a specific jurisdiction must be aware of the legal context in which their practice takes place in order to provide optimal care to their patients and to protect themselves.

Most jurisdictions in North America (state and provincial) will breach confidentiality laws in certain circumstances. For example, most have laws that require a health professional to inform others concerning children in need of protection (which generally include those who are sexually abused).

When, for example, talking to a patient about sexual experiences with children, the health professional should alert the patient *beforehand* of legal reporting requirements. If the particular jurisdiction requires the health professional to report on a child in need of protection because of *current* vulnerability (laws vary on the issue of current and past), one might ask relevant questions of a patient in the following manner (deliberately moving from fantasy to behavior):

Question: "**Do you have sexual fantasies involving children?**"
Answer: "**Yes**"
Statement: "**I'd like to ask you more about this topic but if you tell me about any current experiences with children (rather than fantasies or experiences in the distant past), I have a legal obligation to report them to** _____ (often a **government agency**)."

Behavior that is not illegal or harmful should remain private between the health professional and the patient. However, the presence of a major secret might well inhibit any existing relationship between the health professional and the patient's *partner*, since the former becomes, in effect, an ally of the person with the secret. Under these circumstances, it is best that the two people not be seen as a couple until such time as the patient decides to reveal what is hidden.

> When atypical sexual behavior is discovered, the answers to two questions should be immediately determined: (1) Is this person a physical danger to himself or someone else and (2) is anything occurring that is illegal?

When atypical sexual behavior is discovered, the answers to two questions should be immediately determined:

1. Is this person a physical danger to himself or someone else?
2. Is anything occurring that is illegal?

Obtaining the answers requires that the clinician obtain a detailed description of the problem.

A 47-year-old car salesman, married for 21 years, was referred to a psychiatrist/sex-specialist by his family physician because of a five-year history of sexual involvement with prostitutes at an average frequency of several times each week. The patient was personally distressed by this and wanted to stop. Efforts to do so had so far been unsuccessful. He read about *sexual addiction* and was convinced that the term applied to him.

About once each month, he would have intercourse with his wife. She was unaware of his visits to prostitutes. He never wore a condom with his wife and only did so on about 80% of occasions when he had intercourse with a prostitute. He was never asked the details of his sexual behavior by his family doctor, or the two psychiatrists he saw in the previous two years. He never had a blood test for HIV/AIDS, nor had this been discussed with him by any of the physicians that he consulted. His HIV test was, in fact, negative (a result that he greeted with relief). When he continued to visit prostitutes in the following months (although much less frequently), he regularly used condoms (partly as a result of discussion about the risks to his wife).

A 42-year-old university professor, married for 14 years, was seen together with his wife because of erection problems. When talking with him alone, it became evident that his erection difficulties were situational in that, when alone and occasionally with his wife, he would be fully erect. With some trepidation, he talked of becoming sexually aroused when his wife dressed as a dominatrix in a costume that he purchased for her. She also pretended to whip him (he explicitly disliked pain and viewed the entire sexual process as the acting out of a fantasy). He was embarrassed at asking his wife to engage in this activity and, as a result, did so rarely. After talking with the health professional, he decided to speak more candidly with his wife about the true frequency of his desire for the implementation of his fantasy. While her own sexual preferences were relatively conventional, the two quickly worked out an arrangement whereby they would alternate sexual experiences: one time, "his way," and the next time, "her way." His erectile difficulties disappeared.

Paraphilic Sexual Behaviors: Beyond Screening

The evaluation of paraphilic sexual behavior owes much to the research of Abel and his colleagues.[39] They interviewed convicted sex offenders under conditions that allowed the offenders to talk freely about their experiences without fear of further legal consequence. Two crucial discoveries were made.

First, offenders tend to have a wide variety of atypical sexual experiences, in contrast to the previously held belief that atypical sexual behavior was specific and consistent (e.g., that exhibitionists were not also privately cross-dressing). The clinical application of the finding is that *after any one form of atypical sexual behavior is discovered, it becomes obligatory to ask about others.* Since the varieties of paraphilias seem almost endless, it is obviously necessary to focus questions on those that are more common and more serious (to life and limb).[40]

> If any one form of atypical sexual behavior is discovered, it is obligatory to ask about others.

Suggested Question Regarding Exhibitionism: "**HAVE YOU EVER SHOWN YOUR PENIS TO OTHERS IN A PUBLIC PLACE?**"

Suggested Question Regarding Pedophilia: "**HAVE YOU HAD SEXUAL THOUGHTS OR EXPERIENCES INVOLVING CHILDREN?**"

Suggested Question Regarding Voyeurism: "**HAVE YOU WATCHED OTHER PEOPLE HAVE SEXUAL EXPERIENCES WITHOUT THEM KNOWING?**"

Suggested Question Regarding Fetishism in a Man: "**HAVE YOU DRESSED UP IN WOMEN'S CLOTHES TO BECOME SEXUALLY AROUSED?**"

Suggested Question Regarding Rape: "**HAVE YOU EVER FORCED SOMEONE TO DO SOMETHING SEXUAL WITH YOU?**" (Rape is not listed as a paraphilia in DSM-IV because objections were raised to using rape as a medical diagnosis, which, in turn, could be used to justify this behavior as a legal defense).

Suggested Question Regarding Sexual Asphyxia (tying a ligature around one's neck to lessen the amount of oxygen to the brain and thereby become more sexually aroused): "**HAVE YOU EVER TIED ANYTHING AROUND YOUR NECK TO BECOME MORE SEXUALLY AROUSED?**" (This is also not listed as a paraphilia in DSM-IV, presumably because it appears to be uncommon. It is included here because it may constitute a lifesaving emergency that requires immediate hospitalization).

Second, through the research conducted by Abel and his colleagues, it became apparent that many more sexual offenses occurred than previously were known by legal authorities.[39] The clinical application of this finding is to *assume that what one knows about the frequency of a patient's atypical sexual behavior represents a minimum.* What was said about truth-telling in a sexual history in Chapter 2 was generally accurate (that patients do not usually lie about sexual experiences but rather may not be forthcoming with the truth unless asked). The one exception to this rule is what one might hear from patients who experience paraphilic sexual behavior that could be considered illegal or personally harmful if discovered by others. Such patients will falsify information to conceal it. As a consequence, health professionals should

> One should assume that what one knows about the frequency of a patient's atypical sexual behavior represents a minimum.

> Health professionals should maintain a substantial degree of skepticism about having the whole story, or even one that is entirely accurate, when considering paraphilic behavior.

maintain a substantial degree of skepticism about having the whole story, or even one that is entirely accurate, when considering paraphilic behavior.

Gender Identity Disorders: Sexual Issues and Questions

Definition and Epidemiology of Gender Identity Disorders

Gender identity disorders represent confusion by a person about whether they really belong to the anatomic sex into which they were born, that is, the sex manifested by their secondary sexual characteristics and written on their birth certificate. DSM-IV defines Gender Identity Disorder as requiring "a strong and persistent cross-gender identification" and "persistent discomfort with" one's "sex or sense of appropriateness in the gender role of that sex."[15] The term *transgendered* was introduced recently. It describes "individuals (who) live full- or part-time in the gender role opposite to the one in which they were born. They often seek medical assistance (including hormonal therapy and cosmetic surgery) to more completely approximate the appearance of the gender in which they choose to live. This is especially true of transsexuals, who also usually seek genital reassignment surgery."[41]

When considering only the strictly-defined disorder of Transsexualism, the incidence of such difficulties is quite uncommon among biological males (1:37,000).[42] However, when considering the more liberal term of Gender Dysphoria, which refers to "the whole gamut of individuals who, at one time or another, experience sufficient discomfort with their biological sex to form the wish for sex reassignment"[43] (p.5), the prevalence is estimated to be at least 10 times higher.[40] In contrast to males, the incidence of female-to-male transsexualism is estimated to be 1:100,000.[44] Although the care of such patients tends to be highly specialized, the initial identification may occur on a primary care level, and for this reason the subject is included here.

Gender Identity Disorders and History-taking in Primary Care

Sometimes the presentation of a disorder of gender identity is more subtle than, for example, a man explicitly asking for surgery to change his appearance to that of a woman, and requires a more detailed history. In a man, a gender problem may appear, for example, as a difficulty with sexual function, and in a woman, for example, as an eating disorder.

A 32-year-old single man told his family doctor about a four year history of erectile problems. As a result and with little further information, the patient was referred to a specialist in sexual dysfunctions. The patient described erectile problems in the absence of desire or ejaculatory difficulties. His erections were about 5/10 when awakening, were no different when masturbating, and on the occasional time when he was with a female sexual partner. During the assessment and in response to a question about his reaction to having erectile problems, he commented that he didn't "feel like a man." When the interviewer inquired further into this remark, it became apparent that the patient's meaning was literal (rather than the figurative feelings of demasculinization that plague many men with erectile troubles). He related that since his early teens, he was unhappy about being a male and at times wondered if his life would be easier as a woman.

He previously obtained extensive psychiatric care over several years with several psychiatrists because of substance and child sexual abuse but had never volunteered information about his gender concerns with any health professional. In addition, no such question had ever been asked. He was subsequently referred to a gender clinic for assessment.

A 15-year-old girl appeared with her mother who was concerned about her weight loss. The daughter's intake of food during the past two years was meager, and her weight had drastically decreased from 120 pounds at the age of 12 to 85 pounds at the time of referral. She had been seeing a child psychiatrist for the past one and one half years and her mother was told that her daughter had anorexia nervosa. When seen privately and asked, among other things, about sexual matters (the patient did not discussed this topic with the child psychiatrist), she indicated that her sexual interest was in other girls but added that in her sexual fantasies she thought of herself as a boy. Indeed, for many years she considered herself to be male and to have been born into the wrong body. She said that she lost weight for two reasons:

- To shrink the size of her breasts
- To stop her menstrual periods

She convincingly said that her weight would cease to be a problem after she obtained surgery to become a male. She was referred to a specialist in gender identity disorders.

Suggested Question to be Asked of a Woman (man) in the Context of the History of the Present Illness, a Personal and Social History, or a Review of Systems (ROS): "SOMETIMES AS A CHILD, A GIRL (BOY) IS UNHAPPY ABOUT BEING A GIRL (BOY) AND WANTS TO BE A BOY (GIRL) INSTEAD. DID THIS EVER HAPPEN TO YOU?"

SUMMARY

Questions about sexual issues that appear in the context of medical and psychiatric disorders usually are not asked unless required by the patient's symptoms. The absence of information exists despite public and professional perceptions that physicians and mental health professionals have expertise in this area. In addition to the reasons outlined in previous chapters, one also encounters explanations that relate to the appropriateness of such questions given a patient's current status. An omission is, in fact, reasonable under some circumstances. In the beginning stages of almost any illness, many areas of the history are dropped, since the focus is properly on controlling the acute symptoms. However, after management of the disorder results in some lessening of the patient's symptomatology, the professional returns to completing the history, and, in this context, it is reasonable and fitting to include some sex-related questions. The following seven questions can sensibly be asked in the context of medical and psychiatric illnesses:

1. Has something changed sexually for the patient that would constitute a symptom of the disorder?
2. Is there something related to sexual matters in the patient's developmental history that might help to explain why that person is (1) ill altogether and (2) ill at this particular time?
3. What, if any, relationship is there between the patient's illness and reproduction (e.g., birth control, sexual activity, genetics, maternal and child care)?
4. Is there any relationship between the patient's illness and exposure to STDs.
5. In addition to the medical or psychiatric disorder manifested by the patient, does that person also have a sexual disorder?
6. Has the patient demonstrated any sexual violence in thought or behavior?
7. Is there any aspect of the treatment of the medical or psychiatric disorder that may have some sexual impact on the patient?

Once identified by generalists in the health system, individuals with sexual disorders (apart from sexual dysfunctions), including paraphilias and gender identity disorders, as well as victims of child sexual abuse, are usually cared for by mental health professionals. The identification of such patients requires asking questions that, in context, are neither many nor difficult.

Screening for child sexual abuse should be done in a clear and descriptive way by simply asking if the patient, as a child, had sexual experiences with an adult. This question could be asked without using the phrase "sexual abuse," which so often substitutes for understanding the details of what actually occurred, at what age, and with whom.

Information about paraphilic and nonparaphilic compulsive sexual behaviors (CSBs) is usually not volunteered by patients. Such behavior is disclosed only when discovered by family members or the police. This situation may well involve a primary care health professional, at least for identification and clarification of the problem. When a paraphilia is encountered, the health professional must ensure that no one is at risk of harm (the patient, a family member, or a stranger), and that nothing illegal has occurred. Nonparaphilic CSBs can be enormously disruptive to a patient and his or her family but, since they usually are not illegal, they involve the health (rather then the justice) system. Referral to a mental health professional is justified but should follow a through evaluation at the primary care level. The same can be said of individuals with Gender Identity Disorders. Both disorders can appear in different guises and require careful initial scrutiny.

References

1. Schiavi RC: Chronic alcoholism and male sexual dysfunction, *J Sex Marital Ther* 16: 23-33, 1990.
2. Bullard DG: The treatment of desire disorders in the medically ill and physically disabled. In Leiblum SR, Rosen RC (editors): *Sexual desire disorders*, New York, 1988, The Guilford Press.

3. Schover LR, Jensen SB: *Sexuality and chronic illness: a comprehensive approach*, New York 1988, The Guilford Press.

4. Schover LR: Sexual problems in chronic illness. In Leiblum SR, Rosen RC (editors): *Principles and practice of sex therapy*, ed 2 New York, 1989, The Guildford Press, pp. 319-351.

5. Schover LR, Evans RB, Von-Echenbach AC: Sexual rehabilitation in a cancer center: diagnosis and outcome in 384 consultations, *Arch Sex Behav* 16:445-461, 1987.

6. Bullard DG et al: Sexual health care and cancer: a needs assessment. In Vaeth JM (editor): *Body image, self-esteem, and sexuality in cancer patients*, ed 2 Rev, Basel, 1986, S. Karger AG.

7. Schover LR: *Sexuality and fertility after cancer*, New York, 1997, John Wiley & Sons.

8. Griffith ER, Trieschmann RB: Sexual dysfunctions in the physically ill and disabled. In Nadelson CC, Marcotte DB (editors): *Treatment interventions in human sexuality*, New York, 1983, Plenum Press.

9. Szasz G: Sexuality in persons with severe physical disability: a guide to the physician, *Can Fam Physician* 35:345-351, 1989.

10. Schiavi RC et al: Diabetes mellitus and male sexual function, *Diabetologica* 36: 745-751, 1993.

11. Zola KZ: Communication barriers between 'the able bodied' and 'the handicapped,' *Arch Phys Med Rehabil* 62:356-359, 1981.

12. Elliott S et al: Vibrostimulation and electroejaculation: the Vancouver experience, *J Soc Obstet Gyncol Can* 15: 390-404, 1993.

13. Schover, LR, Jensen SB: *Sexuality and chronic illness: a comprehensive approach*, New York, 1988, The Guilford Press.

14. Maurice WL, Sheps SB, Schechter MT: Physician sexual contact with patients: 2. a public survey of women in British Columbia. Paper presented at the meeting of the Society for Sex Therapy and Research, New York, March 1995.

15. *Diagnostic and statistical manual of mental disorders*, ed 4, Washington, 1994, American Psychiatric Association.

16. Jacobson A, Richardson B: Assault experiences of 100 psychiatric inpatients: evidence of the need for routine inquiry, *Am J Psychiatry* 144:908-913,1987.

17. *Reproductive needs of mentally ill women found to be largely ignored*, November 1995, *Psychiatric News*: newspaper of the American Psychiatric Association, pp. 10-16.

18. Kelly JA et al: AIDS/HIV risk behavior among the chronically mentally ill, *Am J Psychiatry* 149:886-889, 1992.

19. Cournos F et al: Sexual activity and risk of HIV infection among patients with Schizophrenia, *Am J Psychiatry* 151: 228-232, 1994.

20. Barnes TRE, Harvey CA: Psychiatric drugs and sexuality. In Riley AJ, Peet M, Wilson C (editors): *Sexual pharmacology*, New York, 1993, Oxford University Press.

21. Crenshaw TL, Goldberg JP: *Sexual pharmacology: drugs that affect sexual function*, New York, 1996, W.W. Norton & Company, Inc.

22. Wyatt G: Child sexual abuse and its effects on sexual functioning, *Annual Review of Sex Research* 2:249-266, 1991.

23. Browne A, Finkelhor D: Impact of child sexual abuse: a review of the research, *Psychol Bull* 99:66-77, 1986.

24. Watkins B, Bentovim A: Male children and adolescents as victims. In Mezey GC, King MB (editors): *Male victims of sexual assault*, New York, 1992, Oxford University Press, pp. 27-66.

25. Loftus EF, Garry M, Feldman J: Forgetting sexual trauma: what does it mean when 38% forget? *J Consult Clin Psychol* 62:1177-1181, 1994.

26. Green R: Recovered memories of childhood sexual abuse: the unconscious strikes back or therapist-induced madness, *Annual Review of Sex Research* 6:101-121, 1995.

27. Danica E: *Don't: a woman's word*, Charlottetown, 1988, Gynergy Books.

28. Maltz W: *The sexual healing journey*, New York, 1991, Harper Collins Publishers.

29. Travin S: Compulsive sexual behaviors, *Psychiatr Clin North Am* 18:155-169, 1995.

30. Carnes P: *Out of the shadows,* Minneapolis, 1983, CompCare Publishers.

31. Coleman E: The obsessive-compulsive model for describing compulsive sexual behavior, *Am J Prev Psychiatry Neurol* 2:9-14, 1990.

32. Black DW et al: Characteristics of 36 subjects reporting compulsive sexual behavior, *Am J Psychiatry* 154:243-249, 1997.

33. *Diagnostic and Statistical Manual of Mental Disorders,* ed 3, revised, Washington, 1987, American Psychiatric Association.

34. Laumann EO et al: *The social organization of sexuality: sexual practices in the United States,* Chicago, 1994, The University of Chicago Press.

35. Spira A, Bajos N, and the ACSF group: *Sexual behavior and AIDS,* Brookfield, 1994, Ashgate Publishing Company.

36. Johnson AM et al: *Sexual attitudes and lifestyles,* Oxford, 1994, Blackwell Scientific Publications.

37. Robins LN: Lifetime prevalence of specific psychiatric disorders in three sites, *Arch Gen Psychiatr* 41:949-958, 1984.

38. Bland R: Investigations of the prevalence of psychiatric disorders, *Acta Psychiatr Scand* 77 (Suppl 338):7-16, 1988.

39. Abel GG, Rouleau JL, Cunningham-Rathner J: Sexually aggressive behavior. In Curran WJ, McGarry AL, Shah SA (editors): *Forensic psychiatry and psychology: perspectives and standards for interdisciplinary practice,* Philadelphia, 1986, F.A. Davis Company.

40. Money J: *Lovemaps,* New York, 1986, Irving Publishers, Inc.

41. Lawrence AA et al: Health care needs of transgendered patients, *J Am Med Assoc* 276:874, 1996.

42. Brown GR: A review of clinical approaches to gender dysphoria, *J Clin Psychiatry* 51:57-64, 1990.

43. Steiner B, Blanchard R, Zucker K: Introduction. In Steiner B (editor): *Gender dysphoria: development, research, management,* New York, 1985 Plenum Press, pp. 1-9.

44. Roberto L: Issues in diagnosis and treatment of transsexualism, *Arch Sex Behav* 12:445-473, 1983.

Part II

SEXUAL DYSFUNCTIONS IN PRIMARY CARE: DIAGNOSIS, TREATMENT, AND REFERRAL

. . . .most sexual problems are currently considered the net result of a complex interaction among physical, psychological, and interpersonal factors. Increasingly, clinicians are feeling "baffled" about the etiology and treatment of the sexual complaints greeting them....the increased awareness of the dangers as well as the delights of sexuality are dominating popular consciousness and cooling the sexual climate . . . Sexual attitudes in [the] age of AIDS are markedly different from those in the previous "Age of Aquarius!"

LEIBLUM AND ROSEN, 1989[1] (PP. 1-2)

PRIMARY CARE TREATMENT OF COMMON SEXUAL DYSFUNCTIONS: GENERAL CONSIDERATIONS

Health professionals can hardly avoid talking about sexual issues in view of the widespread appearance of sexually transmitted diseases, sexual aggression toward children and adult women, teenage pregnancies, and sexual dysfunctions. Indeed, in some circumstances, it is even hazardous to not talk about these issues (see second case history in the introduction to PART I). The first part of this book explored one of the more common reasons given by health professionals for circumventing the topic of "sex," that is, not being sure of the next questions to ask if the answer to a sex-screening question is 'yes'. PART II examines a second reason: the need for health professionals to know what they can do about a problem *before* a sexual inquiry takes place. *The focus of PART II is on sexual dysfunctions rather than other sexual disorders.* The reasons for the emphasis are twofold. First, sexual dysfunctions are widespread in the community (see Chapter 3 and the epidemiology sections of Chapters 9 through 13). Talking with people about such problems provides almost every health professional the ability to assist those patients directly. Second, talking to people about sexual dysfunctions provides the health professional with an excellent opportunity to rehearse the process of talking to patients about many other sexual issues such as, for example, STDs and their prevention.

Having the capacity to listen to stories of sexual distress and knowing what to do about common sexual problems and when to refer the patient to another health professional, is, for many, a prerequisite to asking sex-related questions. While high-quality guides for the treatment of sexual disorders exist for the specialist health professional,[1,2] there are few guidelines for those working in primary care between those texts and the popular press. PART II attempts to provide this intermediate level of information by reviewing the following five common sexual dysfunctions:

Low sexual desire in women and men (Chapter 9)
Ejaculation/orgasm disorders in men (Chapter 10)
Erectile disorders (Chapter 11)
Orgasmic difficulties in women (Chapter 12)
Intercourse difficulties in women (Chapter 13)

Each is considered from a primary care perspective, providing information about the disorder, diagnostic questions to ask, treatment suggestions, and describing circumstances in which referral might take place.

ASSUMPTIONS

Practice Pattern of the Health Professional

Patterns of practice in primary care vary greatly. Some physicians see patients with their partners if, for example, the couple is retired or flexible work schedules allow for conjoint visits. Others may be seen with other family members or friends, rather than with a partner. When patients are seen alone, a partner may be invited to attend at a later time in response to a request or need. Visits to physicians are often short: 10 to 15 minutes in a family practice setting; the total number of appointments are often limited as a result of other responsibilities, demands, and interests of the professional; and goals of treatment vary from being quite specific to those that are not. With other health professionals such as nurses, psychologists, and social workers visits may be longer and greater in number. However, like physicians, the goals of the other professionals vary substantially.

Classification of Sexual Disorders

One of the "guiding principles" of the primary care version of The Diagnostic and Statistical Manual of Mental Disorders, is that it is "user-friendly . . . with technical jargon removed or explained . . ."[3] (p. xii). It includes a section on "Sexual Dysfunction" within a category of "Disorders That Commonly Present in Primary Care Settings." With a complaint that falls into the area of sexual dysfunctions, the reader is instructed to first consider several issues:

(a) ". . . whether the presenting symptom is due to the direct physiological effects of a general medical condition" (p.5)
(b) ". . . whether the presenting symptom is the direct physiological effect of a drug of abuse (or) a medication side effect. . ." (p. 6)
(c) ". . . whether the symptoms are better accounted for by another mental disorder." (p. 7).

As with the parent version of DSM-IV-PC, readers are directed to use a subclassification scheme in which problems are subdivided into those which are (1) *lifelong* (having always existed) or *acquired* (following a period of unimpaired function) and (2) *generalized* (existing under all sexual circumstances) or *situational* (existing only under specific circumstances).[4] For any health professional, this subclassification provides some direction in thinking about cause(s) and treatment. For example, dysfunctions that are acquired and generalized suggest an alteration in the biological capabilities of the individual. In contrast, the situational occurrence of a sexual dysfunction usually bespeaks the integrity of body systems and points to psychosocial difficulties within the patient or between that person and their partner. However, it is possible for a serious medical illness to appear as a situational sexual dysfunction.[5] In addition, a sexual dysfunction that is generalized may *begin* as one that is situational. In an attempt to overcome diminished sexual response, the patient, for example, may deliberately enhance sexual arousal by various psychological and physical means.

Clinicians should be aware that the diagnoses of some sexual dysfunctions are themselves problematic. First, a patient's subjective concern must be considered, not only objective reality. For example, an erectile dysfunction may objectively exist but be dismissed by the patient as unimportant because of his own sexual disinterest or the uninvolvement of his partner. Second, some definitions on which diagnoses are based are quite unstable in that they ". . . are dependent on social expectations which change over time and across cultures . . . [The DSM-IV system] . . . indirectly acknowledge(s) this by leaving much to the judgment of the therapist . . . ".[6]

Investigation of sexual dysfunctions: History-taking (always), Physical Examination (preferably) and Laboratory Examination (selectively)

The three elements of a medical examination that result in a diagnosis[7] are:

(a) history-taking
(b) physical examination
(c) laboratory examination

In the assessment of a sexual dysfunction conducted by any health professional, the history-taking portion of the examination is essential, so much so that on some occasions it may be all that is necessary diagnostically and therapeutically. The explanation for this is that *sex history-taking can itself be healing*, especially when it involves unburdening oneself of sexual secrets and, in the process, receiving acceptance and reassurance instead of the anticipated news that one is "abnormal."

Physical examination is essential diagnostically if a sexual problem could be the result of a disorder of a body system that itself is integral to the function of the genitalia. Like sex history-taking, a genital examination may also be therapeutic in providing a special opportunity to explain and answer questions about the structure and function of the genitalia (see "Physical Examination" in Chapter 6). Health professionals who for one reason or another do not conduct a physical examination (e.g., mental health professionals) but who wish to integrate concepts related to sexual anatomy and physiology into patient care may use paper and pencil self-drawn schematic diagrams (easy and inexpensive) or plastic/rubber models of genitalia for effective and instructive substitutes.

Laboratory examinations can sometimes be used to add information when a biomedical problem is suspected as a result of the other two parts of the investigation.

Context of the Relationship

Other than masturbation, sexual activity always involves another person. Therefore when sexual function in one partner becomes disrupted the other partner is also affected. One consequence is to view at least some aspects of the solution to a sexual dysfunction in the context of both people (apart from who actually appears with the problem). Correcting whatever difficulty exists, therefore, requires the goodwill, caring, and cooperation of the two people. "Few . . . enjoy the effort or pain [of treatment], but love and commitment can make the work bearable"[8] (p. 92). If these elements are absent (e.g., when one of the partners is secretly sexually involved with another person), the sexual complaint usually becomes an issue of lesser priority than the context within which the sexual activity occurs, that is, the relationship. Treating a sexual dysfunction in primary care (or, indeed, on any level) assumes that the relationship has a reasonably strong foundation.

Therapeutic Focus: Present Versus Past

A treatment approach should be based on (a) specific discovered cause(s). This guideline often seems easier to follow when an exclusively biomedical explanation is evident. However, in thinking about psychosocial causes of a sexual dysfunction, Hawton suggested three groups of factors[9] that one might consider:

1. *Predisposing* factors, including traumatic early sexual experiences and disturbed family relationships (these are issues from the distant past that often require considerable time, effort, and skill in overcoming and as a consequence are best treated by mental health professionals with comfort in this area)
2. *Precipitating* factors, including infidelity and problems related to childbirth (sex-specialists and mental health professionals both see such patients)
3. *Maintaining* factors, including anticipation of sexual failure, poor partner communication, and inadequate information (these are issues related to the present, often seen by a sex-specialist, but usually quite treatable in primary care)

Education/Information as an Element of Treatment

Not long ago, education in the treatment of sexual dysfunctions primarily meant explanation of the following:

1. Aspects of the anatomy and physiology of the genital function of men and women
2. Norms of sexual behavior
3. The epidemiology of sexual problems

Although these are often still necessary, education also now includes other elements such as learning about sexual communication (e.g., partners explaining their sexual desires to one another).

"Self-help" books can be of great educational value in many areas but are best used as an *adjunct* to the health professional rather than as a substitute. The most striking and consistent response of patients to self books is the recognition of "not being alone," that is, there are others with the same problem. Althof and Kingsberg provided health professionals with guidance through the maze of self-help "sex" books for professionals and patients on the subjects of sexual and marital problems.[10] Such books can be specific to a particular problem or generic (such as *In Touch: The Ladder to Sexual Satisfaction*, written by the well-known and popular physician-couple Beryl and Noam Chernick, and available through Sound Feelings Limited, 205-648 Huron Street, London, Ontario, NY5 4J8, phone [519] 672-5420). Specific chapters in this book (*Sexual medicine: primary care*) include suggestions usually located within the 'treatment' sections on self-help books that have been published in recent years or are older but have 'stood the test of time.' Also, Appendix IV lists Web sites that are informative on several sex-related subjects. One must be aware that, in spite of the information available, books (for example) are often not read the very by people who might have the most to gain. Hence the need for the knowledgeable health professional.

Indications for Referral for Consultation or Continuing Care by a Specialist

Although many sexual problems can be handled within primary care, some should be referred to specialists, *but only after an in-depth diagnostic assessment is completed by the primary care clinician.* Referral may be for consultation only (that is, for one or several visits to provide the patient and referring professional with an expert second opinion) or, alternatively, for continuing care (i.e., to transfer the patient's care to another health professional).

Obviously, the purpose in requesting consultation from another health professional is for the consultant to provide the referring person with diagnostic knowledge or skill that he or she does not have. In the inherently multidisciplinary area of the assessment and treatment of sexual problems, consultation can be enormously valuable and should be exploited.

One of the reasons for referral when the purpose is that of transferring care to another health professional is the character of the disorder itself. It makes little sense to attempt treatment within primary care for a problem that sex-specialists, themselves, find management difficult. Such is the case, for example, with the lifelong and generalized absence of sexual desire.

A second justification for referral for continuing care is complexity of the case. Complexities may exist when, for example, there is coexistence of sexual and psychiatric disorders. The intricacies involved in managing two concurrent issues *may* require care that extends beyond the usual pattern of practice, interest, or level of professional expertise found in primary care.

A third opportunity for referral (at least for consultation and possibly for continuing care) is when treatment at the primary care level was attempted but did not help resolve the major concerns of the patient.

The choice of the kind of health professional to whom referral is made depends, obviously, on the reason for the referral. For the evaluation of possible medical contributors to a sexual dysfunction, the opinion of a specialist physician would be desirable. When considering the contribution of psychological factors to a sexual dysfunction, or the integration of biological and psychological issues, consultation with a health professional who has had supervised training and experience in the care of patients with sexual problems and also a background in the behavioral sciences would be advantageous. Such professionals, from several academic health-related areas such as medicine (psychiatrists, gynecologists, urologists, family physicians), psychology, nursing, and social work over the past three decades, established a discipline that is now known as "sex therapy." The skills of these clinicians, and the extent of the field, has developed over the years to include patients with sexual dysfunctions, as well as individuals with various sexual problems associated with medical, psychiatric, and other sexual disorders.

REFERENCES

1. Leiblum SR, Rosen RC: Introduction: sex therapy in the age of AIDS. In Leiblum SR, Rosen SC (editors): *Principles and practice of sex therapy: update for the 1990s,* New York, 1989, The Guilford Press.
2. Bancroft J: *Human sexuality and its problems,* ed 2, Edinburgh, 1989, Churchill Livingstone.
3. *Diagnostic and statistical manual of mental disorders, ed 4, primary care version,* Washington, 1995, American Psychiatric Association.
4. *Diagnostic and statistical manual of mental disorders,* ed 4, Washington, 1994, American Psychiatric Association.

5. Schwartz MF, Banman JE, Masters WH: Hyperprolactinemia and sexual disorders in men, *Biol Psychiatry* 17:861-876, 1982.

6. Binik YM et al: From the couch to the keyboard: psychotherapy in cyberspace. In Kiesler S (editor): *Culture of the Internet*, Mahwah, 1997, Lawrence Erlbaum, pp. 71-100.

7. Hampton JR et al: Relative contributions of history-taking, physical examination, and laboratory investigation to diagnosis and management of medical outpatients, *Br Med J* 2:486-489, 1975.

8. Zilbergeld B, Ellison CR: Desire discrepancies and arousal problems in sex therapy. In Leiblum SR, Rosen SC (editors): *Principles and practice of sex therapy*, ed 1, New York, 1980, The Guilford Press, pp. 65-101.

9. Hawton K: *Sex therapy: a practical guide*, Oxford, 1985, Oxford University Press.

10. Althof SE, Kingsberg SA: Books helpful to patients with sexual and marital problems: a bibliography, *J Sex Marital Ther* 18(1):70-79, 1992.

CHAPTER 9

LOW SEXUAL DESIRE IN WOMEN AND MEN

While something is known about how to generate sexual desire—for example, creation of a new intimacy in a conflicted relationship, education in how to sexually stimulate one another, and provision of permission to engage in sensuous activity—the therapist knows far less than the patient thinks about how to catalyze the appearance of (sexual desire) . . . A sexual desire problem begins as a mystery to both patient and doctor. . .

LEVINE, 1988[1]

THE PROBLEM

A 35-year-old woman described a concern that from the time of her marriage seven years ago until the delivery of her 2½ year old child, she became depressed and irritable the week before her menstrual periods and also lost all interest in anything sexual during that time—thoughts, feelings, or activities. This contrasted with her "normal" sexual desire at other times, which she felt were a rich part of her personal life experience and relationship with her husband. She was sexually active and interested during her pregnancy but since the delivery ceased to be interested in anything sexual. Her husband was distressed and she missed the sexual feelings that had been so important to her in the past.

A 45-year-old man was seen with his 41-year-old wife. They had been married for 17 years. Eleven years before, she developed a bipolar illness and had periods of depression and mania. She was sexually involved with other men on an indiscriminate and impulsive basis during her manic episodes. The couple had no sexual difficulties during the years of their marriage before the onset of her illness but the lack of sexual interest by the husband had become increasingly evident during the previous decade. His loss of sexual desire did not, for example, extend to looking at other women he considered attractive nor to masturbating several times each week when he was alone. He could not explain his diminished sexual interest in his wife. He clearly proclaimed his continuing love for her and his feeling that her sexual liaisons with other men held little meaning.

TERMINOLOGY

Various words and phrases are used as synonyms for sexual desire, including libido,[2] interest, drive, appetite, urge, lust, and instinct. Low sexual desire is variously referred to as: "sexual apathy," "sexual malaise," and "sexual anorexia"[3] (p. 315). For consistency with the DSM system and the wording in most literature sources, the term "sexual desire" is used here.

PROBLEMS IN THE DEFINITION OF SEXUAL DESIRE

Sexual desire disorders are enigmatic and difficult to know how to approach therapeutically, and the entire concept of sexual desire provokes some critical questions, as follows:

- What is "normal" sexual desire? Is it on a bell-shaped curve where, like height or weight, some people have a lot, some people have a little, and most people are in the middle? Kinsey and his colleagues attempted to answer this question in saying ". . . there is a certain skepticism in the profession of the existence of people who are basically low in capacity to respond. This amounts to asserting that all people are more or less equal in their sexual endowments, and ignores the existence of individual variation. No one who knows how remarkably different individuals may be in morphology, in physiologic reactions, and in other psychologic capacities could conceive of erotic capacities (of all things) that were basically uniform throughout a population"[4] (p. 209). Zilbergeld and Ellison suggest that "To say that there is more or less of something . . . necessitates a standard of comparison . . . But there are no standards of sexual desire; we do not know what is right, normal, or healthy, and it seems clear that such standards will not be forthcoming"[5] (p. 67). In a clear and practical, but somewhat contrary, statement, LoPiccolo & Friedman offered the view that "In actual clinical practice . . . most cases [of sexual desire disorders] are so clearly beyond the lower end of the normal curve that definitional issues become moot"[6] (p. 110).
- Is sexual desire the same for men as for women? Bancroft thought not. He speculated "that there may be a genuine sex difference in hormone-behavior relationships, with men showing consistent androgen/behavior relationships across studies (particularly androgen/sexual interest relationships), whereas in women 'the evidence for hormone-behavior relationships is much less consistent, and often seemingly contradictory'."[7]
- Does one measure sexual desire subjectively (by thoughts and feelings), or objectively (by actions), or both? Considering only sexual actions or behavior ignores the fact that, sometimes, nonsexual motives govern sexual activity. For example, a person might engage in sexual activity to please a partner, quite apart from satisfying their own feelings of sexual desire.
- Should sexual desire disorders be classified as sexual dysfunctions as they are in DSM-IV?[8] Are they really on the same level as, for example, physiological difficulties such as erection and orgasm problems, or do they represent a totally different category of sexual disorders? Some patients distinguish the two by using the ubiquitous North American symbol of the car, explain-

> Some patients explain that (1) erection and orgasm problems are like automobile engine troubles and (2) that desire difficulties are more like a problem with the starter in that the engine simply does not turn over.

ing that erection and orgasm problems are like engine troubles, whereas a desire difficulty is more like a problem with the starter in that the engine simply does not turn over.

CLASSIFICATION OF SEXUAL HYPOACTIVE DESIRE DISORDERS

Disorders of sexual desire are classified in DSM-IV as "Sexual Desire Disorders." (SDD).[8] This category contains two conditions:

- Hypoactive Sexual Desire Disorder (HSDD or HSD)
- Sexual Aversion Disorder (SAD)

DSM-IV-PC summarizes the criteria for the diagnosis of HSD as: "persistently or recurrently deficient (or absent) sexual fantasies and desire for sexual activity that causes marked distress or interpersonal difficulty" (p. 115), and criteria for SAD as: "(A) persistent or extreme aversion to, and avoidance of, any genital contact with a sexual partner, causing marked distress or interpersonal difficulty" and "(B) the disturbance does not occur exclusively during the course of another mental disorder . . ."[9](p. 116).

The separation of SDDs into two groupings began with DSM-III,[10] and while Sexual Aversion Disorder has received some attention in the literature, it has not been the subject of much research.[9]

HSD, the focus of this chapter, is often not clinically distinguished from other problems with sexual function seen in primary care settings. Separating the two phenomena and determining the chronology of appearance (i.e., whichever developed first) may be extremely important clinically in considering etiology and treatment.

The assessment of low sexual desire is outlined in Figure 9-1.

SUBCLASSIFICATION OF HYPOACTIVE SEXUAL DESIRE DISORDERS: DESCRIPTIONS

Sexual Desire Discrepancy

Although not categorized as a "disorder" in DSM-IV[8] or DSM-IV-PC,[9] one of the ways that a sexual desire problem becomes apparent is when two partners are sexually interested but not at the same level. Identical levels of sexual desire in sexual partners rarely occur. More usual is the fact that both are interested but one person is more interested than the other. Couples generally "work out" different sexual appetites by mutual acceptance and compromise (or "negotiation"). "Such discrepancies have much in common with other relationship difficulties—how to raise children, how often to dine out or have company in, where to spend the vacation, etc. . ."[5] (p. 68).

> Identical levels of sexual desire in two people rarely occur. Usually both are interested but one person is more interested than the other. Couples generally "work out" different sexual appetites by mutual acceptance and compromise (or "negotiation").

Occasionally, a desire discrepancy becomes a problem so that it results in a concern brought to a health professional. Couples sometimes focus on sexual problems as a way of obscuring other tensions, but then the history of the couple relationship should indicate a change in sexual interest. If the history of discrepancy dates from early in the relationship (not necessarily the beginning when "limerance" (see p. 182) may be prominent), one has to ask: why is it that these two people are unable to do what most

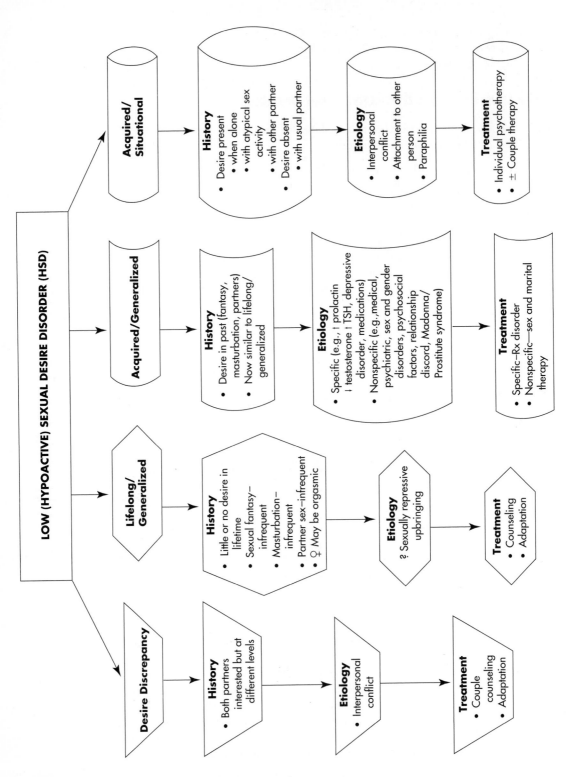

Figure 9-1 Assessment of low sexual desire disorder.

couples seem to do, that is, accept one another and compromise? The search for the answer should begin on a primary care level.

A couple in their mid-50s wanted assistance because of a difference in sexual desire. In talking with them initially together, they candidly said that this discrepancy existed since they married 30 years ago and both agreed that her desire always had been greater than his. When seen alone, he elaborated on his initial statements by saying that, indeed, there had always been a difference in the amount of sexual activity that each preferred. However, he had not been candid with her in the past about particular sexual practices which he fantasized about and, in fact, had enjoyed with other partners before they married. He anticipated resistance from her in telling her now, but, in fact, found the opposite. The quality of their sexual experiences improved greatly in the following months, even though the quantity changed little. When seen in follow-up six months later, the issue of a sexual desire discrepancy had not disappeared but there was much less concern.

Lifelong and Generalized Absence of Sexual Desire

From a clinical viewpoint, this particular form of sexual desire disorder seems to be found more frequently in women than men. The patient shows little, if any, indication of sexual appetite in thought, feeling, or action, now or in the past. Sexual experiences with a partner occur uncommonly and usually on the initiative of the other person. The patient participates out of recognition of the partner's sexual needs rather than a fulfillment of her own. Vaginal lubrication and orgasm may occur but these are not considered momentous. Masturbation to the point of orgasm might also occur occasionally but without enthusiasm. The motivation for masturbation is often other than sexual, such as wanting to diminish feelings of anxiety or as an aid to inducing sleep. Sexual dreams and fantasies are nonexistent and the patient may describe a response to *romantic* stories in books or movies but not a response to depictions of sexual activity in either. During adolescence, the women thought of herself as different from girlfriends in not being interested in boys, easily fending off sexual propositions, and hardly ever thinking about anything sexual. She sums up her present status by saying that she could live the rest of her life without "sex," and may add that the only reason she is seeking consultation is that, implicitly or explicitly, the viability of her relationship is in jeopardy.

A 27-year-old woman was engaged for six months and considering marriage. She was concerned about her lack of sexual interest and wondered if there was something wrong with her. Primarily, she wanted to know if anything could be done to alter her present sexual situation. She experimented sexually to the point of intercourse on two occasions in the past and had become sexually involved with her husband-to-be shortly after they met. It was apparent that she found these experiences to be neither pleasurable nor repellent.

As a teenager she wondered what other girls found so interesting about boys. Sexual urges were not present then or since. Her interest and energy was directed toward scholastic studies, at which she excelled. She eventually became a successful lawyer, specializing in corporate law.

In a separate interview, her fiancee indicated that while sexual experiences were important to him, he was not willing to forsake the relationship because of this difficulty. In the one-year follow-up interval, they married, and while her sexual desire had not changed, she was active from time-to-time as she sensed an increase in his sexual needs. He preferred more sexual activity but he felt as though they had adapted in other ways.

Acquired and Generalized Absence of Sexual Desire

The major difference between the *acquired* and generalized form of a sexual desire disorder and the *lifelong* and generalized form is that the present status represents a considerable change from the past. In the acquired and generalized form of HSD, the patient describes having been sexually interested and active in the past, but relates much the same feelings about "sex" in the present as the person with the lifelong form. That is, she says that in contrast to the past she does not now have sexual thoughts, fantasies, or dreams and is only infrequently sexually active with a partner or by herself through masturbation. She may also say that her interest level is such that life without "sex" does not represent a problem to her directly, although the opposite is usually true for her partner.

A 47-year-old woman, married for 23 years, described feeling diminished sexual desire since her hysterectomy five years earlier. She never experienced sexual difficulties before. Medical history revealed that she had the surgery because of excessive menstrual bleeding associated with fibroids: her ovaries were also removed and she was on hormone replacement therapy (not including testosterone) since then.

Intercourse continued after her hysterectomy but what she liked most was the closeness and affection that was part of this experience. She had little problem becoming vaginally wet when stimulated but found that intercourse ceased to be sexually gratifying. She was regularly orgasmic in the past but was not so in the present. Vaginal pain with intercourse rarely occurred but when it did it was momentary and disappeared with change in position. Testosterone was given because of her ovariectomy (see below) and she found that, as a result, her sexual desire was substantially enhanced.

Acquired and Situational Absence of Sexual Desire

The most striking feature that differentiates a *situational* desire disorder from one that is *generalized* is the continued presence of sexual desire. The sexual feelings that do exist in the present occur typically when the person is alone and manifest either in thought and/or action (through masturbation), rather than in sexual activity with the patient's usual partner. The patient characteristically states that there are sexual themes in his or her thoughts and fantasies, and perhaps attraction to people other than the usual partner. Sexual activity with their partner is considerably less frequent than sexual thoughts in general. In addition, the present level of sexual activity often represents a substantial change from the beginning of the relationship when the frequency was much greater. However, as one reviews other relationships in the past, it may become evident that the same sequence of events occurred before. That is, the interviewer might discover that there was a pattern of initial sexual interest in a partner, followed by a gradual diminution of sexual interest, resulting in relative sexual inactivity.

The 24-year-old wife of a 29-year-old man described a concern about her husband's lack of sexual attention to her. They were married for two years. When they first met, she was relieved and pleased to find that she did not have to fend him off sexually and that he was quite prepared to proceed at her pace. When asked about their premarital sexual experiences with one another, she related having had intercourse on many occasions but also thought that she was probably more sexually interested than he.

After their marriage, the frequency of sexual events dropped precipitously. Her overtures were regularly turned aside, to the point where she stopped asking. She wondered whether his lack of interest was a result of her becoming less sexually appealing to him. When seen alone it became clear that far from being sexually neutral, and unknown to his wife, he masturbated several times each week while looking at magazine pictures of nude women.

Significant issues in the history of his family-of-origin suggested that psychotherapy would be the preferred treatment for this man and he was subsequently referred to a psychiatrist. He accepted this outcome but when they were seen six months later in follow-up he had a myriad of reasons for not having followed through on the referral. She was disappointed at the turn of events, but not surprised. When she then voiced her thoughts about leaving him, he became more determined to put aside his reticence to seek assistance.

EPIDEMIOLOGY OF HYPOACTIVE SEXUAL DESIRE DISORDER

Lack of sexual desire, or sexual disinterest, is probably *the most common sexual complaint heard by health professionals*. Studies of the frequency of sexual disorders tend not to distinguish the different *subcategories* of desire disorders, so that separation into syndromes which are lifelong, acquired, situational or generalized are often based more on clinical experience than research.

> Lack of sexual desire, or sexual disinterest, is probably the most common sexual complaint heard by health professionals.

The survey completed by Laumann and his colleagues was particularly revealing about the subject of sexual interest in the general population (as distinct from specialty clinics).[12] Interviewers asked respondents: "During the last 12 months has there ever been a period of several months or more when you lacked interest in having sex?"

> Interviewers asked respondents: "During the last 12 months has there ever been a period of several months or more when you lacked interest in having sex?" Overall, 33% of women and 16% of men answered 'yes.'

Overall, 33% of women and 16% of men answered 'yes.' The most striking data concerning women revealed that 40% to 45% who were separated, black, did not finish high school, and "poor" answered positively (i.e., lacked sexual interest). The equivalent data concerning men were that 20% to 25% who were in the age group 50-59, never married, black, did not finish high school, and "poor" also answered positively. Positive responses were also related to physical health: women and men in "fair" health, 42% and 25% respectively. Fifty eight percent of women in "poor" health, reported lacking sexual interest. These numbers provoke one to think about the definition of "normal" sexual interest and the apparent role of social, educational, and health factors in influencing sexual desire.

Frank and her colleagues' impressive study of "normal" couples found a rate of sexual "disinterest" almost identical to the overall figures reported by Laumann et al[12]: 35% of wives and 16% of husbands.[13]

In one specialty clinic, the frequency of presentation of low-desire problems rose from about 32% of couples in the mid 1970s to 55% in the early 1980s[6] (p. 112). In these same couples, the sex ratio changed so that in the mid-70s, the woman was the identified patient about 70% of the time; in the early 80s, the man was the focus of concern in 55% of cases. The authors summarized the reason for this shift as follows: "Women's greater comfort with their own sexuality allows them to put sufficient pressure on their low-drive husbands to get the couple into sex therapy; this was not true until the woman's movement legitimized female sexuality."

In a report on the frequency of HSD in a population recruited for a study of sexual disorders generally, 30% of the men had HSD as a "primary" diagnosis.[14] The same authors described the frequency in women as similar to that reported by others: between 30% and 50%, although they found the figure to be 89% in their own study. Over one third of the women and almost one half of the men with a "primary" diagnosis of HSD had another sexual disorder as well. The authors concluded the following:

1. HSD was much more common in women than men
2. Men with HSD were significantly older than women
3. Desire disorders usually coexist with other sexual dysfunctions

Little empirical information exists on the epidemiology of specific HSD syndromes. Among men, Kinsey and his colleagues described 147 men (from about 12,000 interviewed) as "low-rating" (defined as under 36 years of age and whose "rates" [of sexual behavior] averaged one event in two weeks or less[4] (p. 207). Another group of men, about half the number, were described as "sexually apathetic" in that "they never, at any times in their histories, have given evidence that they were capable of anything except low rates of activity" (p. 209). About 2% of women interviewed (of almost 8000) had never by their late 40s "recognized any sexual arousal, under any sort of condition"[12] (p. 512).

On the basis of experience in clinical settings that specialize in the assessment and treatment of sexual problems, the lifelong and generalized form of HSD seems very unusual; the acquired and generalized form appears to be the most common among women. Within men who present with HSD, the acquired and situational form seems to be the most usual.

COMPONENTS OF SEXUAL DESIRE

Attempts to understand the nature of sexual desire (other than desire disorders) have been elusive throughout history. In modern times, Levine conceived of sexual desire as having three parts[16]:

1. *Sexual drive*: "a neuroendocrine generator of sexual impulses [that is] . . . testosterone-dependent . . ."
2. *Sexual wish*: "a cognitive aspiration [that] . . . emphasizes the purely ideational aspect of sexual desire . . . The most important element . . . is the willingness to have sex [which, in turn] . . . is a product of psychological motivation." (An example of a reason why a person would be sexually willing, is to feel connected to another person and less alone. An example of the opposite is, because the person may not yet like anyone enough.)
3. *Sexual motive*: a factor "that depends heavily on present and past interpersonal relationships. [And which] . . . seems to be the most important element of desire under ordinary circumstances" (examples of contributors to sexual motivation include the quality of the nonsexual relationship and sexual orientation)

HORMONES AND SEXUAL DESIRE

Biological factors represent one vital component in the understanding of sexual desire generally (in contrast to disorders of sexual desire). Within the biological domain, knowledge of the hormonal influence on sexual desire is clearly critical—if for no other reason than that many people in the general population firmly believe that alterations in hormones explain changes in sexual behavior. Although this relationship is unequivocally true in subprimates, this view minimizes the huge impact of social learning in humans. The enormous quantity of literature on the significance of hormones on sexual desire in men and women was comprehensively reviewed by Segraves, from which much of the information included immediately below was taken.[17]

Men

Much of the evidence concerning the connection between sexual desire and hormones in men derives from situations that involve decreased androgens resulting from surgical and chemical castration, aging, and hypogonadal states. Surgical castration results in a typical sequence of changes: a sharp drop in sexual drive, subsequent loss of the ability to ejaculate, and then a lessening of sexual activity. Regarding the effect of testosterone loss on erections (see Chapter 11), "It appears that erectile problems are secondary to a decrease in libido and not due to a specific effect of androgen withdrawal on the erectile mechanism"[17] (p. 278). Chemical castration mimics this lack of effect on erections.

   In a study of aging, testosterone, and sexual desire, Segraves observed that while there is " . . . a strong relationship between aging and libido, the relationship between libido and androgen activity (in

> Surgical castration results in a typical sequence of changes: a sharp drop in sexual drive, subsequent loss of the ability to ejaculate, and then a lessening of sexual activity.

> "It appears that erectile problems are secondary to a decrease in libido and not due to a specific effect of androgen withdrawal on the erectile mechanism"[17] (p. 278).

aging men) was low, suggesting that nonendocrinological factors may explain the decline in sexuality with aging"[17](p. 281). Examples of nonendocrine factors include:

- Marital boredom
- Diminished partner attractiveness
- Chronic illness

> The impotence that is seen in hypogonadal men can be explained as "performance anxiety" superimposed on a biogenic desire disorder.

In hypogonadal states, one can witness the effect of testosterone deficiency and subsequently the changes that take place with recovery when a replacement hormone is given. "The clinical literature is consistent in demonstrating a marked reduction in libido and sexual activity in untreated hypogonadal men"[17](p. 281). To the extent that the provision of androgens is successful in hypogonadal men, evidence strongly suggests a primary effect on sexual desire rather than on erectile capacity. The "impotence" that is seen in hypogonadal men can be explained as "performance anxiety" superimposed on a biogenic desire disorder.

> Studies of men who have normal levels of testosterone but who are given an extra amount for the treatment of sexual difficulties suggest that ". . .the effects are subtle and of small magnitude if they exist at all"[17] (p. 284).

Studies of the treatment of hypogonadal men show that the sexual benefits of replacement testosterone disappear as the normal range of blood values is approached, indicating the clinically vital suggestion that treating men who have normal testosterone levels for problems relating to sexual responsivity is likely to be ineffective. In fact, studies of men who have *normal* levels of testosterone but who are given an extra amount for the treatment of sexual difficulties suggest that " . . . the effects are subtle and of small magnitude if they exist at all"[17] (p. 284).

> An attempt to strictly separate sexual problems into "organic" and "psychogenic" etiology may be an exercise in futility. In one study, all of the men with hyperprolactinemia described difficulties with sexual desire, erection, and/or ejaculation dysfunction. Of particular significance is that some of the sexual problems appeared as situational difficulties. Also, all of the men experienced some improvement with sex therapy, which was provided before the hyperprolactinemia was discovered.

Elevated prolactin levels also reveal significant information about hormones and sexual desire in men (and women). One study demonstrates the futility of attempting to strictly separate sexual problems of "organic" and "psychogenic" etiology.[18] All of the hyperprolactinemic men described difficulties with sexual desire, as well as erection and/or ejaculation dysfunction. Of particular significance is that some of the sexual problems of the men in this group appear as situational difficulties (e.g., dysfunction exacerbated by psychological factors, which improved at times of enhanced arousal). *Furthermore all of the men experienced some improvement with sex therapy, which was provided before the hyperprolactinemia was discovered.*

Women

Two areas of investigation help in understanding the influence of hormonal factors on sexual desire in women:

- The impact of endogenous hormones (e.g., changes during the menstrual cycle and with menopause)
- The effect of exogenous hormones (e.g., oral contraceptives)

The possibility that sexual interests change during the menstrual cycle precipitated attempts to discern a relationship between estrogens and progesterone and sexual activity. A correlation has not been found but some evidence shows that average serum testosterone levels across all phases are related to sexual responsivity[17] (p. 290).

Changes in sexual desire associated with menopause have also been investigated. "A minority of women report some decline in sexual activity . . ."[17] (p. 295) but this could relate to factors other than libido (e.g., health and attractiveness of the woman's partner). Some psychophysiological studies report little or no change in subjective sexual arousal of postmenopausal women. Again, in contrast to naturally occurring menopause, Sherwin and her colleagues demonstrated that diminished sexual desire and sexual fantasy accompanies early menopause resulting from surgical removal of a woman's ovaries.[19] The explanation for this observation appears to be decreased testosterone associated with ovariectomy. She also found that in about 50% of instances of naturally occurring menopause, the ovary continues to secrete testosterone; in the other 50%, testosterone secretion is negligible. She suggests the inclusion of testosterone in replacement hormones after a surgically induced menopause, and also that, when diminished sexual desire occurs coincidentally with naturally occurring menopause, it might be reasonable to add testosterone to an estrogen replacement regimen (see "Treatment of Hypoactive Sexual Desire Disorder" below).[20]

On the subject of the impact of oral contraceptives on sexual desire, "The evidence is unclear, but it does not suggest that [they] have a marked effect on libido apart from other side effects" such as nausea and dysphoria[17] (p. 292). Segraves suggests the following guidelines when faced with a patient using oral contraceptives and complaining of low sexual desire:

1. If diminished sexual desire and other side effects persist beyond the second month of use, it might (by implication) be reasonable to change the preparation
2. If diminished sexual desire is a solitary complaint and began after the initiation of oral contraceptive use, it might be sensible to have a trial period off medications
3. If sexual desire returns "off medications," suggest a different drug

ETIOLOGIES OF HYPOACTIVE SEXUAL DESIRE DISORDER

When considering sexual desire difficulties (rather than sexual desire), it seems best to think of these problems as representing a "final common pathway"[6] (p. 116). The linguistic homogeneity implied by the specific diagnosis of "Hypoactive Sexual Desire Disorder" covers a great deal of etiological heterogeneity. There is no reason to assume that (1) HSD in men arise(s) from the same source(s) as in women, (2) a lifelong pattern is caused by the same problems as those which are acquired, or (3) a situational disorder has the same genesis as the other two. Although HSDs in men and women are now usually considered separately, the same cannot always be said of other subcategories.

> When considering sexual desire difficulties (rather than sexual desire), it seems best to think of these problems as representing a "final common pathway"[6] (p. 116). The linguistic homogeneity implied by the specific diagnosis of "Hypoactive Sexual Desire Disorder" covers a great deal of etiological heterogeneity.

The following were noted in a descriptive examination of differences in men and women seen in a "sex clinic" with a sexual desire complaint[21]:

1. Men were described as significantly older (50 years old versus 33)
2. Women reported a higher level of psychological distress, although both groups focused more on the sexual desire concern

3. Men's desire difficulties seemed less affected by relationship discord or dissatisfaction
4. Women reported more domestic stress

Generalized HSD

Biologically related studies of HSD undertaken by Schiavi, Schreiner-Engel, and their colleagues are at the forefront of investigations into the etiologies of HSD and represent important exceptions to the heterogeneity described above. A controlled investigation was completed on a group of men who demonstrated a "generalized and persistent lack of sexual desire" but who were otherwise healthy.[22] The HSD men were found to have significantly lower total plasma testosterone levels when measured hourly throughout the night. (The determination of free testosterone did not show differences between the HSD men and the controls). When Nocturnal Penile Tumescence (NPT) comparisons were made between the HSD men who did and did not have additional erectile difficulties, those who did showed a marked depression in NPT activity when compared to controls in duration, frequency, and degree. The authors speculated that low sex drive results in impaired NPT or that both result from some central biological abnormality.

A companion study of women with generalized HSD (lifelong [38%] and acquired) who were otherwise healthy found no significant differences from controls on hormonal measures (including testosterone) determined over the menstrual cycle.[23] "It is impressive that these two groups of women, who differed so markedly in their levels of sexual desire, had endocrine milieus so similar." The authors summarized by saying that this and other studies failed "to provide convincing evidence that circulating testosterone is an important determinant of individual differences in the sexual desire of eugonadal women."

Medical Disorders and HSD

Many medical conditions are associated with a loss of sexual desire. These are summarized in Box 9-1.

As described in Chapter 8, sexual problems that are in general associated with medical conditions arise from a variety of sources. A loss of sexual desire in particular can be a result of biological, psychological, or social and interpersonal factors[24] (pp. 356-366). Examples of biological factors include the following:

1. Direct physiological effects of the illness or disability
2. Direct physiological effects of medical treatment and management (e.g., steroid treatment of rheumatoid arthritis)
3. Physical debilitation
4. Bowel or bladder incontinence

Examples of psychological factors include:

1. Adopting the "patient" role (as an asexual person)
2. Altered body image
3. Feelings of anxiety, depression, and anger
4. Fears of death, rejection by a partner, or loss of control
5. Guilt regarding behavior imagined as the cause of a disease or disability
6. Reassignment of priorities

Box 9-1

Common Medical Conditions That May Decrease Sexual Desire

A   DISEASES THAT CAUSE TESTOSTERONE DEFICIENCY STATES IN MALES:
castration, injuries to the testes, age-related atrophic testicular degeneration, bilateral cryptorchism, Klinefelter's syndrome, hydrocele, varicocele, cytotoxic chemotherapy, pelvic radiation, mumps orchitis, hypothalamic-pituitary lesions, Addison's disease, etc.
   Conditions requiring anti-androgens drugs, e.g., prostate cancer, antisocial sexual behavior, etc.

IN FEMALES:
Bilateral salpingo-oophorectomy, adrenalectomy, hypophysectomy, cytotoxic chemotherapy, hypothalamic-pituitary lesions, Addison's disease, androgen insensitivity syndrome, etc.
   Conditions requiring anti-androgen drugs, e.g., endometriosis, etc.

B   CONDITIONS THAT CAUSE HYPERPROLACTINEMIA:
pituitary prolactin-secreting adenoma, other tumors of the pituitary, hypothalamic disease, hypothyroidism, hepatic cirrhosis, stress, breast manipulation, etc., and conditions requiring Prl raising medication, e.g., depression, psychosis, infertility, etc.

C   CONDITIONS THAT DECREASE DESIRE VIA UNKNOWN MECHANISMS:
hyperthyroidism, temporal lobe epilepsy, renal dialysis, etc.

D   CONDITIONS THAT CAUSE ORGANIC IMPOTENCE (Indirect cause of low sexual desire in men):
diabetes mellitus, arteriosclerosis of penile blood vessels, venus leak, penile muscular atrophy, Peyronie disease, Lariche's syndrome, steal syndrome, sickle cell disease, priapism, injury to penis, etc.

E   CONDITIONS THAT CAUSE DYSPAREUNIA (Indirect cause of low sexual desire):
IN FEMALES:
urogenital estrogen-deficiency syndrome—normal age-related menopause, surgical menopause, chemical menopause, irradiation of ovaries; endometriosis, pelvic inflammatory disease, vaginitis, herpes, vaginismus, cystitis, etc.
IN MALES:
herpes, phymosis, post-ejaculatory syndrome, etc.

F   ALL MEDICAL CONDITIONS THAT CAUSE CHRONIC PAIN, FATIGUE, OR MALAISE (Indirect cause of low desire):
arthritis, cancer, obstructive pulmonary disease, chronic cardiac and renal insufficiency, shingles, peripheral neuropathy, trigeminal neuralgia, chronic infections, traumatic injuries, etc.

(Modified from Kaplan HS: *The sexual desire disorders*, New York, 1995, Brunner/Mazel, p. 286. Reprinted with permission.)

Examples of social and interpersonal factors include:

1. Communication difficulties regarding feelings or sexuality
2. Difficulty initiating "sex" after a period of abstinence
3. Fear of physically damaging an ill or disabled partner
4. Lack of a partner
5. Lack of privacy

Gynecologic and urologic disorders have a particular association with HSD. Testicular and ovarian disorders can have direct effects on sexual desire (see previous section in this chapter on "Hormones and Sexual Desire" and "Treatment of Hypoactive Sexual Desire" below). Indirect effects on sexual desire can also result from structural disorders occurring in both body systems. Given the fact that one of the major functions of both the gynecologic and urologic systems is sexual, it is hardly surprising that when one function goes awry, sexual function goes awry as well. This may easily result in the patient being discouraged and experiencing a concomitant (but secondary) loss of sexual desire.

Hormonal Disorders and HSD

(See previous section in this Chapter on "Hormones and Sexual Desire" and "Treatment of Hypoactive Sexual Desire Disorder" below.)

Psychiatric Disorders and HSD

The relationship between psychiatric disorders and loss of sexual desire has not been so carefully studied as loss of sexual desire with medical disorders. On a clinical basis, it seems that the association between the two is exceedingly frequent. Of all psychiatric disorders in which a loss of sexual desire is an accompaniment, depression has unquestionably received most attention. Other aspects of depression have been scrupulously scrutinized in the past but this has been only recently true of its sexual ramifications.

> the sexual behavior of the subjects whose depression remitted with treatment did not change but what was altered was the level of satisfaction derived from sexual experiences. Investigators included that ". . . the traditional notion of loss of sexual interest in depressed outpatients is not manifested behaviorally, but rather reflects the depressed patient's cognitive appraisal of sexual function as less satisfying and pleasurable."[25]

The twin issues of depression and sexual desire were carefully studied in 40 depressed men before and after treatment that did not include antidepressant drugs (thus avoiding the potentially confusing factor of the effect of medications).[25] Contrary to the expected diminution in sexual desire, the authors found that the initial level of sexual *activity* engaged in by the subjects was *not* different than the controls. The sexual behavior of those subjects whose depression remitted with treatment, did not change, but what *was* altered was the level of *satisfaction* derived from sexual experiences. They concluded that ". . . the traditional notion of loss of sexual interest in depressed outpatients is not manifested behaviorally, but rather reflects the depressed patient's cognitive appraisal of sexual function as less satisfying and pleasurable." When subjects who did not remit, or only partially remitted, were included in the analysis, there was a "modest" improvement in the level of sexual activity and "drive." The authors found the variability of sexual function in depressed men in this study particularly interesting.

Schreiner-Engel and Schiavi looked at the association of psychiatric disorders and low sexual desire from a different perspective and found that HSD patients (men and women) had significantly elevated lifetime prevalence rates of affective disorder compared to controls.[26] None of the patients or controls had a diagnosable illness at the time of the study and there were no differences found in lifetime diagnoses of anxiety or personality disorders. In 88% of the HSD men, and all of the HSD women, loss of sexual interest occurred at the time of, or following, the onset of the initial episode of depression. The authors speculated on the possibility that central monoaminergic processes were involved in both HSD and depression.

Medications and HSD

The influence of drugs looms large among the various biological factors that can negatively influence sexual desire. This subject has been reviewed in detail by Segraves who acknowledges the limitations in information that often exists,[3] such as:

1. Bias due to dependence on case reports and questionnaire studies
2. Inconsistent use of terminology
3. A focus on the sexual function of men (and relative neglect of women)
4. Reliance on volunteered (rather than requested) information about sexual side-effects
5. Lack of clarity about effects on different phases of the sex response cycle

Drugs that are said to cause HSD are noted in Appendix III and Box 9-2.

Drug-related information seems to change more rapidly than any other material in health care; thus new drugs are promoted for old diseases and side-effects of older drugs become more apparent. The result of the rapid pace of change in information about sexual side effects of drugs is the requirement that health professionals remain informed. An example of this change is the appearance of a negative impact on sexual desire of the Selective Serotonin Reuptake Inhibitors (SSRIs).[27]

Other Sexual and Gender Identity Disorders and HSD

Other sexual and gender identity disorders may be associated with a loss of sexual desire. Of particular significance is the simultaneous occurrence of another sexual dysfunction that may be a cause or a result of HSD. Determining the order of appearance of the two problems is crucial. If the other sexual function difficulty preceded the loss of sexual desire, successful treatment of the former would likely result in disappearance of the latter.

A couple in their late 20s and married for five years was referred because the woman was sexually disinterested. Detailed inquiry of this complaint revealed that, unknown to her husband, she regularly fantasized about sexual activity and masturbated to the point of orgasm using a vibrator several times each month. Her lack of sexual desire was specific to sexual activity with her husband and dated from about two years before. In the first three years of their marriage, both freely initiated sexual activity and she usually become highly aroused but never reached the point of orgasm. She became physically and psychologically uncomfortable, so much so that she decided that "it was better not to start what (she) couldn't finish." By her own description, she refused to become aroused at the *beginning* of their sexual encounters by deliberately "turning off" her sexual desire. Her husband was relieved to discover her interest in masturbation and that she was orgasmic. He was eager to find ways in which that experience could be incorporated into their love-making as a couple.

Box 9-2

Commonly Used Pharmacologic Agents That May Decrease Sexual Desire

A **ANTI-ANDROGEN DRUGS*:**
Cyproterone* and Depo-provera* (for sex offenders), Flutamide* (for prostate cancer in men, virilizing syndromes in women, precocious puberty in boys, etc.), Lupurin,* a gonadotropin releasing hormone analog (for prostrate cancer, used together with Flutamide, also for endometriosis in women); cytotoxic chemotherapeutic agents* (Adriamycin, Methotrexate, Cytotoxin, Fluorouracil, Cisplatin, etc.)

B **PSYCHOACTIVE DRUGS:**
1. *Sedative-Hypnotics:* loss of desire dose-related: in low doses, disinhibition may cause increase in desire; high doses and chronic use reduce desire. Alcohol; Benzodiazepines (Valium, Ativan, Xanax, Librium, Halcion, etc); Barbiturates (phenobarbital, amytal, etc.); Chlorol hydrate, Methaqualone, etc.
2. *Narcotics** (Heroin, Morphine, Methadone, Meperidine, etc.)
3. *Anti-Depressants:* (Dopamine blocking and serotonergic) SSRIs* (Prozac, Zoloft, Paxil); Tricyclics (Tofranil, Norpramin, Amitriptyline, Aventyl, Clomipramine*); MAOIs* (Nardil, Marplan), Lithium carbonate, Tegretol.
4. *Neuroleptics (increase Prl):* Phenothiazine (Thorazine,* Thioridazine) Prolixin,* Stelazine, Mellaril, etc.); Haldol,* Sulpiride.*
5. *Stimulants:* loss of desire is dose-related: low, acute doses may stimulate libido; high doses and chronic use reduce sex drive. (Dexadrine, Methamphetamine, Cocaine).

C **CARDIAC DRUGS:**
1. *Antihypertensives:* (Hydrochlorothiazide,* Chlorthalidone,* Methyldopa,* Spironolactone,* Reserpine,* Clonidine, Guanethidine,* etc.)
2. *Cardiac Drugs:* Beta adrenergic blockers* (Inderal, Atenolol, Timolol, etc.); Calcium blockers** (Nifedipine, Verapramil, etc.)

D **DRUGS THAT BIND WITH TESTOSTERONE:**
1. Tamoxifen, Contraceptive agents, etc.

E **MISCELLANEOUS DRUGS:** Cimetidine* (for peptic ulcer); Pondimin* (serotonergic appetite suppressor); Diclorphenamine, Methazolamide (for glaucoma); Clofribrate, Lovastatin (anticholesterol); Steroids (chronic use for inflammatory conditions), (Prednisone, Decadron, etc.).

All the drugs listed have been reported to result in the loss of sexual desire and/or in erectile problems. However, the frequency with which sexual side effects occur varies considerably, and the drugs that have a very high incidence of decreased libido have been marked with.
**Long-acting calcium channel blockers are more likely to decrease desire and impair erection than the short-acting preparations.
(Modified from Kaplan HS: *The sexual desire disorders,* New York, 1995, Brunner/Mazel, p. 287. Reprinted with permission.)

Psychosocial Issues and HSD

Psychosocial causes of low sexual desire include the following[6] (pp. 119-129):

1. Religious orthodoxy (a factor that is "oversimplified at best")
2. Anhedonic or obsessive-compulsive personality style (accompanied by usual difficulties of displaying emotion and discomfort with close body contact)
3. Primary sexual interest in other people of the same sex
4. Specific sexual phobias or aversions (after sexual assault as an adult or child[28])
5. Masked paraphilia (perversion)
6. Fear of pregnancy
7. "Widower's syndrome" (sexual function difficulties, usually in the areas of desire or erection, in a man after his wife has died, resulting from attachment to his wife or the unfamiliarity of sexual activity with a new partner)
8. Relationship discord (cause, effect, or coexistence with HSD may be difficult to determine)
9. Lack of attraction to a partner
10. Poor sexual skills in the partner ("lousy lover")
11. Fear of closeness and inability to fuse feelings of love and sexual desire (especially in men [see "Acquired and Situational Absence of Sexual Desire" above])

Relationship Discord and HSD

On the basis of clinical impression, relationship discord and HSD seem to be frequently related to each other. When two sexual partners who love each other and have *no* sexual concerns are engaged in a dispute, it is commonplace to declare a sexual moratorium until the conflict resolves. It is as if one says to the other, 'I'm angry at you and don't feel like going to bed with you while I have these feelings'. It is logical to theorize that some instances of acquired HSD that are nonspecific in origin may represent submerged anger about which the person is unaware. Experimental evidence exists for the idea of suppressed sexual desire in the presence of anger.[29] Such theorizing may provide direction for clinical care. This observation about anger may, in some instances, relate to the finding that when woman with and without HSD were compared, the former "reported significantly greater dissatisfaction with nearly every reported relationship issue."[30]

> It is logical to theorize that some instances of acquired HSD that are nonspecific in origin may represent submerged anger about which the person is unaware.

In the concluding chapter to their multi-authored book on the subject of Sexual Desire Disorders, Leiblum and Rosen summarized the views of contributors generally, saying that " . . . relationship conflicts are viewed by the majority of our contributors as the single most common cause of desire difficulties"[31] (p. 452). From personal clinical experience, they found that women partners "were more aware of and less willing to tolerate relationship distress, and consequently that desire in women is more readily disrupted by relationship factors" (p. 449). At the same time, humility was suggested with treatment because all-too-often less marital discord resulted without any accompanying change in sexual desire (p. 451).

Madonna/Prostitute Syndrome and HSD

Freud described a man choosing one woman for love and another for sexual activity and seemingly unable to fuse the two.[2] He referred to this idea as the Madonna/Prostitute syndrome. It seems especially applicable today to many young men who relate experiences consistent with an acquired and situational form of HSD.

Multiple Etiological Factors in HSD

Sometimes HSD seems to result from the operation of only one of the factors described above: a hormone deficiency or the onset of a debilitating illness. More often than not, the onset (especially of the acquired form) can probably best be explained by multiple factors.[32]

A couple in their late 20s explained that during the two years before their marriage and the three years before she became pregnant their sexual experiences were mutually initiated, frequent, pleasurable, and free of problems. After the delivery of her child, attempts at intercourse were painful for her. Her husband knew of this but persisted in approaching her sexually. After telling him of her discomfort on one occasion, she felt she had little alternative but to "put up with it," until finally she became quite disinterested and "shut down."

Both partners described her as a person who could not candidly and frankly talk about her feelings, especially when she was angry. Being forthright was discouraged in her family-of-origin, particularly by her alcoholic father who was verbally abusive to her when she said something he found unpleasant. It seemed that the current sexual difficulties were superimposed on some issues concerning her personality and problems in their relationship as a couple. The treatment program centered on her expressiveness, as well as "communication" and sexual issues. Her ability to talk openly about her feelings improved dramatically. Her husband was upset with himself as he discovered the extent of her vaginal and psychological discomfort and his own insensitivity. As their sexual experiences resumed, she discovered that her dyspareunia disappeared. However, although lovemaking was more frequent than before, her previous sexual urge did not return.

INVESTIGATION OF HYPOACTIVE SEXUAL DESIRE DISORDER

> Given the etiological heterogeneity and therapeutic complexity of HSD, *careful investigation of the complaint and establishing the correct subcategory is often the most important contribution that can be made by a primary care clinician.*

Given the etiological heterogeneity and therapeutic complexity of HSD, careful investigation of the complaint and establishing the correct subcategory is often the most important contribution that can be made by a primary care physician.

Scrutinizing the history of the patient and couple is usually the most revealing part of the examination. Concerns about sexual desire usually surface in the context of a couple's relationship. The patient often appears unruffled, and the partner seems the one who is more distressed. The patient becomes upset secondarily if the partner is implicitly or explicitly threatening to dissolve the relationship. Sexually interested women who are partners of disinterested men may also describe doubts about themselves and wonder if they are the source of the difficulty, thinking (for example) that they are sexually unappealing. The disinterested person often does not express worry about himself or herself but more about the unfulfilled sexual needs of the partner.

Occasionally, the disinterested partner seeks help. The reason is often a feeling of sexual abnormality because such patients compare themselves, for example, to (1) how they felt in the past, (2) friends and partners, and (3) depictions of "sex" on TV and the movies.

Complaints about sexual desire are infrequent in patients without partners. One exception is when a person believes that their lack of sexual interest contributed to a disrupted previous relationship and is apprehensive about it happening again.

History

Comprehensive assessment of a complaint about sexual desire involves asking an initial open-ended question, followed by specific inquiry concerning at least three areas:

- Sexual behavior
- Psychological manifestations of sexual stimuli
- Body changes in response to sexually arousing stimuli

Specific issues to inquire about, and suggested questions include the following:

1. Duration (see Chapter 4, "lifelong versus acquired")

Suggested Question: "HAS A FEELING OF LOW SEXUAL DESIRE ALWAYS BEEN PART OF YOUR LIFE OR WAS THERE A TIME WHEN THIS WAS NOT A PROBLEM?"

2. Sexual behavior with the usual partner (see Chapter 4, "generalized versus situational")

Suggested Question when Talking with a Heterosexual Man/Woman: "ABOUT HOW OFTEN ARE YOU AND SHE/HE SEXUALLY INVOLVED WITH EACH OTHER?"

Additional Suggested Question when Talking with a Heterosexual Man/Woman: "WHAT KIND OF THOUGHTS DO YOU HAVE BEFORE OR DURING YOUR SEXUAL EXPERIENCES?"

3. Sexual behavior with other partners of the opposite sex (see Chapter 4, "generalized versus situational")

Suggested Question: "HAVE YOU HAD SEXUAL EXPERIENCES WITH OTHER WOMEN/MEN SINCE YOU'VE BEEN IN THIS RELATIONSHIP?"

4. Sexual behavior with other partners of the same sex (see Chapter 4, "generalized versus situational")

Suggested Question: "ARE YOU SOMETIMES SEXUALLY AROUSED BY THOUGHTS OF OTHER MEN/WOMEN?

Additional Suggested Question if the Answer is, "yes": "APART FROM THOUGHTS, HAVE YOU HAD SEXUAL EXPERIENCES WITH OTHER MEN/WOMEN?"

5. Sexual behavior through masturbatory sexual activity (see Chapter 4, "generalized vs. situational")

Suggested Question: "HOW FREQUENTLY DO YOU STIMULATE YOURSELF OR MASTURBATE?"

6. Psychological manifestations—fantasy (see Chapter 4, "generalized versus situational")

Suggested Question: "HOW OFTEN DO YOU HAVE SEXUAL DAYDREAMS (OR FANTASIES)?"

Additional Suggested Question: "WHAT DO YOU FANTASIZE ABOUT WHEN MASTURBATING?" ALSO: "WHAT DO YOU FANTASIZE ABOUT WHEN YOU'RE IN THE MIDST OF A SEXUAL EXPERIENCE WITH ANOTHER PERSON?"

7. Psychological manifestations—response to pictures with a sexual theme (see Chapter 4, "generalized versus situational")

Suggested Question: "WHAT DO YOU THINK ABOUT AND FEEL SEXUALLY WHEN YOU SEE A PICTURE OR MOVIE THAT HAS A SEXUAL THEME?

8. Psychological manifestations—response to stories in literature (see Chapter 4, "generalized versus situational")

Suggested Question: "WHAT DO YOU THINK ABOUT AND FEEL SEXUALLY WHEN YOU READ STORY IN WHICH SOMETHING SEXUAL OCCURS?"

9. Body change—genital swelling [erection or vaginal lubrication] (see Chapter 4, "description")

Suggested Question when Talking with a Man/Woman: "WHEN YOU THINK ABOUT SOMETHING SEXUAL, WHAT HAPPENS TO YOUR PENIS/VAGINA?"

Additional Suggested Question: "DOES IT BECOME HARD/DO YOU BE-COME WET?"

10. Psychological accompaniment (see Chapter 4, "patient and partner's reaction to problem")

Suggested Question: "WHEN YOU ARE SEXUALLY UNINTERESTED, WHAT THOUGHTS ARE GOING THROUGH YOUR MIND?"

Addition Question: "HOW DOES YOUR WIFE (HUSBAND, PARTNER) REACT?"

Patients who regard answers to questions about sexual desire as private should *not* be expected to discuss these aspects of the topic (at least initially) in the presence of their partner (see Chapter 6). When a couple is interviewed together and someone is asked a question about something generally regarded as private, the fact of not answering the question might, itself, be revealing (i.e., if one partner does not want to answer a question about masturbation, the non-answer might convey to the other partner that there is secret information). Under such circumstances, it is best to avoid the question altogether. The clinician must be careful not to unwittingly coerce someone to disclose private information to a partner. Information that was obtained when someone was seen alone may emerge at a later time when a couple is seen together but this should occur only if the patient who previously asked for privacy takes the initiative.

Questions about thoughts and sexual fantasies (with masturbation or with a partner) are often regarded by patients as even more private than actual behavior. As a result, there may be obvious reticence to talk about what occurs in one's mind. Information about thoughts and sexual fantasies can be enormously revealing from a diagnostic point of view, since it may, for example, indicate a complete absence of sexual thought, a sexual desire for someone else, or, a different sexual orientation than what the person's behavior may have suggested.

Physical Examination

The potential significance of the physical examination in HSD is signaled by the patient's history. Considering the four subcategories described above, the acquired and generalized *loss* of sexual desire is the principal form in which a diagnostic physical examination is required. The major contrasting element separating the acquired/generalized pattern from the others is widespread change. Ordinarily one would not expect to find physical abnormalities with the other three forms because of the absence of such change: discrepancy in sexual desire, as well as situational and lifelong/generalized disorders. With a desire discrepancy, interest continues to exist by both partners in the present as it was in the past, but it is nevertheless problematic because the two people function at different levels. Where sexual desire is situationally absent, interest continues as before except for one particular situation. In the lifelong/generalized form, if a physical abnormality existed it would also have been lifelong, a circumstance that is possible (e.g., a congenital disorder) but at the same time usually obvious.

> The acquired and generalized loss of sexual desire is the principal form in which a diagnostic physical examination is required.

If a physical examination is part of the evaluation of acquired and generalized loss of sexual desire, what does one look for? Before attempting to answer this question, one must ask what loss of sexual desire represents. Is it, in fact, a disorder? Or is it a syndrome (a collection of symptoms resulting from several causes)? In most instances, the answer seems to be the latter. In that sense, loss of sexual desire resembles other phenomena such as loss of appetite for food, or fatigue (both are accompaniments of many different medical and psychiatric disorders from cancer to depression and neither are associated with any *specific* physical findings on examination).

When the complaint is loss of sexual desire and the history does not suggest a specific cause, one looks for evidence of generalized and previously unrecognized disease (e.g., renal or cardiac disease) in a physical examination. One would search also for the physical changes associated with abnormalities in endocrine function. The main endocrine disorders would be hypoandrogen states and hypothyroidism. Physical signs of low testosterone in men are often delayed; in women, they are often absent. Signs of hypothyroidism may be subtle. Since generalized disease and endocrine disorders can coexist, the presence of the former does not necessarily mean that the explanation for sexual desire loss has been found and that a search for an accompanying endocrine disorder is, therefore, unnecessary.

Laboratory Studies

Since HSD is occasionally a result of a hormonal deficiency, laboratory studies usually become part of the evaluation process. In men, this should always involve a determination of the patient's serum testosterone and prolactin levels. Segraves[17] (p. 285) justifies this policy in the following ways:

- Low cost
- Possibility of overlooking treatable cause of a low desire complaint
- Difficulty in distinguishing psychological from endocrinological causation on the basis of history alone
- Negligible risk (i.e., venipuncture)

He further emphasizes the importance of too quickly attributing the cause of low desire to interpersonal discord, since low sexual desire may, itself, *result* in relationship conflict. In an effort to determine the cause of a low testosterone level and because of the negative feedback loop in relation to the pituitary gland, a follow-up test should be performed to determine the patient's Luteinizing Hormone (LH) status. Other clinicians propose a somewhat different format. Kaplan suggests that LH testing should coincide with testing for testosterone, free testosterone, prolactin, total estrogens, and thyroid status (for men)[33] (p. 289). Kaplan, and Rosen & Leiblum, suggest that Follicle Stimulating Hormone (FSH) be measured as well.[32,33]

On the subject of laboratory investigation of sexual desire complaints in women, Segraves suggested that " . . . extensive endocrinological assessment of every case of inhibited sexual desire in females is not indicated"[17] (pp. 298-99). He adds that, since many gynecological conditions may interfere with sexual desire in nonspecific ways (e.g., causing dyspareunia), correction of the condition may be sufficient to reverse the sexual problem. As well, low sexual desire might occur in postmenopausal women as a result of uncomfortable or painful intercourse associated with the diminished vaginal lubrication. This symptom commonly accompanies atrophic vaginitis and is caused by lack of estrogen stimulation to a woman's vagina (see Chapter 13). The unusual patient with the complaint of diminished sexual desire but who also describes absent menstrual periods and galactorrhea should have a serum prolactin determination test performed. Kaplan differed from Segraves in suggesting that the hormone profile described in the previous paragraph be used in women as well as men; the one exception being that estradiol be determined instead of total estrogens[33] (p. 289).

Unrecognized, untreated, or uncontrolled medical and psychiatric disorders may become evident during the investigation of a sexual problem. Common sense dictates that, ordinarily, attention to the sexual problems be delayed until these other disorders are under control. Examples include the following[6]:

- Depression
- Alcohol or drug dependence
- Spouse abuse
- Active extramarital relationships
- Severe marital distress with imminent separation or divorce

TREATMENT OF HYPOACTIVE SEXUAL DESIRE DISORDER

In many circumstances, the most important role of the primary care health professional is to carefully delineate the subcategory of desire difficulty and the possible etiology. While carrying out this task, patients with HSD, regardless of cause, will usually appreciate the primary care clinician's initial step of encouraging them to agree to temporarily stop struggling with attempts at *sexual experiences* (no matter how favorable the circumstances) and to simply enjoy being *affectionate* with their partner. The history of the couple often reveals that affectionate exchanges were common in the past but abandoned with the onset of the desire difficulties, since affection was interpreted as a prelude to an unwanted (and often refused) sexual encounter. Affection without the "threat" of any sexual consequence is usually a relief and something that is highly desired by the disinterested partner. This arrangement is easily accomplished in primary care, and the agreement is best made with both partners together so that there is no misinterpretation of directions or mutual blame.

> Patients with HSD usually appreciate the primary care clinician's initial step of encouraging them to temporarily stop struggling with attempts at sexual experiences and to simply enjoy being affectionate with their partner.

Specific Treatment Approaches

Specific treatment of a sexual desire disorder will result from the discovery of a specific cause. Limits to the involvement of a particular health professional depends on that person's skills and pattern of practice. An illustration of a specific cause is that of testosterone deficiency. For example, Sherwin showed that testosterone is beneficial in the loss of sexual desire associated with surgically induced menopause as a result of bilateral oophorectomy.[19] Also, testosterone may be helpful in medically induced menopause that results from the use of some cytotoxic agents and radiation in treatment of various cancers.[34-36] A second and more complex example of a specific etiology is the discovery and treatment of prostate cancer. In this instance, sexual counseling has a major role in program of care and would likely focus on "here-and-now" issues. The treatment program may involve the coordinated work of a nonpsychiatric physician and sex-specialist or mental health professional with interest and skills in the area of sexual rehabilitation. A third and potentially even more intricate example of a specific cause is loss of sexual desire after sexual trauma. Counseling is pivotal in treatment and might well extend to past issues in the patient's life. The ongoing care of such a patient would optimally be undertaken by a health care professional with psychotherapy skills and comfort in talking about sexual issues.

Nonspecific Treatment Approaches

Nonspecific methods for the treatment of a sexual desire disorder must be used if, as is often the case, specific explanatory factors cannot be pinpointed. Some clinicians and patients find that self-help books are useful in the initial care of a patient with nonspecific HSD.[37] Unfortunately, few such books exist.

The subcategory of HSD should be considered in nonspecific treatment objectives and methods.

Sexual Desire Discrepancy

Differences in sexual desire among sexual partners are so common as to possibly be universal. Considered from that perspective, one might then consider such differences to be "normal" rather than "pathological." The epidemiology of discrepancies in sexual desire should be conveyed to patients—not to delegitimize their complaint but to help them understand that other nonsexual issues may be significant contributors to the problem.

Primary care health professionals can assist partners in the following ways:

1. Understanding the role of extraneous influences on their sexual experiences (e.g., fatigue and preoccupation, especially in relation to the parenting of young children)
2. Talking candidly about the sexual expectations that each may have of the other
3. Appreciating the significance of "transition activities" (see following paragraph)
4. "Negotiating" a sexual activity compromise

Even before attempting to alter facets of sexual desire, attention should be paid to the role of "transition activities" (e.g., sporting activities or dinners alone). "It is no secret that modern living produces tremendous tension which often inhibits sexual interest, excitement, and performance . . . The type of transitions employed are of little moment, the important thing being that they help move [the patient] from a tense, pressured state to one which feels more comfortable and in which he or she is more open to sexual stimuli . . . When [transition activities] are done together [with a partner], they can function as a bridge into a shared building of arousal and enjoyable sexual activity"[5] (p. 95).

Viewing sexual desire discrepancies in the same way as other relationship discrepancies " . . . suggests a focus on both partners, rather than the more common practice of working only on the partner with less interest . . . we (try) to increase the desire of the one while at the same time trying to decrease that of the other"[5] (p. 68).

Careful history-taking sometimes reveals that a difference in sexual desire actually represents a *diminution* on the part of one partner. This apparent decrease may actually represent a lowering of sexual desire to the patient's usual level after an initial period of "limerance," (the passionate intensity of a new romantic relationship). A sexual desire discrepancy may then appear as a desire disorder that is acquired and generalized.

Lifelong and Generalized Absence of Sexual Desire

Altering a lifelong absence of sexual desire is exceedingly difficult at any level of care, primary or otherwise. If the major treatment purpose is one of substantially enhancing the patient's level of sexual desire, an approach at any level will likely, in ordinary circumstances, not be productive. However, one reasonable treatment objective is the reversal of any concomitant sexual dysfunction. For example, a woman patient with this form of HSD may also be anorgasmic. While becoming orgasmic may not result in much change in her sexual desire level, sexual events may become more pleasurable for her and as a result cause less tension in the couple's relationship. (In instances of low sexual desire, disappointment usually follows an expectation that an improvement in the *quality* of sexual experiences results in an increase in the *quantity*). In the absence of an associated sexual dysfunction, treatment to help the couple *adapt* to this situation could be potentially quite beneficial. Even accomplishing this objective can be difficult and time-consuming and is probably best undertaken by a sex-specialist with counseling skills, or a mental health professional comfortable and skilled in talking about sexual and relationship issues.

Acquired and Generalized or Situational Absence of Sexual Desire

PSYCHOLOGICAL TREATMENT METHODS

Nonspecific treatment methods for HSD are usually psychologically based, involve counseling or psychotherapy, and involve individuals or couples. Techniques vary and include:

- Psychodynamic and interpersonal approaches[16,39,40]
- Cognitive and behavioral methods[6,41,42]
- Systems and interactional approaches[43,44]

Unfortunately, little consensus exists concerning treatment approaches to nonspecific HSD. Also, not all health professional groups have the requisite interest, knowledge, or training in the use of these various treatment techniques. The situational absence of sexual desire requires psychologically-based treatment methods only.

HORMONAL TREATMENT: MEN

Hormonal treatments have been used for nonspecific HSD. For example, some men who complain of "impotence" have an HSD rather than an erectile difficulty. Physicians will sometimes attempt a trial of testosterone for their male patients with the general concern of "impotence" without ascertaining whether a desire disorder exists and is, in fact, primary. Segraves is unequivocal in his opinion: "Some physicians routinely prescribe exogenous testosterone to men with sexual complaints without determining baseline values or even monitoring the serum testosterone response to exogenous androgens. There is little justification for such an approach"[17] (p. 288). Beyond this opinion, physicians must be concerned about exogenous testosterone accelerating the growth of an existing but occult prostatic cancer or the risk of prostate cancer development.[45]

HORMONAL TREATMENT: WOMEN

There is considerable controversy over the use of androgens in the treatment of a sexual desire disorder in postmenopausal women. (Kaplan is adamant in saying that testosterone "has no place in the treatment of *premenopausal* women" (italics added) with normal testosterone levels)[33] (p. 278).

Other than specific research, Sherwin speculates that testosterone may be helpful to women who report diminished libido *beginning* in the perimenopausal time period.[20]

Kaplan also suggests that physiological doses (of testosterone) present little risk and that "a brief trial is justified in postmenopausal women with a global loss of libido whose T (testosterone) levels are abnormally low . . . or in the low-normal ranges. (She considered 20-25 ng/dl to be the lower limit of normal levels according to her clinical experience and a survey of medical texts)[33] (p. 279).

In contrast to the encouragement of Sherwin and Kaplan, Segraves regards the use of testosterone in the care of women with a sexual desire disorder to be "clearly exper-imental"[17] (pp. 294-5) and suggests caution for the following reasons:

1. The studies have not been properly controlled
2. Doses used exceed physiological levels
3. Side effects can be unpleasant
4. There is lack of clarity about the effect on sexual desire of variations in andro-gens within the normal physiological (versus subphysiological) range that women experience

Others have also been circumspect about promoting testosterone for the care of post-menopausal women with a sexual desire disorder because of evidence for its possible role in the development of breast cancer. Dorgan and her colleagues conducted a prospective study that involved examining blood that was donated up to 10 years before. Women who subsequently developed breast cancer (compared to healthy con-trols) had significantly higher serum levels of the adrenal androgens dehy-droepiandrosterone (DHEA), its sulfate (DHEAS), and its metabolite 5-androstene-3β,17β-diol (ADIOL).[46,47]

There is concern about the role of sex steroids in the etiology of cardiovascular dis-ease in postmenopausal women, particularly over the potentially negative effect of testosterone on lipid levels. Sherwin et al. reviewed the literature on this subject and concluded that "the evidence that testosterone decreases HDL (high density lipopro-tein cholesterol) and increases LDL (low density lipoprotein cholesterol) is impres-sive." She nevertheless found a different result in her own subjects.[48] She compared the effect of different hormone treatment approaches on the lipoprotein lipid profiles of three groups of women who had undergone total hysterectomy and bilateral salpingo-oophorectomy: a combined estrogen-androgen preparation (containing 150 mg of testosterone enanthate), estrogen alone, and an untreated group. She reported "no between-group differences in total cholesterol, triglycerides, high-density lipoprotein, or low-density lipoprotein values. Nor was the low density/high density lipoprotein ratio significantly different between groups. . . ."

Research findings on the effect of testosterone on lipids in postmenopausal women are contradictory. Phillips and his colleagues found that free testosterone (in contrast to total testosterone) was significantly related (positively) with coronary artery disease in a group of 60 postmenopausal women undergoing coronary angiography.[49] The authors speculated that an elevated free testosterone level might be a risk factor for coronary atherosclerosis.

In her research on women who experienced surgically induced menopause, Sherwin considered the possibility of an equal and opposite effect of each hormone (estrogen and androgens) that masked the effect of testosterone alone.[48] Another study found that testosterone prevented (to a small degree) the rise in HDL cholesterol that was seen in oophorectomized women given estrogen alone.[50] The same authors found in yet another study that testosterone decreased LDL cholesterol.[51] The complexity of the issue was further illustrated by the unpublished finding that estrogen alone and estrogen-testosterone implants resulted in lower LDL and increased HDL cholesterol but that estrogen-testosterone implants in heavy smokers produced a fall in HDL cholesterol.[52] Some speculate that the mode of administration of the hormones may have a role in explaining the contradictory findings.[48]

In summary, testosterone seems beneficial to women with an androgen deficit as a result of surgically (and probably medically) induced menopause and diminished sexual desire. There is *no* reported evidence that testosterone is useful in the treatment of sexual desire difficulties in men or postmenopausal women who have experienced a naturally occurring menopause. Some evidence exists that it may be harmful.

> Testosterone seems beneficial to women with an androgen deficit as a result of surgically (and probably medically) induced menopause and diminished sexual desire. There is no reported evidence that testosterone is useful in the treatment of sexual desire difficulties in men or postmenopausal women who have experienced a naturally occurring menopause. Some evidence exists that it may be harmful.

TREATMENT OUTCOME OF HYPOACTIVE SEXUAL DESIRE

Despite the enormity of the problem of HSD in extent (in the general population) and depth (in the individual), the voluminous scientific literature on the subject, and the many treatment approaches that have been described (often with confidence in their utility), there is not a great deal of information concerning treatment results. The two existing long-term follow-up studies of treatment of low sexual desire are generally quite discouraging. De Amicis et al. found that three years after treatment, "desire for sexual contact and frequency of sexual contact, clearly demonstrate a lack of sustained success for both men and women."[53] Despite the absence of change in the specific problem, both men and women reported continued improvement in "satisfaction in [the] sexual relationship," and women also reported persistent improvement in the "frequency of orgasm through masturbation and genital caress." Hawton et al. reported on a prospective follow-up study of sex therapy undertaken for various sexual disorders.[54] Treatment occurred between one and six years earlier and at least one partner was interviewed in 75% of cases. The effects of treatment in instances of "female impaired sexual interest," "showed a *marked deterioration* (italics added) . . . when compared with post-treatment outcome. This finding is accentuated by the fact that even post-treatment outcome for this problem was relatively modest."

There are only a handful of controlled treatment studies of HSD. O'Carroll reviewed the only eight that he could find that met his (gradually expanding) inclusion criteria for his search.[7] These included two psychotherapy studies, three drug or hormone studies, and three studies that combined the two methods. Of this review, he concluded that "if only studies which had specified (and analyzed) a discrete subject group who presented with low sex interest had been accepted, one would have been left with a single controlled treatment study which used only ten subjects!"

The one study about which O'Carroll wrote compared ten men with HSD to ten men with erectile dysfunction.[55] All initially had normal testosterone levels and all were treated with high-dosage testosterone or placebo using a double-blind crossover design. The HSD men responded with a significantly increased level of frequency of sexual thoughts. O'Carroll concluded that "high dosage testosterone treatment may have a modest role to play in the treatment of some eugonadal men who present with low sex interest."[7]

Leiblum and Rosen reviewed factors associated with treatment outcome found by those who presented case histories in their multi-authored book "Sexual Desire Disorders."[56] Success was particularly linked (p. 453) to desire problems affecting men who were in their 30s, 40s, and 50s and who reported concomitant sexual dysfunctions (especially erectile difficulties) and, in the case of couples, commitment to the marriage (despite relationship discord) and the treatment process (p. 454). Unsuccessful outcome of treatment was especially evident (p. 454) when there were secrets in the marital relationship, history of chronic alcoholism, religious orthodoxy, history of depression, organic erectile dysfunction, and "major body image problems."

INDICATIONS FOR REFERRAL FOR CONSULTATION OR CONTINUING CARE BY A SPECIALIST

Etiological heterogeneity of HSD means that therapeutic versatility is a necessity. The required range of skills will not likely be in the armamentarium of all primary care clinicians. Referral may become necessary and the kind of health professional to whom a referral is made will depend on the knowledge and skills of each and the apparent cause of the disorder.

Specific Causes of HSD

The capabilities of the primary care clinician may or may not encompass the treatments required for patients with specific causes of HSD. One or several visits with a consultant from a different discipline may be needed and may be all that is necessary. However, in complex circumstances it may also be advisable to complement one's own care (over an extended time period) with that of another health professional who has different skills.

- One example of a specific cause of HSD that sometimes requires only a consultation is the diagnosis of major depression. While most patients with this diagnosis are entirely cared for by primary care health professionals, in some instances, physicians in primary care might provide antidepressant medication and psychotherapy to the patient after consultation and advice from a psychiatrist or psychotherapist.
- Another example of a specific cause of HSD that may require more than simple consultation is the loss of sexual desire associated with the diagnosis and treatment of prostate cancer. This situation may require asking the advice of a medical specialist and the continuing cooperative efforts of the primary care clinician and a sex-specialist with counseling skills.
- A third example of a specific cause of HSD that may involve ultimate transfer of the patient to another health professional is that of sexual trauma (see "Sexual Sequelae of Child Sexual Abuse in Adults: Sexual Issues and Questions" in Chapter 8). A primary care professional may

provide acute care but the needs of the patient may require ongoing intensive care from a mental health professional who has psychotherapeutic skills and is also comfortable with sexual topics.

Nonspecific Causes of HSD

The care of an individual or couple where HSD is a concern, and for which no explanation has become apparent after investigation, reasonably suggests referral—at least for brief consultation, and often for continuing care. Despite the great frequency of the problem in the general population, nonspecific HSD is, *generally, not a disorder amenable to care at the generalist level. Careful subclassification and investigation are the most important responsibilities of the primary care clinician when considering nonspecific HSD, and they will determine the direction of referral.* In most instances, the most helpful professional is a sex therapist or sexual medicine specialist with counseling skills.

- Desire discrepancies occasionally do not respond to intervention at the primary care level. Consideration might then be given to referral to a mental health professional who is also comfortable with couples and in talking about sexual issues. Even then, referral should probably be reserved for circumstances that, if they continue, may threaten the continuity of the relationship.
- HSD that is lifelong and generalized often presents with questions about the continuity of a current relationship. Care of the patient or couple who appear in these complex and potentially turbulent circumstances should be undertaken by a sex therapist or sexual medicine specialist with a mental health professional background.
- The acquired and generalized form of HSD arises from several sources (see above) and the apparent origins (there may be more than one) influence the direction of referral. Because (1) the nature of such complaints are perplexing and intricate, (2) etiological clarity is often lacking, (3) disappointment and (often) anger is generated by the sexual change, and (4) because the partners are usually disappointed when they discover that expectations of return to previous sexual desire status often is not realized, treatment at the primary care level is not suggested. In most instances sex therapists or sexual medicine specialists, should be involved in treatment, at least on a consultation level if not in the continuing care of such individuals or couples.
- HSD that is acquired and situational occurs for a multiplicity of reasons and each one requires a different referral approach. For example, some instances are clearly a result of relationship discord, and the appropriate person to be caring for such a couple would be a mental health professional interested in relationship therapy. Other instances may represent a disorder such as the Madonna/Prostitute Syndrome (discussed earlier in this chapter), for which treatment is quite intricate and warrants referral to a mental health professional for continuing care. Yet other cases are a result of sexual issues specific to a couple (e.g., odors) and in that instance, should be referred to a sex therapist.

SUMMARY

The problem of low sexual desire or Hypoactive Sexual Desire Disorder (HSD) requires subclassification into syndromes that denote at least four possibilities:

- A desire discrepancy
- A disorder that is lifelong and generalized
- A disorder that is acquired and generalized
- A disorder that is acquired and situational

In general, low or absent sexual desire is the most common sexual complaint heard by health professionals, and about one third of women and one sixth of men answering a community survey report having had this experience for several months during the last year. Testosterone seems to be the "libido hormone" for men and women in that withdrawal of this substance has profound effects on sexual desire in both. Elevated Prolactin has a similar effect. HSD seems to arise from many different sources, hence the application of the term: *final common pathway*. When compared to normal controls, biologically related studies of healthy people with HSD have found some testosterone determinations and nocturnal penile tumescence differences in men, but no differences in women. HSD is associated with the following:

- A variety of general medical conditions
- Gynecologic and urologic disorders
- Psychiatric disorders
- Substance abuse
- Other sexual and gender identity disorders
- Intrapersonal difficulties
- Relationship discord

The investigation of HSD requires history-taking, physical examination for generalized disorders, and selective laboratory studies. The most valuable contribution of primary care professionals to patients with HSD is correct subclassification and investigation of the etiology. Treatment of HSD depends on the reason for the disorder. The more specific the etiology, the more specific the treatment, and the more specific the treatment, the more might be reasonably undertaken in primary care—alone or together with another health professional. Nonspecific HSD (apart from the problem of a desire discrepancy) generally requires referral to a health professional who specializes in the counseling and therapy of people with sexual difficulties.

REFERENCES

1. Levine SB: *Sexual life: a clinician's guide*, New York, 1992, Plenum Press.
2. Freud S: The transformations of puberty: [3] the libido theory. In Freud S: *On sexuality: three essays on the theory of sexuality and other works*, Middlesex, 1905/1977, Penguin Books, pp. 138-140.
3. Segraves T: Drugs and desire. In Leiblum SR, Rosen RC (editors), *Sexual desire disorders*, New York, 1988, The Guilford Press, pp. 313-347.

4. Kinsey AC, Pomeroy WB, Martin CE: *Sexual behavior in the human male*, Philadelphia and London, 1949, W.B. Saunders.

5. Zilbergeld B, Ellison CR: Desire discrepancies and arousal problems in sex therapy. In Leiblum SR, Pervin LA (editors): *Principles and practice of sex therapy*, ed 1, New York, 1980, The Guilford Press, pp. 65-101.

6. LoPiccolo J, Friedman JM: Broad-spectrum treatment of low sexual desire: integration of cognitive, behavioral, and systematic therapy. In Leiblum SR, Rosen RC (editors): *Sexual desire disorders*, New York, 1988, The Guilford Press, pp. 107-144.

7. O'Carroll R: Sexual desire disorders: a review of controlled treatment studies, *J Sex Res* 28:607-624, 1991.

8. *Diagnostic and statistical manual of mental disorders*, ed 4, Washington, 1994, American Psychiatric Association.

9. *Diagnostic and statistical manual of mental disorders*, ed 4, *primary care version*, 1995, Washington, American Psychiatric Association.

10. *Diagnostic and statistical manual of mental disorders*, ed 3, 1980, Washington, American Psychiatric Association.

11. Kaplan HS: *Sexual aversion, sexual phobias, and panic disorder*, New York, 1987, Brunner/Mazel, Inc.

12. Laumann EO et al: *The social organization of sexuality: sexual practices in the United States*, Chicago, 1994, The University of Chicago Press, pp. 35-73.

13. Frank E, Anderson C, Rubenstein D: Frequency of sexual dysfunction in normal couples, *N Engl J Med* 299:111-115, 1978.

14. Segraves KB, Segraves RT: Hypoactive sexual desire disorder: prevalence and comorbidity, *J Sex Marital Ther* 17:55-58, 1991.

15. Kinsey AC et al: *Sexual behavior in the human female*, Philadelphia and London, 1953, W.B. Saunders.

16. Levine SB: Intrapsychic and individual aspects of sexual desire. In Leiblum SR, Rosen RC (editors): *Sexual desire disorders*, New York, 1988, The Guilford Press, pp. 21-44.

17. Segraves T: Hormones and libido. In Leiblum SR, Rosen RC (editors): *Sexual desire disorders*, New York, 1988, The Guilford Press, pp. 271-312.

18. Schwartz MF, Bauman JE, Masters WH: Hyperprolactinemia and sexual disorders in men, *Biol Psychiatry* 17:861-876, 1982.

19. Sherwin BB, Gelfand MM, Brender W: Androgen enhances sexual motivation in females: a prospective, crossover study of sex steroid administration in the surgical menopause, *Psychosom Med* 47:339-351, 1985.

20. Sherwin BB: Menopause and sexuality, *Can J Obstet/Gynecol Women's Health Care* 4:254-260, 1992.

21. Donahey KM, Carroll RA: Gender differences in factors associated with hypoactive sexual desire, *J Sex Marital Ther* 19:25-40, 1993.

22. Schiavi RC et al: Pituitary-Gonadal function during sleep in men with hypoactive sexual desire and in normal controls, *Psychosom Med* 50:304-318, 1988.

23. Schreiner-Engel P et al: Low sexual desire in women: the role of reproductive hormones, *Horm Behav* 23:221-234, 1989.

24. Bullard DG: The treatment of desire disorders in the medically ill and physically disabled. In Leiblum SR, Rosen RC (editors): *Sexual desire disorders*, New York, 1988, The Guilford Press, pp. 348-384.

25. Nofzinger EA et al: Sexual function in depressed men, *Arch Gen Psychiatry* 50:24-30, 1993.

26. Schreiner-Engel P, Schiavi RC: Lifetime psychopathology in individuals with low sexual desire, *J Nerv Ment Dis* 174:646-651, 1986.

27. Segraves T: Overview of sexual dysfunction complicating the treatment of depression, *J Clin Psychiatry* 10:4-10, 1992.

28. Becker JV: *Impact of sexual abuse on sexual functioning*. In Leiblum SR, Rosen RC (editors): *Principles and practices of sex therapy: Update for the 1990s*, ed 2, New York, 1989, The Guilford Press, pp. 298-318.

29. Bozman AW, Beck JG: Covariation of sexual desire and sexual arousal: the effects of anger and anxiety, *Arch Sex Behav* 20:47-60, 1991.

30. Stuart FM, Hammond DC, Pett MA: Inhibited sexual desire in women, *Arch Sex Behav* 16:91-106, 1987.

31. Leiblum SR, Rosen RC (editors): *Sexual desire disorders*, New York, 1988, The Guilford Press.

32. Rosen RC, Leiblum SR: Hypoactive sexual desire, *Psychiatr Clin North Am* 18:107-121, 1995.

33. Kaplan HS: *The sexual desire disorders: dysfunctional regulation of sexual motivation*, New York, 1995, Brunner/Mazel.

34. Kaplan HS, Owett T: The female androgen deficiency syndrome, *J Sex Marital Ther* 19:3-24, 1993.

35. Feldman JE: Ovarian failure and cancer treatment: incidence and interventions for the premenopausal woman, *Oncol Nurs Forum* 16:651-657, 1989.

36. Chapman RM: Effect of cytotoxic therapy on sexuality and gonadal function, *Semin Oncol* 9:84-94, 1982.

37. Williams W: *Rekindling desire: bringing your sexual relationship back to life*, Oakland, 1988, New Harbinger Publications Inc.

38. Nichols M: Low sexual desire in lesbian couples. In Leiblum SR, Rosen RC (editors): *Sexual desire disorders*, New York, 1988, The Guilford Press, pp. 387-411.

39. Scharff DE: An object relations approach to inhibited sexual desire. In Lieblum SR, Rosen RC (editors): *Sexual desire disorders*, New York, 1988, The Guilford Press, pp. 45-74.

40. Apfelbaum B: An ego-analytic perspective on desire disorders. In Leiblum SR, Rosen RC (editors), *Sexual desire disorders*, New York, 1988, The Guilford Press, pp. 75-104.

41. Rosen RC, Leiblum SR: A sexual scripting approach to problems of desire. In Lieblum SR, Rosen RC (editors): *Sexual desire disorders*, New York, 1988, The Guilford Press, pp. 168-191.

42. Lazarus AA: A multimodal perspective on problems of sexual desire. In Leiblum SR, Rosen RC (editors): *Sexual desire disorders*, New York, 1988, The Guilford Press, pp. 145-167.

43. Schwartz MF, Masters WH: Inhibited sexual desire: the Masters and Johnson Institute treatment model. In Leiblum SR, Rosen RC (editors): *Sexual desire disorders*, New York, 1988, The Guilford Press, pp. 229-242.

44. Verhulst J, Heiman JR: A systems perspective on sexual desire. In Leiblum SR, Rosen RC (editors): *Sexual desire disorders*, New York, 1988 The Guilford Press, pp. 243-267.

45. Gann et al: Prospective study of sex hormone levels and risk of prostate cancer, *J Natl Cancer Institute* 88: 1118-1126, 1996.

46. Dorgan JF et al: Relation of prediagnostic serum estrogen and androgen levels to breast cancer risk, *Cancer Epidemiol Biomarkers Prev* 5:533-539, 1996.

47. Dorgan JF et al: Relationship of serum dehydroepiandrosterone (DHEA), DHEA sufate, and 5-androstene-3β,17β-diol to risk of breast cancer in postmenopausal women, *Cancer Epidemiol Biomarkers Prev* 6:177-181, 1997.

48. Sherwin BB et al: Postmenopausal estrogen and androgen replacement and lipoprotein lipid concentrations, *Am J Obstet Gynecol* 156:414-419, 1987.

49. Phillips GB, Pinkernell BH, Jing T-Y: Relationship between serum sex hormones and coronary artery disease in postmenopausal women, *Arterioscler Thromb Vasc Biol* 17: 695-701, 1997.

50. Farish E et al: The effects of hormone implants on serum lipoproteins and steroid hormones in bilaterally oophorectomized women, *Acta Endocrinol* 106: 116-120, 1984.

51. Fletcher CD et al: Long-term hormone implant therapy- effects on lipoproteins and steroid levels in postmenopausal women, *Acta Endocrinol* 111:419-423, 1986.

52. Sands R, Studd J: Exogenous androgens in postmenopausal women, *Am J Med* 98(suppl 1A):76S-79S, 1995.

53. De Amicis LA et al: Clinical follow-up of couples treated for sexual dysfunction, *Arch Sex Behav* 14:467-489, 1985.

54. Hawton K: Long-term outcome of sex therapy, *Behav Res Ther* 24:665-675, 1986.

55. O'Carroll R, Bancroft J: Testosterone therapy for low sexual interest and erectile dysfunction in men: a controlled study, *Br J Psychiatry* 145:146-151, 1984.

56. Leiblum SR, Rosen RC: Conclusion: Conceptual and clinical overview. In Leiblum SR, Rosen RC (editors): *Sexual desire disorders*, New York, 1988, The Guilford Press, pp. 446-458.

CHAPTER 10

EJACULATION/ORGASM DISORDERS

T hree disorders of ejaculation/orgasm are most common in primary care: Premature Ejaculation [PE], Delayed Ejaculation/ Orgasm [DE/O], and Retrograde Ejaculation [RE]. Three others are found infrequently: Anejaculation, Painful Ejaculation, and Anorgasmic Ejaculation. The six conditions are discussed in order of frequency.

PREMATURE EJACULATION

Time and time again premature ejaculators of many years' standing not only lose confidence in their own sexual performance but also, unable to respond positively while questioning their own masculinity, terminate their sexual functioning with secondary impotence. This stage of functional involution is, of course, the crowning blow to husband and wife as individuals and usually to the marital relationship.

MASTERS & JOHNSON, 1970[1]

The Problem

A couple in their late 20s and married for three years was concerned about the man's ejaculation. For religious reasons, they had not attempted intercourse before marriage. Since they were married, he regularly ejaculated before attempts at vaginal entry. As a result, their union had not been "consummated." Her sexual desire diminished considerably over the three years of their marriage. Apart from embarrassment and diminished sexual pleasure that they both experienced, they wanted to have children and for her to become pregnant in the "natural way." Ejaculating quickly was not a new problem for him. Since the first time he attempted intercourse at the age of 14, he was unable to accomplish vaginal entry except on one occasion, and, then, he ejaculated in a matter of seconds. Since the "squeeze technique" described by Masters & Johnson[1] was tried and found not helpful, the couple felt desperate and anticipated separation and divorce if another way to help them could not be found.

A couple in their mid-50s and married for 25 years was seen because of erectile and ejaculation problems. Sexual difficulties began about five years before and were gradually becoming worse. The husband was aware of the association between sexual dysfunctions and diabetes (a disease with which he lived in the previous 20 years) but until recently had not volunteered information to his physician about his sexual difficulties. He believed that the onset of his (generalized) erectile problems preceded his ejaculation difficulty by about one year. He described ejaculating rapidly after a frantic process of gaining vaginal entry and before any softening of his erection made continued containment impossible.

Terminology

Patients often use the word "come" to describe an ejaculation/orgasm and "Premature Ejaculation" when this process happens too quickly. When the term, *Premature Ejaculation* (PE), is used by health professionals, some consider it to be pejorative and value laden. Preferring a more descriptive term, McCarthy has suggested *Early Ejaculation* as an alternative[2] (p. 144). Others have also used the term, *Rapid Ejaculation*.[3,4] These terms indicate that speed of ejaculation is on a continuum from slow to fast rather than a normal/abnormal dichotomy. For reasons of consistency with DSM-IV[5] and DSM-IV-PC[6] nomenclature, as well as the inclusion of the concept of control in the definition (see immediately below), the term, *Premature Ejaculation*, will be used in this chapter.

Definition

Definition problems abound in attempts to clarify PE. Does one use a time element? (Critics say that no one carries a stopwatch to bed.) Or is it better to specify the number of movements or thrusts? (One might legitimately ask: just what is the "correct" number?) Should one follow the Masters and Johnson suggestion that the woman be "satisfied" 50% of the time when intercourse occurs?[1] (p. 92) (On the presumption that "satisfaction" means "orgasm," of what relevance is the Masters and Johnson definition to a man who is having intercourse with a woman who comes to orgasm only with direct clitoral stimulation and not with intercourse?)

Usually no one debates the issue of the definition of prematurity when a heterosexual man ejaculates before, during, or immediately after vaginal entry. Definition problems arise with lengthening of the amount of time after penetration. It is conceivable that two syndromes exist: (1) ejaculation before, during, or immediately after vaginal entry and (2) ejaculation after vaginal entry but with little or no control over the timing. It may be that the former has "premature ejaculation" and the latter is simply quite fast and would be reasonably described as having "rapid ejaculation."

Grenier and Byers suggest a different way of considering the definition of PE: there should be two criteria for the diagnosis. One is based on the extent of voluntary control experienced by the man and the other is based on "latency," or the amount of time from vaginal entry to ejaculation.[3]

Does PE apply to men who are sexually active with other men? The literature is unclear on this subject. Masters and Johnson found that PE "rarely represents a serious problem to interacting male homosexuals . . . [since] . . . neither man is dependent upon the other's ejaculatory control to achieve sexual satisfaction"[7] (p. 239). However, another study declared that 19% of a convenience sample of 197 gay men reported "ejaculating too soon/too quickly."[8]

If the definition of PE includes only the speed of ejaculation, the definition doubtless applies to men sexually active with other men. However, if the definition also includes control, the answer is not so clear. It might depend on the kind of sexual practices between the two men. For example, some men might ejaculate rapidly and out of control during anal intercourse but rapidly and in control with mutual masturbation.

Classification

DSM-IV-PC summarizes the criteria for the diagnosis of PE as follows: "Persistent or recurrent ejaculation with minimal stimulation before, on, or shortly after penetration and before the person wishes it, causing marked distress or interpersonal difficulty."[6] (This statement introduces a subjective element by using the phrase "wishes it"). The clinician is further instructed to " . . . take into account factors that affect the duration of the sexual excitement phase, such as age, novelty of the sexual partner or situation, and frequency of sexual activity." As with other sexual dysfunctions, clinicians are also asked to specify if the problem is lifelong or acquired, or situational or generalized. The assessment of premature ejaculation is outlined in Figure 10-1

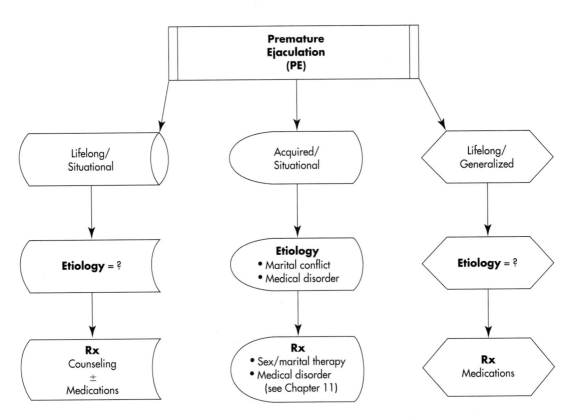

Figure 10-1   Assessment of premature ejaculation.

Description

The majority of men who ask for assistance describe a lifelong pattern of ejaculating quickly and without any control in attempts at intercourse. This process usually contrasts with ejaculation with masturbation, the timing of which is described as entirely in their control.

History reveals increasing concern about ejaculation in intercourse after an initial period in which the man seemed unaware of possible dissatisfaction of previous sexual partners ("no one ever said anything"). His sexual activities tend to focus on intercourse. On a time scale, the man often ejaculates within seconds after vaginal entry. While ejaculation is pleasurable, the total sexual experience is anything but, since it is filled with worry and trepidation about 'the same thing taking place that occurred the last time.' Various attempts at controlling ejaculation (including distracting oneself by nonsexual thoughts or masturbating before a sexual encounter) have been tried and found wanting. The patient is apologetic to his partner and privately self-deprecatory. The current partner is often angry because her sexual arousal is repeatedly interrupted. Her interest in sexual activities may decline. Sometimes a woman in this situation believes that the man deliberately chooses not to control the timing of his ejaculation. Resulting intra- and interpersonal tensions can be substantial.

Some men describe difficulties with the timing of ejaculation of relatively recent onset and after a lengthy period in which this was not considered to be a problem by him or his partner(s). The distinction between this acquired form and its lifelong counterpart is important from etiological and therapeutic viewpoints.

Epidemiology

Some information about "normal" latency was provided by Kinsey and his colleagues in their survey of men in the general population[9] (pp. 579-581). While they did not seem to consider PE to be a disorder, curiosity about speed of ejaculation (rather than definition of the problem) resulted in them asking about ejaculation latency (that is, the estimated average time for ejaculation to occur after vaginal entry). The time was two minutes for about three fourths of the men studied.

Laumann and his colleagues asked those who were surveyed: "during the last 12 months has there ever been a period of several months or more when you came to a climax too quickly?"[10] pp.368-375) Twenty-nine percent of the men answered "yes"—the most common sexual complaint, by far, of the men surveyed. Positive answers were greatest in men who were under the age of 40 and over the age of 54, married and divorced (compared to those who had never married), less educated (i.e., received less than high school education), black, in poor health, and unhappy.

> Question: "During the last 12 months has there ever been a period of several months or more when you came to a climax too quickly?" Twenty-nine percent of the men surveyed answered, "Yes." (This is, by far, the most common sexual complaint of the men surveyed.)

PE has varied from 15% to 46% of presenting complaints at sexual problem clinics in a review of studies completed between 1970 and 1988.[11] Furthermore, for unknown reasons, PE may be decreasing over time as the principal sexual concern of men who appear at the clinics.

The acquired form of PE (sometimes referred to as "secondary") is characterized by: (1) an older man, (2) a briefer interval of time existing between beginning of the difficulty and seeking professional assistance, and (3) erectile difficulties preceding the onset.[12]

Etiology

The variety of psychologically and biologically based etiological hypotheses for PE have been thoroughly reviewed[3] and include the following:

1. Psychodynamic theories (excessive narcissism or a virulent dislike of women)
2. Early experience (conditioning based on haste and nervousness)
3. Anxiety (causing activation of the sympathetic nervous system or distraction from worry resulting in lack of awareness of sensations premonitory to ejaculation)
4. Low frequency of sexual activity
5. Not using techniques that other men have learned to control the timing of ejaculation
6. Not considering rapidity of ejaculation to be a disorder, since it is a superior trait from an evolutionary viewpoint
7. Easier arousal
8. Greater sensitivity to penile stimulation
9. Malfunctioning of the normal ejaculatory reflex[3]

Theories about PE represent etiological speculations concerning men who are otherwise healthy. However, PE has also been reported in association with trauma to the sympathetic nervous system during surgery for aortic aneurysm, pelvic fracture, prostatitis, urethritis[4] and neurological diseases such as multiple sclerosis[2] (p. 148).

> Many men (perhaps most) who ejaculate unpredictably with a partner are able to control the timing of their ejaculation when masturbating.

While the presence of anxiety often seems to be associated with PE, the direction of the relationship (cause or effect) is unclear. What is striking, however, is the fact that many men (perhaps most) who ejaculate unpredictably with a partner are able to control the timing of their ejaculation when masturbating. (A few men who appear to be otherwise healthy ejaculate spontaneously and without control in the presence of any kind of sexual stimulation.) Assuming a relationship between anxiety and ejaculatory control, anxiety is helpful as an explanation for the occurrence of PE only in relation to intercourse (since men are considerably less anxious when masturbating[13]).

> Speed of ejaculation was compared in premature and nonpremature ejaculating men when masturbating. Assessment of latency to ejaculation showed that when at home the men with PE ejaculated in about half the time as their conterparts (three minutes versus six minutes).

One of the more compelling hypotheses for PE is that it "may be, at least in part, the result of a physiologically determined hypersensitivity to sexual stimulation," that is, PE may be a reflection of a lower ejaculatory threshold. In a study that adds support to this idea, speed of ejaculation was compared in premature and nonpremature ejaculating men when masturbating. Assessment of latency to ejaculation showed that when at home the men with PE ejaculated in about half the time as their counterparts (three minutes versus six minutes).[11] The authors of this study suggest a diathesis-stress model in which "some individuals with a particularly strong somatic vulnerability may require little, if any, anxiety in order to manifest their low orgastic threshold."

Investigation into the etiology of the acquired form of PE suggests separation into two groups: (1) one in which the patients had a "demonstrable organic cause" (e.g., erectile dysfunction as a result of diabetes) and (2) one in which the men were involved in disturbed relationships.[12]

Investigation

History

The history is the key to the diagnosis of PE in a man who is otherwise healthy. While history can be obtained from the man alone, the effect of this syndrome on both sexual partners is best gauged by talking directly with each. Issues to inquire about and suggested descriptive questions (asked of heterosexual men, although easily adapted to gay men as well) include:

1. Duration of ejaculatory difficulty (see Chapter 4, "lifelong versus acquired")

Suggested Question: HAS EJACULATING QUICKLY ALWAYS BEEN A PROBLEM FOR YOU OR WAS THERE A PERIOD OF TIME WHEN THIS DID NOT OCCUR?"

2. Subjective feeling before ejaculation (see Chapter 4, "generalized versus situational")

Suggested Question: "IF YOU COMPARE YOUR EJACULATION WHEN HAVING INTERCOURSE TO MASTURBATING, HOW MUCH WARNING DO YOU HAVE THAT EJACULATION IS ABOUT TO OCCUR IN EACH SITUATION?"

3. Timing of ejaculation (see Chapter 4, "description")

Suggested Question: "DO YOU EJACULATE BEFORE, DURING, OR AFTER VAGINAL ENTRY?"

4. Speed of ejaculation (see Chapter 4, "description")

Question if Answer is "After": "ON THE BASIS OF TIME, HOW LONG DOES IT TAKE YOU TO EJACULATE AFTER ENTRY?"

Additional Question: "ON THE BASIS OF NUMBERS OF MOVEMENTS OR THRUSTS, HOW MANY OCCUR BEFORE YOU EJACULATE?"

5. Methods used to control ejaculation (see Chapter 4, "description")

Suggested Question: "HAVE YOU TRIED TO CONTROL THE TIMING OF YOUR EJACULATION?"

If the Answer is "Yes," Follow-up Suggested Question: "WHAT METHODS HAVE YOU USED TO DO THIS?"

Additional Question: "FOR EXAMPLE, MANY MEN STOP MOVING (OR USE CONDOMS, ANESTHETIC CREAMS OR OILS, OR THINK OF SOMETHING NONSEXUAL) IN AN ATTEMPT TO PREVENT THEMSELVES FROM GETTING CLOSE. IS THAT SOMETHING YOU'VE TRIED TO DO?"

6. Subjective feeling of orgasm (see Chapter 4, "description")

Suggested Question: "ALTHOUGH ORGASM IS DIFFICULT TO DESCRIBE, CAN YOU EXPLAIN WHAT IT FEELS LIKE WHEN YOU EJACULATE?"

Additional Possible Question: "IS IT A PLEASANT OR UNPLEASANT EXPERIENCE FOR YOU?"

7. Description of emission (see Chapter 4, "description")

Suggested Question: "MEN USUALLY EXPERIENCE REPEATED OR RHYTHMIC CONTRACTIONS WHEN THEY EJACULATE SO THAT THE SEMEN COMES OUT IN SPURTS. DO YOU NOTICE THESE CONTRACTIONS WHEN YOU EJACULATE?"

Additional Suggested Question: "WHEN EJACULATION OCCURS, DOES THE SEMEN COME OUT IN SPURTS OR DOES IT DRIBBLE OUT?"

(Comment: There is less force to ejaculation when there is some obstruction [e.g., prostatic hypertrophy or urethral stricture] neurological disorder, and in the aging process[14] [pp. 257-259].)

8. Psychological accompaniment (see Chapter 4, "patient and partner's reaction to problem")

Suggested Question: "WHEN YOU HAVE TROUBLE WITH EJACULATION, WHAT'S GOING THROUGH YOUR MIND?"

Additional Question: "WHAT DOES YOUR WIFE (PARTNER) THINK?"

Physical and laboratory examinations

In otherwise healthy men, these investigations add little useful information.

Treatment

> Given the prevalence of lifelong Premature Ejaculation, the focus on history-taking as the principal diagnostic technique, the etiological concentration on the present rather than the past, and the usefulness of some brief approaches, treatment of this disorder is well within the purview of primary care.

Given the substantial frequency of lifelong Premature Ejaculation in the community, the focus on history-taking as the principal diagnostic technique, the etiological concentration on the present rather than the past, and the usefulness of some brief approaches, treatment of this disorder is well within the purview of primary care.

Masters and Johnson described a talk-oriented treatment method for PE that provides an "overall failure rate" of 2.7%[1] (pp. 92-115 and 367). Perhaps as a result of the reported benefits, little else was suggested therapeutically for some time after. Others also reported positive effects after treatment but when long-term follow-up studies were done considerably less robust results were found. A three-year follow-up study (for example) reported dramatic changes at the end of treatment for PE in the duration of intercourse. However, pretreatment levels returned after three years.[15] (Interestingly, significant improvements in the duration of *foreplay* reported at the end of treatment were found in this study to have persisted at follow-up.)

Counseling and medications are presently the mainstays of treatment for lifelong PE. Obviously, drug prescription is available only to physicians. However, cooperative relationships between all professionals in the health care system increasingly reflect changes toward improvement in the quality of patient care.

Pharmacotherapy

Evidence for the utility of drug treatment of PE is increasing. In case reports and single blind studies, psychotropic drugs are noted to interfere with ejaculation as a side effect.[16] Some investigators reason that this observation could be turned to advantage, suggesting that a side effect is not necessarily an *adverse* effect. The antidepressants paroxetine,[17] sertraline,[18] and clomipramine[4] have undergone double-blind testing for their usefulness in the treatment of PE (often in smaller doses than that used in the treatment of depression). (Paroxetine [Paxil] and sertraline [Zoloft] are selective serotonin reuptake inhibitors [SSRIs], and clomipramine [Anafranil] is a chemical hybrid of a tricyclic and SSRI).

Waldinger and his colleagues conducted a double-blind, randomized, placebo-controlled study of paroxetine (40 mg/day for five of the six weeks of the study [higher than what is usually prescribed in treating depression]) in the treatment of PE in 17 men.[17] Patients and partners were questioned separately. The improvement was described as dramatic and began in the first days of treatment (suggesting that the effect was not a result of diminished psychopathology). No anticholinergic side effects (a possible problem with clomipramine, depending on the dose) or effect on erection function was reported.

Mendels and his colleagues randomly assigned 52 heterosexual males to an eight week study of either sertraline or a placebo administered in a double-blind fashion.[18] The drug was given daily and the dose varied from 50 to 200 mg, depending on the beneficial response and adverse experiences of the patient. Sertraline was judged to be significantly better than placebo in (1) prolongation of time to ejaculation and (2) number of successful attempts at intercourse.

Althof and his colleagues completed a double-blind placebo-controlled crossover trial of clomipramine in a group of 15 otherwise healthy men with lifelong PE who were also married or cohabiting with a woman for at least six months.[4] Partners participated in the study. Results of the study are as follows:

1. Mean ejaculatory latency increased almost threefold at a dose of 25 mg/day and over five-fold at the other studied dose of 50 mg/day
2. Both partners reported statistically significant greater levels of sexual satisfaction
3. Some of the women who reported never previously experiencing orgasm with intercourse became coitally orgasmic
4. Over half of the 10 women who previously reported orgasm during intercourse indicated that it now happened more frequently
5. The men reported greater emotional and relationship satisfaction

However, when the drug was discontinued, sexual function returned to the level that existed before the study.

The use of clomipramine on an "as needed" basis was examined[19] in another study. Using a double-blind, placebo-controlled, crossover design, eight men with PE, six men with PE and erectile dysfunction, and eight control men were studied. Partners did not participate in the study. Subjects took 26 mg of clomipramine or placebo 12 to 24 hours before anticipated sexual activity. In contrast to the marked beneficial effect in the men with "primary" (i.e., lifelong) PE, the authors report that the drug was not useful in men who had PE and erectile dysfunction. This result affirms the importance of subclassification.

A 28-year-old man and his 32-year-old wife were seen because of his difficulty with regular ejaculation before vaginal entry. This pattern of ejaculation had existed since the beginning of his attempts at intercourse as a teenager. His wife was becoming sexually disinterested and questioned her commitment to the relationship, particularly because "the biological clock was ticking" and she wanted to begin a family. The couple had undergone a Masters and Johnson-type of treatment program about one year earlier and found that the initial gains were short-lived.[1] A one-visit assessment was conducted with them together, and clomipramine was prescribed. The couple was seen again two weeks later, when substantial improvement was reported in the following:

- His ejaculation latency
- Their sexual relationship
- Other aspects of their life as a couple

Much to the wife's pleasure, she became pregnant within two months of the first visit. The man was seen for a third time alone because the wife was unable to accompany him for the visit. He reported continued improvement in sexual and nonsexual areas of their life. Telephone contact was periodically maintained for the purpose of medication refills.

In a review of pharmacologic studies into the treatment of PE, Althof asks the following serious questions.[4]

1. Should drugs be the first line of treatment?
2. How should drugs be used? (daily? the day of intercourse? a duration of weeks? months? lifetime?)
3. What are the indications and contraindications? (Used only in the lifelong form? The acquired form? Prescribed only for men who do not ejaculate before, during, or immediately after entry but want to "last longer?")
4. What should be the relationship between drug treatment and psychotherapy?

Althof concludes that all of these questions require empirical research and are therefore difficult to answer at the present time. Some of these questions are considered below, and the information given is based more on clinical judgment and experience than research data.

Should drugs be the first line of treatment? Drugs may well be used immediately, as follows:

- A man who persistently ejaculates in an uncontrolled manner with any form of sexual stimulation and particularly before vaginal entry
- A couple when talk-oriented treatment methods are not helpful
- Many single men without partners
- When talking to a couple is unproductive even if a couple relationship exists (e.g., in the case of a couple raised in a culture where gender roles dictate that the woman is subservient to the man and both subscribe to this philosophy—a situation that is functionally the same as talking with the man by himself)

How should drugs be used? Daily and ad hoc (e.g., clomipramine four hours before intercourse is expected to occur) administration methods have been found helpful.

What are the contraindications? There are two reasons why drug treatment should not be used in men who have the acquired form of PE based on relationship discord. First, PE in this situation is clearly symptomatic and it makes little sense to treat the symptom and not the "disease" (i.e., the relationship discord). Second, the problem of PE may well be reversed with attention given to the disrupted relationship. Furthermore, in acquired PE associated with erectile problems, clomipramine treatment has been shown to be ineffective.[17] On the subject of contraindications, Althof also counseled that considerable caution be exercised in response to requests from men who want "boundless intercourse or designer orgasmic capabilities."[4]

What should be the relationship between drug therapy and psychotherapy? Althof states that there should not be an either/or attitude to the use of these treatment methods and that both may be desirable or necessary.[4] "The two treatment approaches are not to be compared solely in terms of economics or ejaculatory latency. Psychotherapy educates, clarifies, and often addresses other issues not perceived when the diagnosis was originally made." Indeed, if the physician's approach to medications is such that psychotherapy is *not* used in conjunction, then, by experience so far, the man is implicitly being told that he must take this medication for, perhaps, a lifetime. The implications of such a treatment decision are substantial, especially given that many of the men presenting with the lifelong and situational form of PE are young and in the early stages of their sexual experience.

> If the physician's approach to medications is such that psychotherapy is not used in conjunction, the man patient is implicitly being told that he must take this medication for (perhaps) a lifetime. The implications of such a treatment decision are substantial, especially since many men presenting with the lifelong and situational form of PE are young and in the early stages of their sexual experience.

Counseling

The talking part of the treatment of someone with PE includes at least four components:

- Information
- Specific techniques
- Adaptation
- Attention to psychological issues

Some are easily incorporated into primary care practice.

INFORMATION

PE-related self-help books seem to be particularly useful in providing two elements of counseling[20-22]:

- Information (in this instance about men and sexual issues)
- Specific advice (in this example about controlling ejaculation)

The extent to which these two elements are therapeutically helpful is unclear, since men who benefit greatly from such books would not be likely to seek assistance from health professionals. Judging by the reaction of patients to whom such books are suggested, many find the content to be at least informative and reassuring and some follow the specific treatment methods suggested. Apart from specific issues around ejaculation control, Zilbergeld, in particular, interests male readers when discussing the powerful and influential sexual "myths" that so often determine how men think and behave sexually—in their own eyes and in those of their sexual partners.[20,22] This is "sex education" as it should be, that is, the description of body parts and their function and the discussion of sex-related aspects of human relationships. Kaplan's book includes information about PE and specific techniques for ejaculatory control (see immediately below).[21]

SPECIFIC TECHNIQUES

A second element in counseling, more applicable to couples, is directed at specific techniques to control the speed of ejaculation. Two approaches were described in the past: "stop-start"[23] and the "squeeze technique"[1] (pp. 102-104). The stop-start technique is more popular among sex therapists because it is easier for health professionals to explain and for patients to use. The stop-start approach involves an exercise in "communication" and comprises at least four steps:

1. Both partners initially agree not to attempt intercourse on at least several occasions (this is essential)
2. The woman stimulates the man's erect penis until he is close to ejaculation at which point he signals her to stop
3. This happens three or four times on any one sexual occasion before he eventually ejaculates
4. The couple then integrates this into intercourse experiences with frequent "pauses"

ADAPTATION

An additional facet of counseling, also more directed to couples, is incorporated into the concept of adaptation. Even if little change develops in the timing or speed of ejaculation as a result of talking forms of treatment, a considerable shift may occur in the sexual experiences of the couple such that the timing of the man's ejaculation becomes a lesser or even nonissue. For example, if the usual "order" of sexual events is such that the man ejaculates before his partner is stimulated, this process can be altered so that attention is given to the woman's satisfaction and (possibly) orgasm, before or after vaginal entry occurs. The notion of adaptation is consistent with some results found at follow-up, namely that treatment of PE may change aspects of foreplay rather than ejaculatory control.[12]

PSYCHOLOGICAL ISSUES

Ignoring concurrent psychological issues in the counseling process decreases the potential for a good outcome.

A couple in their late 30s, married for 15 years, was referred because the man regularly ejaculated immediately after vaginal entry, a pattern that existed throughout all of his life. In the process of initially talking with both (together and separately) it became clear that she was angry and "at the end of (her) rope." She was seriously considering separation for sexual and nonsexual reasons. Sexually, her level of interest was similar to her husband's (i.e., substantial) but her sexual arousal was interrupted continually by his ejaculation. She was orgasmic with direct clitoral stimulation before intercourse but this was irregular and unpredictable. Her animosity toward her husband about nonsexual concerns related to his inclination to continually avoid talking about contentious issues (including their sexual troubles). It was evident that simply delaying his ejaculation by using pharmacotherapy would not circumvent the discord between the two. Thus deliberate decision was made to treat this couple using traditional counseling methods.

Psychological issues may be particularly important in the solo male. A man might ask for solo treatment for several reasons:

1. He may not have a partner
2. Confidentiality and trust issues may prevent the involvement of a new partner
3. A partner may be unwilling or unable to participate in the process (this is less frequent than many men report)

In such circumstances, it is usually best to explain that although much can be accomplished diagnostically in seeing him alone, the absence of a sexual partner is often therapeutically limiting. Some aspects of the multifaceted treatment approach described above can be applied to the solo male, including the provision of information and learning specific techniques such as stop-start while masturbating.

When the limitations of solo (versus couple) treatment are discussed, clinicians frequently meet with a "catch-22" response in which the man says that the very existence of this problem prevents establishment of a relationship. He is, in effect, saying that speed of ejaculation is a determining force in relationships between men and women— a suggestion that (to say the least) not everyone supports. The fact that a partner is not present to possibly refute this argument puts the health professional in the difficult position of presenting a different point of view to the patient and potentially disrupting the professional relationship in the process. Psychotherapy might be helpful to the extent that the man is prepared to examine *all* aspects of a failed relationship, sexual and otherwise.

Indications for Referral for Consultation or Continuing Care by a Specialist

1. Consultation with a physician is required when pharmacotherapy is considered and the health professional is trained in a different discipline.
2. In the acquired form of PE associated with relationship discord, the ejaculation issue is likely symptomatic and treatment would involve relationship therapy— a process that is best undertaken on a continuing care basis by those in the health care system with clinical experience in this area, that is, mental health professionals.
3. In the acquired form of PE associated with an erectile disorder, managing both problems may be complex. Therefore referral to a sex-specialist for continuing care may be necessary.
4. Care of the solo man, beyond the use of drugs, often presents a dilemma. Men who are unwilling to use pharmacotherapy or who continue to have inter- or intrapersonal difficulty despite slower ejaculation are best seen for continuing care by a mental health professional who is comfortable with sexual issues.
5. Unsuccessful treatment at the primary care level should result in referral to a sex-specialist, at least for consultation, and possibly for continuing care.

Summary

Premature Ejaculation (PE) in heterosexual men is difficult to define precisely except in situations where ejaculation occurs persistently before, during, or immediately after vaginal entry. Control over the process of ejaculation appears to be a significant element in the definition, as well as the duration of time between vaginal entry and ejaculation. Most men with this disorder describe a lifelong pattern. "Coming to a climax too quickly" was the most common sexual complaint registered by men in a substantial survey of sexual behavior. An unreplicated study suggests an appealing hypothesis for the etiology of the lifelong form of PE, namely, that it is partly related to a "physiologically determined hypersensitivity to sexual stimulation." The acquired form seems to be the result of relationship discord or medical illness. The focus of investigation into the lifelong form of PE is particularly on history-taking (rather than physical examination or laboratory studies). Counseling and medications are the mainstays of treatment of this disorder. The latter has demonstrated great value, although many details concerning drug treatment have yet to be elaborated.

Long term follow-up studies of counseling alone show modest results. The potential value of combining the two treatment forms has not been investigated. Intuitively, medications may be considered a short-term intervention, and psychotherapy may be included toward the long-term goal of permanent change. Referral for consultation with a physician is required when drug therapy is undertaken by a health professional from another discipline. Referral for continuing care is particularly reasonable in the acquired form of PE and when slowing of ejaculation in a man seen alone has resulted in limited success in allowing him to develop intimate relationships.

DELAYED EJACULATION/ORGASM

Terminology

This syndrome has been variously called:

- Ejaculatory Incompetence[1]
- Retarded Ejaculation[24]
- Male Orgasm Disorder[5,6]

An evident problem with the terms is the confusion about whether this is a disorder of ejaculation, of orgasm, or both. These two phenomena are separate from a neurophysiological viewpoint although usually tightly interwoven. The separateness is evident in the normal development of preadolescent boys who are able to come to orgasm but who cannot ejaculate because the mechanism is not fully developed. The term, *Delayed Ejaculation/Orgasm* (DE/O), is preferred because it is entirely descriptive and DE/O refers to a delay in both ejaculation *and* orgasm.

Definition

Defining DE/O presents problems similar to PE, namely, the question of how much time constitutes a delay? In one form, the definition of time is not a problem, since the man can ejaculate without difficulty when alone (without any delay), but usually not at all when with a partner. When ejaculation is truly delayed, it is slow in *all* situations—regardless of the sexual activity and the nature of the partnership. In fact, ejaculation/orgasm may be so delayed that the person stops trying. In either case (delayed or absent) the definition is usually provided by the patient as he, for example, compares his present experience to that of the past or receives complaints from a sexual partner who may become vaginally uncomfortable because of a lengthy period of intercourse.

Classification

In DSM-IV-PC, orgasm difficulties for men and women are classified similarly[6] (p. 117). "Male Orgasmic Disorder" is defined as: persistent or recurrent delay in, or absence of, orgasm after a normal sexual excitement phase. This can be present in all situations, or present only in specific settings, and causes marked distress or interpersonal difficulty. Additional clinical information is provided: "In diagnosing Orgasmic Disorder, the clinician should also take into account the person's age and sexual experience. . . . In the most common form of Male Orgasmic Disorder, a male cannot reach orgasm during intercourse, although he can ejaculate with a partner's manual or oral stimulation. Some males. . . . can reach coital orgasm but only after very prolonged and intense noncoital stimulation. Some can ejaculate only from masturbation. When a man has hidden his lack of coital orgasm from his sexual partner, the couple may present with infertility of unknown cause." Determining the subclassification as lifelong or acquired, generalized or situational can be crucial to determining etiology and treatment.

The assessment of Delayed Ejaculation/Orgasm is outlined in Figure 10-2.

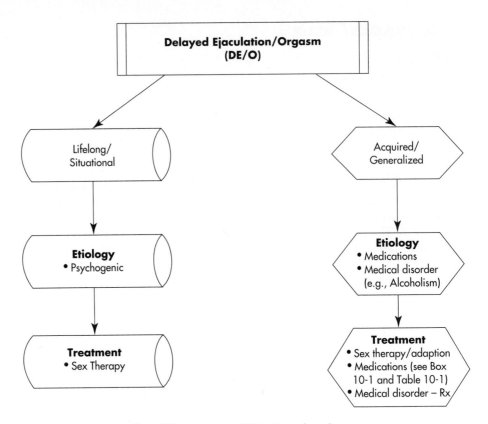

Figure 10-2   Assessment of delayed ejaculation/orgasm.

Description

DE/O presents clinically in one of two forms:

- Situational
- Generalized

When situational, the problem is usually lifelong rather than acquired. When generalized, it is much more likely to be acquired.

In the situational form, the history is usually one of ejaculation without difficulty when alone but inability to ejaculate with partners generally or during a specific sexual activity, typically intercourse. The request for assistance often can be traced to the partner and characteristically results from vaginal discomfort, concerns about reproduction, or both. Sometimes the man describes a method of masturbation that is difficult to transfer to sexual activity with a partner (e.g., rubbing his penis against a firm surface rather than using his hand).

Two gay men in their 20s were seen because one was unable to ejaculate in the presence of the other while having no such difficulty when masturbating alone.

Strains in their relationship became apparent when the sexually functional partner let it be known that he considered his partner's inability to ejaculate to be a form of rejection. History revealed that the man with DE/O experienced this pattern of ejaculation in previous brief sexual relationships as well as the three he considered long-term. Treatment using the approach described by Masters and Johnson was unsuccessful at reversing the pattern[1] (pp. 129-133). One-year follow-up revealed that the relationship had dissolved.

In the generalized form (lifelong or acquired), history reveals that the man is experiencing substantial delay or absence of ejaculation/orgasm in all circumstances. Typically, the history is brief and clearly indicates that this is acquired and dates from the onset of the use of a particular medication (see "Etiology" below in this chapter). Occasionally this may be life long. Cultural or religious beliefs may also be a critical factor.

On some occasions, the history reveals a hybrid form, that is, one that has characteristics of both syndromes. Ejaculation is possible but only during masturbation. When ejaculation does occur in such circumstances, vigorous and lengthy penile stimulation is usually required—much more so than can be provided by vaginal intercourse.

A 35-year-old single man described an inability to ejaculate with a partner in spite of intercourse lasting up to one hour. Women partners initially enjoyed the experience and would find themselves repeatedly orgasmic. However, this attitude was soon replaced by one of impatience as the pleasure was superseded by the vaginal discomfort accompanying the long duration of intercourse. He described being able to ejaculate only with masturbation in a process that required about 15 minutes and great physical exertion in which he "worked" so hard he would sweat. He forcefully rubbed his penis against a hard surface while fantasizing about himself dressed as a woman.

Epidemiology

In the Laumann study, 8% of men reported being "unable to orgasm"[10](pp. 370-374). (The investigators did not apparently distinguish between ejaculation/orgasm that was delayed and that which was entirely absent.) The age category in which this syndrome was reported with greatest frequency was the 50 to 54 year old group (14%). Inability to come to orgasm was also reported more commonly in "Asian/Pacific Islander" men (19%), as well as those who were poorly educated (13%—less than high school), and financially poor (16%). As with other dysfunctions, the percentages of affected men increased with diminished health (18% of those whose health was "fair") and happiness (23% of men who were "unhappy most times").

In the Lauman study,[10] 8% of men reported being "unable to orgasm." (The investigators did not apparently distinguish between ejaculation/orgasm that was delayed and that which was entirely absent.)

"Male Orgasm Disorder" accounted for 3% to 8% of cases presenting for treatment in a review of clinical studies.[11]

Etiology

In the situational and hybrid forms, it is evident that specific sexual and/or psychosocial factors are central to etiological speculations[25] (pp.179-185); [1](p. 126). Theories include:

1. That some men are highly reactive genitally
2. That some men are fearful of dangers associated with ejaculation
3. An inhibition reflex
4. Religious orthodoxy
5. Male fear of pregnancy
6. Sexual interest in other men
7. A psychologically traumatic event

In the acquired and generalized form, there is often a history of recent use of a medication that is known to interfere with ejaculation/orgasm (see Appendix V) or the presence of a neurological disorder such as multiple sclerosis.

> All drugs approved for treatment of depression or obsessive-compulsive disorder in the United States with the exception of nefazodone and bupropion are reported to be associated with ejaculatory or orgasmic difficulty.[26]

"All of the drugs approved for the treatment of depression or the treatment of obsessive-compulsive disorder in the United States, with the exception of nefazodone and bupropion, have been reported to be associated with ejaculatory or orgasmic difficulty."[26] Prevalence figures for any one of the drugs varies as a result of different sources (manufacturer or published report) or variations in methodology (spontaneous reports or direct inquiry). Ejaculatory problems (delay or inhibition) have been reported in patients taking the following drugs:

- Imipramine (30%)
- Phenelzine (40%)
- Clomipramine (96%)
- Fluoxetine (24% to 75%)
- Sertraline (16%)
- Paroxetine (13%)
- Venlafaxine (12%)

Some antihypertensive drugs also interfere with ejaculation/orgasm. One of the problems in investigating the extent of this problem is that hypertension can cause sexual difficulties apart from the drugs used in its treatment. "Ejaculatory dysfunction" was not found at all in two studies that included normotensives, but was associated with 7% to 17% of untreated, and 26% to 30% of treated patients[27] (p. 204). Antihypertensive drugs that can cause sexual difficulties were reviewed[27]: and, in relation to delayed ejaculation, specifically included the following:

- Reserpine (p. 216)
- Methyldopa (p. 219)
- Guanethidine (p. 224)

- Alpha$_1$ blockers (p. 235)
- Alpha$_2$ agonists (p. 237)
- Calcium channel blockers (p. 245)

Notably missing from this list were the following:

- Diuretics (p. 210)
- Beta-blockers (p. 227)
- ACE inhibitors (p. 242)

Investigation
History

1. Duration (see Chapter 4, "lifelong versus acquired")

Suggested Question: "HAS EJACULATION DIFFICULTY BEEN A PROBLEM ALL YOUR LIFE OR IS IT A PROBLEM THAT DEVELOPED RECENTLY?"

2. Ejaculation with a partner (see Chapter 4, "generalized versus situational")

Suggested Question: "DO YOU EJACULATE AT ALL NOW WHEN YOU ARE WITH A PARTNER?"

Additional Question if the Answer is "No": "HAVE YOU EVER EJACULATED WITH A PARTNER?"

Additional Question if the Answer to Either Previous Question is "Yes": "WHAT KIND OF SEXUAL ACTIVITY RESULTED IN YOUR EJACULATION (E.G., INTERCOURSE OR ORAL STIMULATION)?"

3. Ejaculation with masturbation (see Chapter 4, "generalized versus situational")

Suggested Question: "DO YOU EJACULATE NOW WHEN YOU MASTURBATE?"

Additional Question if the Answer is "No": "HAVE YOU EVER EJACULATED WHEN YOU MASTURBATED?"

4. Feeling prior to ejaculation/orgasm (see Chapter 4, "description")

Suggested Question: "DO YOU SOMETIMES FEEL THAT YOU ARE CLOSE TO EJACULATION/ ORGASM BUT THEN THE FEELING DISAPPEARS?"

Additional Question: "WHEN WITH A PARTNER, DO YOU EVER PRETEND THAT YOU HAVE COME TO ORGASM?"

Physical and Laboratory Examinations

In an otherwise healthy man, no particular physical or laboratory examinations are required.

Treatment

In the care of men with the situational form of DE/O, reported series are few. Masters and Johnson described their treatment format and their five-year follow-up of 17 men and reported a treatment failure rate of 17.6%[1] (pp. 116-136, p.357). Another three-year follow-up study in the United States described the treatment of five men[15] who reported themselves as:

Three men	Improved
One man	The same
One man	Worse

A one to six year follow-up study conducted in the United Kingdom described two cases of "ejaculatory failure" and reported that in one there was no change, and in the other, the problem was resolved although still experienced.[28] No other case studies involving large numbers of patients have been published.

> Men with DE/O usually do not ask for treatment until they are pressured into it by a sexual partner. By then, many sexual experiences may have taken place, resulting in a firmly established pattern of ejaculation that may be difficult to change.

On the basis of impression rather than data, the occasional man with DE/O asks for care in his teens, and soon after intercourse experiences have begun. Such men may be amenable to the reassurance and provision of information that often comes with history-taking alone. The health professional might be justifiably optimistic about the result in such circumstances. Unfortunately, in most instances, men with DE/O do not ask for treatment until years later when they are pressured into it by a sexual partner. By that time, many sexual experiences have taken place (either alone or with partners) with a particular method of ejaculation, a pattern that may have become crystallized and difficult to change.

In the generalized form of DE/O, and when there is reason to suspect the use of a medication in the etiology, the following treatment "strategies" are suggested:

1. Maintain dosage of the medication and wait for tolerance to develop
2. Reducing the dosage
3. Change the regimen (e.g., the use of a "drug holiday")[29]
4. Change to an alternative medication (e.g., when the sexual side effects of sertraline and nefazodone were compared in the treatment of depression, nefazodone was said to have no inhibitory effects on ejaculation)[30]
5. Administer a second medication to counter the sexual side-effect of the first (see immediately below)[26]

Two potential problems exist when using other medications at the same time: the clinician must ensure that the second medication does not counteract the *therapeutic* impact of the first, and sexual spontaneity inevitably diminishes somewhat when planning precedes the sexual event (although often an exaggerated patient concern).

Segraves described seven medications that have been used in an effort to control the sexual side-effects of antidepressants (mostly SSRIs): bethanechol, cyproheptadine, yohimbine, amantadine, bupropion, dextroamphetamine, and penoline.[26] Methylphenidate has been suggested[31] also, as well as intermittent nefazodone[32] (Box 10-1 and Table 10-1).

Box 10-1

Strategies in Treating Delayed Ejaculation/Orgasm due to Antidepressant Drugs

1. Wait for tolerance to develop
2. Decrease dosage
3. Change regimen (e.g., "drug holiday")
4. Use alternate drugs
5. Use additional drugs ("antidotes")

Table 10-1 Drug Treatment of Delayed Ejaculation/Orgasm Due to Antidepressant Medications

DRUG	DOSAGE
Bethanecol	10-20 mg 1-2 hours pre IC
Cyproheptadine	4-8 mg 1-2 hours pre IC
Yohimbine	5.4-10.8 mg as needed
Amantadine	100-400 mg as needed
Bupropion	75 mg per day
Penoline	18.75 mg per day
Methylphenidate	5-25 mg as needed
Dextroamphetamine	5 mg sublingual 1 hr pre sex activity
Nefazodone	150 mg 1 hour pre IC

IC, Intercourse

Since outcome research has not subclassified patients, one can only provide clinical impressions about the generalized and lifelong form of DE/O. Given that biological factors likely explain the etiology, helping the patient adapt through the provision of information seems the optimal approach.

Indications for Referral for Consultation or Continuing Care by a Specialist

1. Situational DE/O: If this pattern of ejaculation has existed for some years, referral for sex therapy for the purpose of continuing care may be most beneficial
2. Acquired and generalized DE/O: where medications seem etiologically significant but the symptom has not altered with the strategies outlined in Box 10-1, it is reasonable to ask for advice (consultation) from a physician who has expertise in the use of the particular class of drugs
3. Lifelong and generalized DE/O: if the provision of information and reassurance about the likely positive outcome proves insufficient, referral to a sex therapist for continuing care is the next logical step

Summary

Delayed Ejaculation usually represents a disorder (delay or absence) of both ejaculation and orgasm, hence the use of the abbreviation, "DE/O." The disorder appears in two forms:

- Situational, in that the man can come to ejaculation/orgasm without problem when alone but has great difficulty when a partner is present
- Generalized in the sense that the man has difficulty under all circumstances (with a partner or when alone with masturbation)

While unusual, the problem of delayed ejaculation is by no means rare (8% of men in one community survey indicated inability "to orgasm"). Etiologies are as follows:

1. The situational form includes significant psychosocial factors
2. The lifelong and generalized form includes biological factors that have not yet been defined
3. The acquired and generalized form can usually be explained by the use of medications (especially medications used in Psychiatry and in the control of hypertension) or the onset of a neurological disorder

The effects of treatment in the situational form seem better when the duration of the problem is brief. Several approaches are suggested for the generalized and acquired form where the etiology is related to medications. Treatment for the lifelong and generalized form can generally be undertaken initially on a primary care level through the provision of information and reassurance. Men with the acquired and generalized form who have never ejaculated in the waking state require care from a specialist.

RETROGRADE EJACULATION

Definition

Retrograde ejaculation (RE) "is the propulsion of seminal fluid from the posterior urethra into the bladder".[33] What is usually referred to as "ejaculation" actually comprises three separate events[34] (p. 423):

- First, "emission"
- Second, closure of the "bladder neck"
- Third, "ejaculation"

Emission involves the deposition of seminal fluid from the vas deferens, the seminal vesicles, and prostate gland into the posterior urethra. Ejaculation refers to the expulsion of semen from the penis, which, in turn, requires simultaneous closure of the muscular valve at the junction between the urethra and bladder (the bladder "neck"). This blockage prevents the semen from traveling backward into the bladder instead of going forward out the end of a man's penis. The expulsion of semen (true ejaculation) also involves intermittent relaxation of the "external sphincter"; there are three to seven contractions about 0.8 seconds apart (see Figure 10-3).

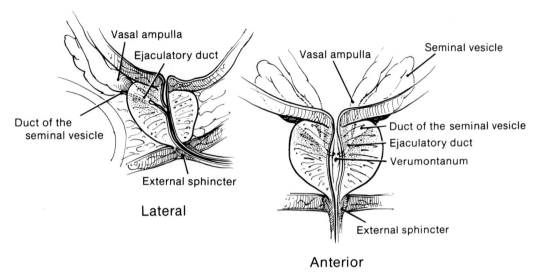

Figure 10-3   Anatomy of male accessory sex organs. (From Shaban SF, Seaman EK, Lipshultz LI: Treatment of abnormalities of ejaculation. In Lipshultz LI, Howards SS (editors): *Infertility in the male,* ed 3, St. Louis, 1997, Mosby.)

The final portion of this process comprises rhythmic contractions of the bulbospongiosus and ischiocavernosus muscles, resulting in forward movement of seminal fluid through the anterior urethra and emerging from the penile meatus. Orgasm is considered a cerebral event that occurs together with emission or ejaculation and associated with unknown physiological mechanisms[35] (p. 155).

Emission and bladder neck closure appear to be predominantly under the control of the sympathetic portion of the autonomic nervous system, and the expulsion of semen is predominately under the influence of the somatic nervous system[35] (pp. 165-166). "Any interference (anatomical, traumatic, neurogenic or drug-induced) with (the integrity of these systems) may result in abnormal function of the internal sphincter of the urethra, and favor retrograde ejaculation (RE) as the path of least resistance".[36]

Etiology

One way of considering etiological factors in RE is to separate them into (1) ones that disrupt the anatomy of the sphincter at the bladder neck and (2) ones that interfere with this sphincter's function[37] (p. 383). The best example of an anatomical disruption of this sphincter is a transurethral prostatectomy (TURP). Examples of factors that interfere with function of this sphincter include the following:

1. Retroperitoneal lymph node dissection (RPLND) or total lymphadenectomy in the treatment of some testicular cancers
2. Diabetes
3. Abdominopelvic surgery
4. Spinal cord injury

Some medications can induce a pharmacologic "sympathectomy" resulting in failure of emission and/or bladder neck closure (see Appendix V). These drugs[34] (p. 427) include the following antipsychotics (e.g., chlorpromazine and Haldol), antidepressants (e.g., amitriptyline and SSRIs), antihypertensives (e.g., guanethidine, diuretics and prazosin), and others (including alcohol).

Epidemiology

RE seems to be common as a complication of TURP but the actual frequency is not entirely clear. In one study of men before and after surgery, 24% who had no presurgical difficulty with ejaculation answered "yes" to the following question after surgery: "Do you have difficulty with getting the sperm out?"[38] However, 37% of the men who had no presurgical difficulty also said that they had no ejaculatory problem afterward.

Given the frequency with which RE seems to occur as a result of TURP, the aging of the population (assuming TURP continues to be medically popular as a treatment of benign prostatic hypertrophy) might well result in an increase in the prevalence of RE.

RE seems to be infrequent as a cause of infertility in men (up to 2%)[37] (p. 383).

Investigation

History reveals that the patient reports not ejaculating while (in the majority of cases) continuing to experience orgasm ("dry orgasm"). The definitive diagnosis is made by laboratory examination of the man's urine immediatly after orgasm, and finding spermatozoa in the sample.

Treatment

> Most men who develop RE as a consequence of TURP accept this situation and do not ask for treatment. When care is required (usually because of infertility), RE is best managed by physicians. The focus of infertility treatment is on attempting to induce antegrade ejaculation by increasing sympathetic tone at the bladder neck or diminishing parasympathetic activity.[33]

Most men who develop RE as a consequence of TURP accept this situation and do not ask for treatment. When care is required (usually because of infertility), RE is best managed by physicians. The focus of infertility treatment is on attempting to induce antegrade ejaculation by increasing sympathetic tone at the bladder neck or diminishing parasympathetic activity.[33] Alpha-adrenergic agents are commonly used to enhance sympathetic tone. In a detailed study of one patient who stopped ejaculating as a result of lymphadenectomy, four such drugs were used[39] and all seemed equally efficacious:

1. Dextroamphetamine sulphate, 5 mg four times daily
2. Ephedrine, 25 mg four times daily
3. Phenylpropanolamine, 75 mg twice daily
4. Pseudoephedrine, 60 mg four times daily

The study concluded that long-term treatment was consistently more effective than a single dose. Elliott (personal communication, 1997) found that in patients who have RE as a result of a spinal injury the effects of pseudoephedrine, in particular, can diminish if used continuously for more than four days, and that it may be more useful to use it on an "as needed" basis Anticholinergics have also been used successfully (brompheniramine 8 mg twice daily) and imipramine (25 to 50 mg daily). Surgery has also been suggested.[33]

When antegrade ejaculation can not be restored the treatment of infertility involves inseminating the woman with sperm cells taken from the urine by the process of centrifugation. In one group of eight patients with RE, the combination of alkalinization of the urine, immediate removal of sperm cells from the urine, and the implementation of artificial insemination techniques resulted in a "fecundity rate" of 45%[40] (p. 440).

When psychological concerns exist, they often relate to surprise and apprehension if, for example, a patient who has undergone a TURP was not forewarned about not seeing semen when he ejaculates. Psychological concerns may also be about other accompanying factors such as the possible presence of erectile or orgasmic difficulties and infertility. These other issues can have powerful repercussions.

Indications for Referral for Consultation or Continuing Care by a Specialist

As an isolated issue, RE does not appear to be a cause of further sexual difficulties. To the extent that sexual concerns are related to information, primary care treatment is usually sufficient. Consultation with a sexual medicine specialist may be useful in instances when RE is associated with other sexual difficulties. When infertility concerns result from RE (generally younger men of reproductive age who have experienced retroperitoneal lymph node dissection or total lymphadenectomy for the treatment of testicular cancer), continuing care should be undertaken by an expert physician.

Summary

Retrograde ejaculation (RE) is usually reported by a man as an orgasm without the associated emergence of semen ("dry orgasm"). Semen travels "backward" into the bladder and the definitive diagnosis can be made by the finding of spermatozoa in the urine. The most common cause of RE is the TURP procedure for benign prostatic hypertrophy. For most men, information is the only treatment needed. When fertility is a concern, medical treatment focus is on the attempt to enhance sympathetic tone at the bladder neck by using alpha-adrenergic agents or diminishing parasympathetic activity. Specialist care is required only in those instances where there are associated sexual difficulties or concerns about infertility.

INFREQUENT EJACULATION/ORGASM DISORDERS

Infrequent ejaculation/orgasm disorders include painful ejaculation, anejaculation and anorgasmic ejaculation. The assessment of infrequent ejaculation/orgasm disorders is outlined in Figure 10-4.

Reports of genital pain associated with ejaculation are uncommon. The following four causes are known:

1. Some of the tricyclic antidepressants (amoxapine [related to loxapine], imipramine, desipramine, clomipramine)[41,42]
2. Seminal vesicle calculi[43]
3. Urological surgery
4. Vacuum erection devices (VEDs)

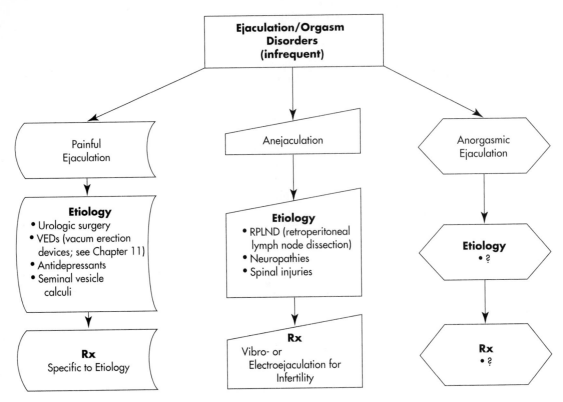

Figure 10-4   Assessment of infrequent ejaculation/orgasm disorders.

The first two explanations may not be immediately apparent. When associated with tricyclic antidepressants, ejaculatory pain is dose-related so that it diminishes when the dose is decreased and disappears when the medication is discontinued.[42]

The absence of ejaculation, or anejaculation (antegrade or retrograde), occurs as a result of peripheral sympathetic neuropathy[44] (pp. 404-6). It occurs in men with spinal cord injury, men who had retroperitoneal lymph node dissection (RPLND) for testicular cancer, and in neuropathies such as those seen in multiple sclerosis and diabetes. Diagnosis is based on the absence of seminal fluid in postejaculatory urine to eliminate the possibility of RE. Emission/ejaculation and subsequent pregnancy can result from the use of specialized procedures such as vibratory stimulation or electroejaculation.[45]

Ejaculation without orgasm is quite unusual judging from the literature and clinical experience. The etiology is unknown.

A 47-year-old man was seen with the complaint of ejaculating without the sensation of orgasm. He vividly recalled the powerful feeling of orgasm in the past and hoped that it would return. The sensation of orgasm tapered during the past three years so that it was virtually absent at the present time—regardless if he ejaculated with masturbation or with a partner. He had previously been married for 12 years and had experienced premature ejaculation throughout all of the marriage. In four of the seven years after his divorce, his sexual experiences with other women were described with relish, particularly since he was then free of any ejaculatory difficulty. His general health was unimpaired, his sexual desire was as strong as ever, and he never experienced any erectile difficulties. When seen one year after his initial consultation, the problem had not changed.

REFERENCES

1. Masters WH, Johnson VE: *Human sexual inadequacy*, Boston, 1970, Little, Brown and Company.
2. McCarthy BW: Cognitive-behavioral strategies and techniques in the treatment of early ejaculation. In Leiblum SR, Rosen RC (editors): *Principles and practice of sex therapy: update for the 1990s*, ed 2, New York, 1989, The Guilford Press, pp. 141-167.
3. Grenier G, Byers ES: Rapid ejaculation: a review of conceptual, etiological, and treatment issues, *Arch Sex Behav* 24:447-472, 1995.
4. Althof SE: Pharmacologic treatment of rapid ejaculation. In Levine S (editor): *Psychiatr Clin North Am* 18:85-94, 1995.
5. *Diagnostic and statistical manual of mental disorders*, ed 4, revised, Washington, 1987, American Psychiatric Association.
6. *Diagnostic and statistical manual of mental disorders*, ed 4, primary care version, Washington, 1995, American Psychiatric Association.
7. Masters WH, Johnson, VE: *Homosexuality in Perspective*, Boston, 1979, Little, Brown and Co.
8. Simon Rosser BR et al: Sexual difficulties, concerns, and satisfaction in homosexual men: an empirical study with implications for HIV prevention, *J Sex Marital Ther* 23:61-73,1997.
9. Kinsey AC, Pomeroy WB, Martin CE: *Sexual behavior in the human male*, Philadelphia and London, 1949, W.B. Saunders.
10. Laumann EO et al: *The social organization of sexuality: sexual practices in the United States*, Chicago, 1994, The University of Chicago Press.
11. Spector IP, Carey MP: Incidence and prevalence of the sexual dysfunctions, *Arch Sex Behav* 19:389-408, 1990.
12. Godpodinoff ML: Premature ejaculation: clinical subgroups and etiology, *J Sex Marital Ther* 15:130-134, 1989.
13. Strassberg DS et al: The role of anxiety in premature ejaculation: a psychophysiological model, *Arch Sex Behav* 19:251-257, 1990.
14. Masters WH, Johnson VE: *Human Sexual Response*, Boston, 1966, Little, Brown and Co.
15. De Amicis LA et al: Clinical follow-up of couples treated for sexual dysfunction, *Arch Sex Behav* 14:467-489, 1985.
16. Balon R: Antidepressants in the treatment of premature ejaculation, *J Sex Marital Ther* 22:85-96, 1996.
17. Waldinger MD, Hengeveld MW, Zwinderman AH: Paroxetine treatment of premature ejaculation: a double-blind, randomized, placebo-controlled study, *Am J Psychiatry* 151:1377-1379, 1994.
18. Mendels J, Camera A, Sikes C: Sertraline treatment for premature ejaculation, *J Clin Psychopharmacology* 15:341-346, 1995.
19. Haensel SM et al: Clomipramine and sexual function in men with premature ejaculation and controls, *J Urol* 156:1310-1315, 1996.
20. Zilbergeld B: *Male sexuality*, New York, 1978, Bantam Books.
21. Kaplan HS: *PE:how to overcome premature ejaculation*, New York, 1989, Brunner/Mazel, Inc.
22. Zilbergeld B: *The new male sexuality*, New York, 1992, Bantam Books.

23. Semans JH: Premature ejaculation: a new approach, *South Med J* 49:353-358, 1956.

24. Kaplan HS: *The new sex therapy: active treatment of sexual dysfunctions*, New York, 1974, Brunner/Mazel.

25. Apfelbaum B: Retarded ejaculation: a much-misunderstood syndrome. In Leiblum SR, Rosen RC (editors): *Principles and practice of sex therapy: update for the 1990s*, ed. 2, New York, 1989, The Guilford Press, pp. 168-206.

26. Segraves RT: Antidepressant-induced orgasm disorder, *J Sex Marital* Ther 21:192-201, 1995.

27. Crenshaw TL, Goldberg, JP: *Sexual pharmacology: drugs that affect sexual function*, New York, 1996, W.W. Norton & Company.

28. Hawton K et al: Long-term outcome of sex therapy, *Behav Res Ther* 24:665-675, 1986.

29. Rothschild AJ: Selective serotonin reuptake inhibitor-induced sexual dysfunction: efficacy of a drug holiday, *Am J Psychiatry* 152:1514-1516, 1995.

30. Feiger A et al: Nefazodone versus sertraline in outpatients with major depression: focus on efficacy, tolerability, and effects on sexual function and satisfaction, *J Clin Psychiatry* 57(Suppl 2):53-62, 1996.

31. Bartlik BD, Kaplan P, Kaplan HS: Psychostimulants apparently reverse sexual dysfunction secondary to selective serotonin reuptake inhibitors, *J Sex Marital Ther* 21:264-271, 1995.

32. Reynolds RD: Sertraline-induced anorgasmia treated with intermittent Nefazodone (letter), *J Clin Psychiatry* 58:89, 1997.

33. Hershlag A, Schiff SF, DeCherney, AH: Retrograde ejaculation, *Hum Reprod* 6:255-258, 1991.

34. Shaban SF, Seaman EK, Lipshultz LI: Treatment of abnormalities of ejaculation. In Lipshultz LI, Howards SS (editors): *Infertility in the male*, ed 3, St. Louis, 1997, Mosby, pp. 423-438.

35. Benson GS: Erection, emission, and ejaculation: physiological mechanisms. In Lipshultz LI, Howards SS (editors): *Infertility in the male*, ed 3, St. Louis, 1997, Mosby-Year Book, Inc., pp. 155-172.

36. Yavetz H et al: Retrograde ejaculation, *Hum Reprod* 93:381-386, 1994.

37. Oates RD: Nonsurgical treatment of infertility: specific therapy. In Lipshultz LI, Howards SS (editors): *Infertility in the male*, ed 2, St. Louis, 1991, Mosby - Year Book, Inc., pp 376-394.

38. Thorpe AC et al: Written consent about sexual function in men undergoing transurethral prostatectomy, *Br J Urol* 74:479-484, 1994.

39. Proctor KG, Howards SS: The effect of sympathomimetic drugs on post-lymphadenectomy aspermia, *J Urol* 129:837-838, 1983.

40. Gilbaugh JH: Intrauterine insemination. In Lipshultz LI, Howard SS (editors): *Infertility in the male*, ed 3, St. Louis, 1997, Mosby, pp. 439-449.

41. Kulik FA, Wilbur R: Case report of painful ejaculation as a side effect of Amoxapine, *Am J Psychiatry* 139:234-235, 1982.

42. Aizenberg D et al: Painful ejaculation associated with antidepressants in four patients, *J Clin Psychiatry* 52:461-463, 1991.

43. Corriere JN Jr: Painful ejaculation due to seminal vesicle calculi, *J Urol* 157:626, 1997.

44. Hakim LS, Oates AD: Nonsurgical treatment of male infertility: specific therapy. In Lipshultz LI, Howards SS (editors): *Infertility in the male*, ed 2, St. Louis, 1997, Mosby.

45. Elliott S et al: Vibrostimulation and electroejaculation: the Vancouver experience, *J Soc Obstet Gyncol Can* 15:390-404, 1993.

CHAPTER 11

ERECTION DISORDERS

*Despite the current rhetoric. . . . about sex and intimacy's involving more than penile-vaginal inter-
course, the quest for a rigid erection appears to dominate both popular and professional interest. Moreover, it seems likely that our diligence in finding new ways for overcoming erectile difficulties serves
unwittingly to reinforce the male myth that rock-hard, ever-available phalluses are a necessary component of male identity. This is indeed a dilemma.*

ROSEN AND LEIBLUM, 1992[1]

GENERAL CONSIDERATIONS
The Problem

A 49-year-old widower described erection difficulties for the past year. His 25-year
marriage was loving and harmonious throughout but sexual activity stopped after
his wife was diagnosed with ovarian cancer six years before her death. Their sexual
relationship during the period of her illness had been meager as a result of her lack
of sexual desire. Although he missed her greatly, he felt lonely since her death
three years before and, somewhat reluctantly at first, began dating other women. A
resumption of sexual activity soon resulted but much to his chagrin he found that
in contrast to when he would awaken in the morning or masturbate, his erections
with women partners were much less firm. He felt considerable tension, particularly because some months before, he had developed a strong attachment to one
woman in particular and was fearful that the relationship would soon end because
of his sexual troubles. As he discussed his grief over the loss of his wife and talked
about his guilt over his intimacy with another woman, his erectile problems began
to diminish.

A 67-year-old man, married for 39 years, and having a history of angina prior to a
coronary by-pass operation three years before was referred to a "sex clinic"
together with his wife because of his erectile difficulties. Sexual experiences had
been enjoyable and uncomplicated for both until he developed angina at the age
of 62. Orgasm provoked his chest pain. Nitroglycerin was prescribed but he used
it only occasionally because it resulted in headache. His angina during sexual activity was frightening to his wife who, nevertheless, recognized the importance of

sexual experiences in his life and supported his desire to continue being sexually active. Cardiac surgery resulted in the disappearance of his chest pain. However, some months before his operation, he began to experience difficulty becoming fully erect at any time, and would frequently lose whatever fullness he had before vaginal entry occurred. His erectile difficulties with his wife had become persistent and when questioned, it was apparent that his morning erections were not different. Sildenafil (Viagra) was dismissed as a treatment possibility because of his occasional use of nitroglycerin. He was referred to a urologist for intracavernosal injections.

Terminology

The phrase "erectile dysfunction" has provided competition for the more popular word "impotence." The latter has a tenacity for usage that does not exist for the female equivalent and now rarely-seen word, "frigidity." Both words have similar deficiencies: they are so broad in usage they (1) incorporate disorders of desire and function and (2) imply something pejorative about the patient's personality quite apart from their sexual expression.[2]

The social confusion surrounding the word "impotence" is, perhaps, exemplified by the first recommendation of the National Institutes of Health Consensus Statement on Impotence, which was to change the term *impotence* to *erectile dysfunction* as a way of characterizing "the inability to attain and/or maintain penile erection sufficient for satisfactory sexual performance."[3] (Interestingly, no conference was necessary to change usage of the word "frigidity").

Mechanism of Erection

The fundamental element in the development of an erection is the trapping of blood in the penis. The mechanism by which this occurs was described by Lue and Tanagho (Figure 11-1). A human penis has three cylinders: Paired corpora cavernosa (CC) on the dorsal surface, and the completely separate corpus spongiosum (CS), which carries the urethra and is responsible for the ventral bulge.

The CS anatomically includes the glans of the penis. The CC are each surrounded by an inflexible envelope of fibrous tissue: the tunica albuginea (TA). The CS has a much thinner TA and is connected to the glans, which has almost none.

> As an erection develops, the smooth muscle around the arterial tree and walls of the sinusoids relaxes, increasing the inflow of blood into the penis and allowing more blood to remain. While expansion occurs, the venules are compressed between the sinusoids and TA, thereby stopping the outflow and in effect trapping blood in the sinusoids of the penis.

Blood is carried to the penis by the two internal pudendal arteries and within the penis by paired cavernosal arteries. The latter subsequently divide into smaller vessels (arterioles), which are surrounded by smooth muscle. The same can be said of the helicine arteries (small spiral shaped arteries). In the CC and CS, blood is then carried to interconnecting sinusoids (microlakes, which have the appearance of a sponge when filled but are mostly collapsed when a penis is flaccid), which are also surrounded by smooth muscle. Small veins (venules) carry blood away to the emissary veins, which in turn pierce the TA.

As an erection develops, there is relaxation of the smooth muscle around the arterial tree and walls of the sinusoids, increasing the inflow

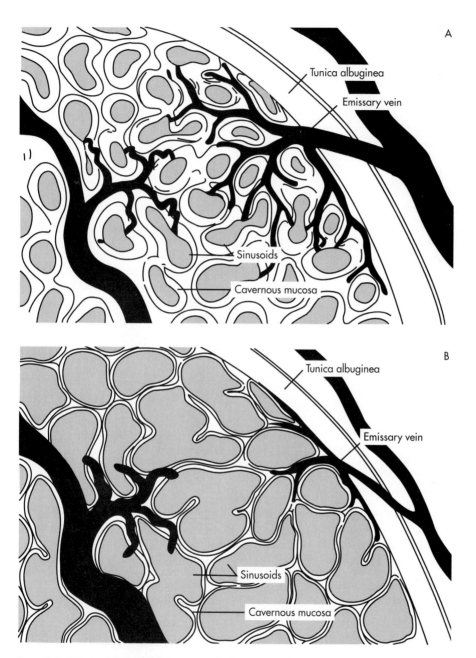

Figure 11-1   The mechanism of penile erection. In the flaccid state (**A**), the arteries, arterioles, and sinusoids are contracted. The intersinusoidal and subtunical venular plexuses are wide open, with free flow to the emissary veins. In the erect state (**B**), the muscles of the sinusoidal wall and the arterioles relax, allowing maximal flow to the compliant sinusoidal spaces. Most of the venules are compressed between the expanding sinusoids. Even the larger intermediary venules are sandwiched and flattened by distended sinusoids and the noncompliant tunica albuginea. This effectively reduces the venous capacity to a minimum. (From Lue TF: *Male sexual dysfunction.* In Tanagho EA, MaCninish JW: *Smith's general urology,* Stamford, 1992, Appleton & Lange, p. 669.)

of blood into the penis and allowing more blood to remain. While expansion occurs, the venules are compressed between the sinusoids and TA, thereby stopping the outflow and in effect trapping blood in the sinusoids of the penis. "The smooth muscles in the arteriolar wall and trabeculae surrounding the sinusoids are the controlling mechanism of penile erection."[4]

(Biochemical aspects of erection are discussed in the treatment section of " Generalized Erectile Dysfunction: Organic, Mixed, or Undetermined Origin" below in this chapter).

Definition

The main difficulty with the definition of erectile dysfunction is whether the diagnosis of erectile problems should refer only to the hardness or softness of a man's erection or if it should also include a behavioral component. For example, should a man who has erections that are persistently partial but whose penis is sufficiently enlarged to regularly engage in intercourse be designated as having an "erectile disorder?" If that same man designates himself as "impotent," what should be the diagnostic position of the health professional? Should there be a subjective component to an erectile disorder: does it make any difference what the man (or his partner) thinks? Is the fullness of a man's penis in intercourse all that matters? Is intercourse the only sexual activity on which the definition is based? What about erections with other sexual practices? These, and other questions, are not intellectual exercises but daily clinical quandaries.

Classification

> Erectile dysfunction in all situations, including the lack of nocturnal erections, strongly suggests that a general medical condition or substance use is the cause.[5]

DSM-IV-PC summarized the criteria for the diagnosis of "Male Erectile Disorder" as follows: "persistent or recurrent inability to attain, or to maintain until completion of the sexual activity, an adequate erection, causing marked distress or interpersonal difficulty"[5](p. 116). The clinician is further instructed to "especially consider problems due to a general medical condition . . . such as diabetes or vascular disease, and problems due to substance use . . . such as alcohol and prescription medication. *Erectile dysfunction in all situations, as well as lack of nocturnal erections, strongly suggests that a general medical condition or substance use is the cause*"(italics added).

The subclassification of Erectile Disorders used in this chapter is summarized in Figure 11-2.

Epidemiology

The Massachusetts Male Aging Study (MMAS) provided revealing information about erectile function, dysfunction, and "potency" in middle-aged and older men.[6] The study was conducted in the late 80s, was concerned with health and aging in men, was community-based, and involved a random sample of noninstitutionalized men 40 to 70 years old. Individuals who completed a self-administered questionnaire on sexual function and activity included 1290 (75%) of the 1709 MMAS subjects. "Potency" was subjective in that it was defined by those who completed the questionnaires. Defined as "satisfactory functional capacity for erection," "potency" could "coexist with some

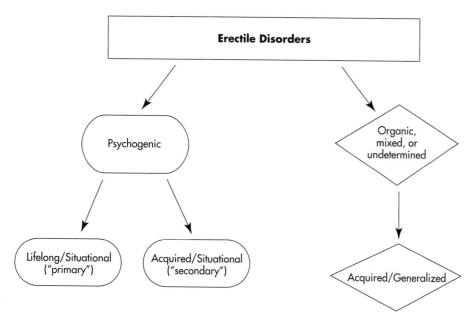

Figure 11-2 Classification of erectile disorders.

degree of erectile dysfunction in the sense of submaximal rigidity or submaximal capability to sustain the erection." Four degrees of "impotence" were described:

- None
- Minimal
- Moderate
- Complete

The overall prevalence of impotence in this study was found to be 52%, with 15% defined as minimal, 25% moderate, and 10% complete. Prevalence was highly related to age with the probability of moderate impotence doubling from 17% to 34% and complete impotence tripling from 5% to 15% between subject ages 40 to 70 years. Looking at this from the opposite perspective, 60% of men were *not* impotent at age 40 years, compared to 33% *not* impotent at age 70 years.

> Sixty percent of men were not impotent at age 40 compared to 33% not impotent at age 70 years.

The frequency of erectile problems found in health care settings seems to depend somewhat on the clinical context. That is, different percentages can be found in various clinical settings: medical outpatients, urology, and sex therapy[7] (p. 11). In a review of the frequency of sexual problems presented to "sex clinics" between the mid-70s to 1990, 36% to 53% of men complained of "male erectile disorder."[8] Masters and Johnson subcategorized this diagnosis into "primary" and "secondary".[9] The former referred to a man who had never had intercourse (p. 137), and the latter referred to a man who had been able to have intercourse at least once in the past (p.157). Of all the men with "impotence" who consulted Masters & Johnson, 13% had the primary form (p. 367).

Etiology

"Repeatedly bandied about is the hackneyed declaration that in the 1970s, mental health professionals pronounced 90% of impotence to be psychogenic; more recently urologists proclaim that 90% of impotence is organic. Both sides are wrong, not just for the disrespectful attitudes toward one another, but for failing to develop more sophisticated notions of etiology."[10]

LoPiccolo saw clinical limitations to the either/or approach and suggested an alternative way of thinking about the etiology of erectile dysfunctions: that organic and psychogenic factors be viewed as two "separate and independently varying dimensions" and that *both* should be examined in *each* instance.[11] To support this position, he reported on 63 men with erectile difficulties who were carefully and thoroughly investigated in both areas. Ten men were found to have a purely psychogenic etiology, and three men were found to have a purely organic etiology. The majority of men in this study (50/63) displayed a mixture of factors, indicating that a "two-category typology was . . . inappropriate." Furthermore, almost one third of the men (19/63) had "mild organic impairments" but "significant psychological problems." These men might have been considered "organic" in a two-part etiological scheme, however, they might also have been sufficiently responsive to psychological intervention such that physical treatment may not have been necessary.

In a diagnostic and a therapeutic sense, the implication of LoPiccolo's approach is quite serious. It means that even if a factor that is of *potential* etiological significance is found (biological or psychological), it is not necessarily *the* factor. Or, in other words, "the detection of some possible etiological factor . . . does not mean that the cause . . . has been fully explained. Such a factor may even be coincidental, of no (actual) etiological significance."[12]

The possible nature of the interrelationship between biological and psychological factors was suggested as the following: "When any one (organic factor) occurs in isolation, it may serve to make erections more vulnerable to emotional disturbances and sympathetic overactivity, facilitating the vicious circle of performance anxiety that maintains ED."[12]

Investigation

History

History-taking is an indispensable element in the investigation of erectile disorders and provides direction for further exploration and treatment. Issues to inquire about and questions to ask include:

1. Duration (see Chapter 4, "lifelong versus acquired")

Suggested Question: "HAVE YOU ALWAYS HAD DIFFICULTIES WITH ERECTIONS OR IS THIS A RELATIVELY NEW PROBLEM?"

2. Partner-related erections (see Chapter 4, "generalized" versus "situational")

Suggested Question: "WHAT ARE YOUR ERECTIONS LIKE WHEN YOU ARE WITH YOUR WIFE (PARTNER)?"

3. Sleep [including morning] erections (see Chapter 4, "generalized versus situational")

Suggested Question: "WHAT ARE YOUR ERECTIONS LIKE WHEN YOU WAKE UP IN THE MORNING?"

Additional Question: "DO YOU WAKE UP AT NIGHT FOR ANY REASON?"

Additional Question if the Answer is Yes: "WHAT ARE YOUR ERECTIONS LIKE WHEN YOU WAKE UP AT NIGHT?"

(Comment: the assessment value of asking about sleep-related erections is generally recognized but not universally accepted.[13] When full sleep-related erections exist, the information seems highly useful from a diagnostic viewpoint. However, partial or nonexistent sleep erections are not necessarily meaningful since this situation may coexist with daytime erections firm enough for intercourse.)

4. Masturbation erections (see Chapter 4, "generalized versus situational")

Suggested Question: "WHAT ARE YOUR ERECTIONS LIKE WHEN YOU STIMULATE YOURSELF (OR MASTURBATE)?"

5. Fullness of erections (see Chapter 4, "description")

Suggested Question: "ON A SCALE OF ZERO TO TEN WHERE ZERO IS ENTIRELY SOFT AND TEN IS FULLY HARD AND STIFF, WHAT ARE YOUR ERECTIONS LIKE WHEN YOU ARE WITH YOUR WIFE (PARTNER)?"

Additional Question: "USING THE SAME SCALE, WHAT ARE YOUR ERECTIONS LIKE WHEN YOU WAKE UP IN THE MORNING?"

Additional Question: "IF YOU WAKE UP DURING THE NIGHT, USING THE SAME SCALE, WHAT ARE YOUR ERECTIONS LIKE AT THAT TIME?"

Additional Question: "USING THE SAME SCALE, WHAT ARE YOUR ERECTIONS LIKE WITH SELF-STIMULATION OR MASTURBATION?"

Additional Question Under All Three Circumstances: "ABOUT HOW LONG DO YOUR ERECTIONS LAST?"

(Comment: Even though erections may be full under all three circumstances, the duration of erections may be important. Erections may consistently be short-lived—a matter of diagnostic significance, since that observation may indicate a "venous leak").[13]

6. Psychological accompaniment (see Chapter 4, "patient and partner's reaction to problem")

Suggested Question: "WHEN YOU HAVE TROUBLE WITH YOUR ERECTION, WHAT'S GOING THROUGH YOUR MIND?"

Additional Question: "WHAT DOES YOUR WIFE (PARTNER) SAY AT THESE TIMES?"

Physical Examination

> In men with erectile difficulties, physical examination is essential even if the "yield is low."[12] Many patients feel that they have not been properly assessed or taken seriously if there is no physical examination, and they may refuse a psychogenic diagnosis as a result.[12]

In men with erectile difficulties, physical examination is essential even if the "yield is low."[12] "Without it many patients feel that they have not been properly assessed or taken seriously and they may refuse a psychogenic diagnosis as a result".[12] The physical examination concentrates particularly on the endocrine, vascular and neurologic systems, as well as local genital factors.

Signs of hormonal abnormalities include the following[14] (p. 85):

1. Testicular atrophy
2. Gynecomastia
3. Galactorrhea
4. Visual field abnormalities
5. Sparse body hair
6. Decreased beard growth
7. Skin hyperpigmentation
8. Signs of thyroid abnormalities
9. Low energy level and lack of "well-being"

Signs of vascular disease include the following[14] (p.91):

1. Weak pulses in legs or ankles
2. Hair loss on lower legs
3. Unusually cool temperature of penis or lower legs
4. High lipid levels
5. High cholesterol levels
6. Duputyren's contractures [Peyronie's disease only]
7. Fibrosis of outer ear cartilage [Peyronie's disease only]

Signs that indicate neurological factors include the following[14] (p. 93):

1. Weak or absent genital reflexes (bulbocavernosus, cremasteric, scrotal, internal anal, and superficial anal)
2. Neurological abnormalities in the S2 to S4 nerve root distribution
3. Reduced penile sensory thresholds to light touch electrical stimulation or vibration

An investigation conducted in a medical outpatient clinic found that the physical examination rarely helped to differentiate various etiological factors with two exceptions[15]:

- Small testes in patients with primary hypogonadism
- Peripheral neuropathy in patients with diabetes

Laboratory Investigation

The extent of a clinician's use of the laboratory in the investigation of erectile dysfunction depends on the results of the history and physical examination (see "Investigation" below in this Chapter in the sections on "Situational ['psychogenic'] Erectile Dysfunction" and "Generalized Erectile Dysfunction: Organic, Mixed, or Undetermined Origin."

Treatment

As LoPiccolo has shown, psychological and physiological factors are present in the vast majority of men with an erectile disorder.[11] "Psychological" factors include social, cultural, religious, and interpersonal elements, and those within the person. Since *all* sexual behavior of men is influenced to a great degree by these issues, it is reasonable to assume that these factors are present in the context of erectile difficulties as well. The logical result of LoPiccolo's research is the concept that regardless of the etiology of a man's erectile difficulties, a health care clinician must always attend to universally concomitant psychological issues. That is: "Given the critical role of psychological factors, even in cases with clearcut organic etiology, *the failure to attend to psychological issues is indefensible* (italics added). The potential impact of erectile difficulties on mood state, self-esteem and self-efficacy, as well as on the couple's relationship cannot be overemphasized."[16]

> Failure to attend to psychological issues is indefensible. The potential effect of erectile difficulties on mood state, self-esteem, and self-efficacy (as well as the couple's relationship) cannot be overemphasized.[16]

SITUATIONAL ("PSYCHOGENIC") ERECTILE DYSFUNCTION

The assessment of situational erectile disorders is summarized in Figure 11-3.

Description

Lifelong ("Primary") Erectile Disorders

In this unusual syndrome, the man reveals that all, or most, attempts at intercourse result in diminution of his erection before attempts at vaginal entry. Levine reasonably suggested that the definition of the disorder be "liberalized" to include men who gain vaginal entry "occasionally"[17] (p. 208), Typically, the man has no difficulty obtaining full erections when alone, with masturbation, or when awakening. Ejaculation and orgasm have been similarly unimpaired. The sexual desire phase may have been problematic if thoughts associated with sexual arousal were atypical (as is often the case), such as fantasies related to paraphilias. Since behavior connected to such fantasies is often easier to carry out alone, such men tend to avoid intimate relationships and may depend on prostitutes (with whom they can be more candid) for partner-related sexual experiences. Even then, intercourse rarely, if ever, occurs.

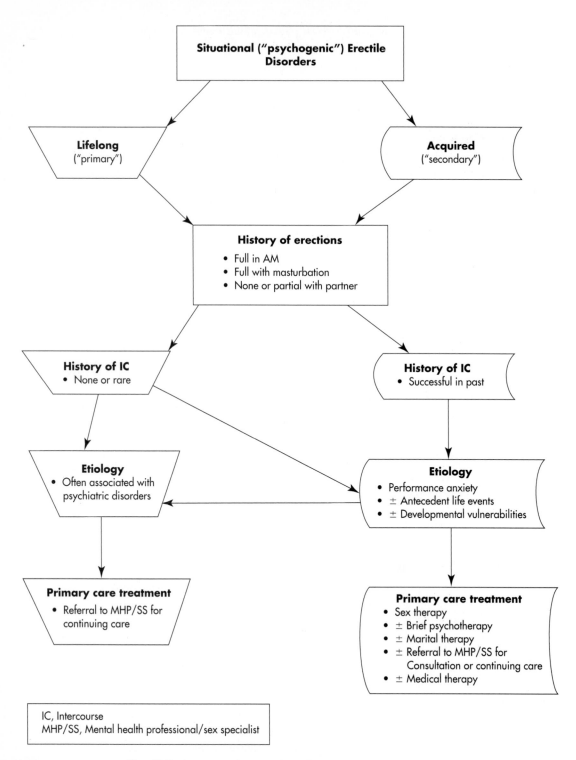

Figure 11-3   Assessment of situational erectile disorders.

Pressure from a (non-prostitute) partner may be a major factor in seeking treatment. When this occurs, the patient may not be particularly forthcoming about his thoughts and feelings.

A 32-year-old man was seen with his 29-year-old wife. They were married for two years and despite being sexually active with one another several times each week, intercourse never occurred. (They previously agreed not to engage in intercourse before they married.) She was aware of the fact that he had never experienced intercourse in the past. His erection predictably diminished whenever he moved close to her vagina. She wanted to become pregnant and felt the "biological clock ticking."

Her desire for pregnancy and her love for her husband resulted in a single-minded pursuit of her attempts at solving their sexual difficulties. He was less enthusiastic. Attempts at psychotherapy with him alone and sex therapy as a couple proved unhelpful. Since he was a shy person and spontaneously revealed little about himself, he never previously told anyone about having been repeatedly sexually assaulted as a child by his mother. Nor had he ever discussed his current sexual fantasies (about which he was quite ashamed) that involved the insertion of a knife into a woman's vagina. He was again referred for individual psychotherapy and accepted the need for candor with his therapist concerning his sexual experiences as a child and his current sexual thoughts and feelings.

Acquired ("Secondary") Erectile Disorders

In contrast to the lifelong form of situational erectile dysfunction, the patient reports having had intercourse in the past, perhaps on many occasions for many years. However in the present, full erections might occur with his partner before clothes are removed but the fullness may diminish after he reaches the bed or after the commencement of sexual activity. Intercourse might occur sometimes but this seems unpredictable. Characteristically, he never had a problem obtaining full erections after a period of sleep and with masturbation and, as well, describes no difficulty with ejaculation and orgasm now or in the past. History reveals that when younger, he frequently had erection troubles with partners on the first few occasions when sexual intercourse was attempted. However, when in a long-term relationship, he functioned well sexually although erectile difficulties occasionally reappeared at times of "stress." After a relationship of many years, doubts about his sexual "performance" developed. There may have been a marked diminution of sexual activity in spite of his partner's attempts at reassurance. She believed him not to be sexually interested, and wondered about her own attractiveness to him. Questioning revealed that his apparent sexual disinterest is actually avoidance. He remains privately interested but feels that he is not "a man" anymore with his wife.

A 51-year-old rather shy man was seen together with his 49-year-old outspoken wife. They were married for 23 years. Sexual activity had never been a problem until about five years ago when his erections sometimes became soft after vaginal entry, so much so that intercourse could not continue. This sequence of events, and erectile loss even before intromission, gradually occurred more often and culminated in the complete lack of intercourse in the previous six months. His sexual desire, while never as strong as that of his wife, had not changed and he would masturbate (without erectile problem) and ejaculate about once or twice each month. He thought that the origin of his erection troubles were mainly related to his age but he also wondered if his substantial use of alcohol for the previous 25 years was also a factor. His heavy drinking stopped completely about five years ago when he joined AA. This was about the same time that his erection problems began. After discussion of possible etiological factors, he understood that much of his erectile difficulty was connected to his feelings about his wife. They were referred to a treatment program that focused on both their marriage and their sexual relationship.

Etiology
Lifelong ("Primary") Erectile Dysfunction

This syndrome is "often, though not invariably, associated with a diagnosable major [psychiatric] condition"[18] (p. 133). Masters and Johnson described a group of 31 men with "Primary Impotence," eleven of whom were in unconsummated marriages[9] (pp. 137-156). Factors they considered to be of etiological significance were multiple and included the following:

1. Homoerotic desire
2. Mother/son incest
3. Strict religious orthodoxy
4. Psychologically damaging attempts at first intercourse with a prostitute (sometimes associated with drugs or alcohol)

Other investigators also reported associated paraphilias and gender identity disorders[18] (pp. 133-135);[19] (p. 245).

Acquired ("Secondary") Erectile Dysfunction

> In almost all men with acquired erectile dysfunction, the etiology involves a combination of factors[17] in three areas:
>
> 1. Performance anxiety
> 2. Antecedent life events
> 3. Developmental vulnerabilities

Most men with a clearly situational erectile dysfunction also indicate that it is acquired.

In almost all such men, the etiology involves some combination of factors[17](p. 200) in the following three areas:

1. Performance anxiety
2. Antecedent life events
3. Developmental vulnerabilities

The "phase of time" for each of these three is, respectively, here-and-now lovemaking, months to years ("recent" history), and childhood/ adolescence ("remote" history).

A major here-and-now issue is "performance anxiety," a concept introduced by Masters and Johnson to describe the worry that a patient may have about his or her sexual function and whether it will be similarly impaired on a current occasion as it was at a previous time.[9] Performance anxiety is partner related and probably universal in men with erectile difficulties. From a primary care perspective, performance anxiety is an important target of the treatment of "psychogenic impotence" in both solo men and couples. However, this component explains only part of the etiology of this syndrome, since eliminating performance anxiety does not always result in cure.

Antecedent life events and developmental vulnerabilities may be of therapeutic significance also, but they are difficult to consider in detail in a primary care setting.

The former "typically fall into one of five categories"[17] (p.202):

1. Deterioration in the nonsexual relationship with a spouse or partner
2. Divorce
3. Death of a spouse
4. Vocational failure
5. Loss of health

Developmental vulnerabilities include such issues as child sexual abuse and impairments in sexual identity.[17]

On a clinical level, one frequently has the impression of a link between psychogenic erection difficulties and difficulty with expression of anger. In the MMAS study, the suppression and expression of anger was assessed. "Men with maximum levels of anger suppression and anger expression showed an age-adjusted probability of 35% for moderate impotence and 16% to 19% for complete impotence, both well above the general level (9.6%)."[6] The MMAS study did not subcategorize men with "impotence" according to whether the origin was "psychogenic," "organic," mixed," or "undetermined." It may certainly be possible that problems with anger may also potentiate some of the etiological factors associated with erectile difficulties of organic, mixed or undetermined origin discussed below.

| Performance anxiety is partner related and probably universal in men with erectile difficulties. |

| Eliminating performance anxiety does not always result in cure. |

| Antecedent life events typically fall into one of five categories[17]:
1. Deterioration in the nonsexual relationship
2. Divorce
3. Death of a spouse
4. Vocational failure
5. Loss of health |

| Developmental vulnerabilities include child sexual abuse and impairments in sexual identity.[17] |

Laboratory Investigation

If in instances where the man reports being otherwise healthy, the history clearly indicates the situational nature of the man's erectile dysfunction, there is no sign of any contributory physical abnormality, and there are no other sexual symptoms (such as lack of sexual desire), little needs to be done to obtain additional specific laboratory data.

Treatment

"It is fortunate for many psychologically impotent men that a complete understanding of the causes is not necessary. Some men spontaneously get over their problem

Areas to be addressed include:

1. Genital anatomy and physiology
2. The sex response cycle
3. Masturbation
4. Male-female differences in sexual response
5. Effects of aging, illness, and medication on sexual desire, arousal, and orgasm

Easily-available, comprehensible and comprehensive, inexpensive, and up-to-date self-help books can be used as an adjunct in this educational process.[20]

The "gold standard" of erectile function for many men is what occurred in their teenage years. The folly of "living in the past" becomes evident to a man in his (for example) 40s when he is asked to provide another example of a part of his body that functions in the present as it did when he was a teenager.

within a short period of time without any therapy"[17] (p. 202). For those whose problem is not solved, an approach is proposed that concentrates on five themes that have been identified in a review of the literature (Box 11-1).[16] Most importantly for generalist health professionals, some of these five themes listed in Box 11-1 can be easily integrated into primary care.

The first theme is accurate information and realistic ideas and expectations regarding sexual performance and satisfaction—all of which is a problem in many men with erectile difficulties (and their women partners).

Areas to be addressed include:

1. Genital anatomy and physiology
2. The sex response cycle
3. Masturbation
4. Male-female differences in sexual response
5. Effect of aging, illness, and medication on sexual desire, arousal, and orgasm

Comprehensive, inexpensive, and up-to-date self-help books are easily vailable and can be used as an adjunct in this education process.[20] The provision of information can correct unrealistic ideas and expectations—thoughts that could, themselves, significantly interfere with erectile function. For example, the "gold standard" of erectile function for many men is what occurred in their teenage years. The folly of "living in the past" becomes evident to a man in his (for example) 40s when he is asked to provide another example of a part of his body that functions in the present as it did when he was a teenager. In addition, it could be pointed out to him that he is, in effect, basing his sexual expectations for his 60 years of adult sexual function (approximate life expectancy minus 15 years of pre- and early adolescence) on the five (or so) years of erectile experience as a teen! Other examples of ideas and expectations that might be discussed with a patient include his thoughts when he or his partner is initiating sexual activity and when his penis is becoming firmer or softer.

Box 11-1

Themes in the Treatment of Situational ("Psychogenic") Erectile Dysfunction

- INFORMATION, including realistic ideas and expectations concerning sexual performance and satisfaction
- PERFORMANCE ANXIETY RELIEF through use of "sensate focus"
- "SCRIPT" MODIFICATION ('who does what to whom')
- ATTENTION TO RELATIONSHIP ISSUES (e.g., intimacy, control, conflict resolution, trust)
- RELAPSE PREVENTION

Yet another example of the therapeutic value of information is that of the sexual changes associated with aging. The educational effect on the treatment of erectile dysfunction was studied in a group of heterosexual couples between the ages of 55 and 75.[21] Investigators found that a four-hour workshop resulted in increased knowledge, especially about the normal changes that occur with age, thereby allowing participants to have more realistic expectations of themselves and their partners. Sexual satisfaction also increased despite the presence of associated organic factors.

The second theme is the relief of "performance anxiety." Diminishing or eliminating this frequently appearing factor involves inducing sexual response in the man (in this instance, erection) while he paradoxically avoids sexual invitations for intercourse. Masters and Johnson described this approach to the treatment of performance anxiety[9] (pp. 193-213). The method involves couple oriented touching "exercises" and concentrates on *sensate focus,* a term they coined (pp. 71-75) to denote a focus on immediate sensation rather than sexual goals of, for example, intercourse. Briefly, the exercises occur in stages and initially exclude intercourse and touching of breasts (in the woman) and genitalia, then include touching of the previously barred areas (while maintaining the exclusion of intercourse), and finally include unrestricted touching and intercourse. Couples do not move to the next level of the exercise until the previous one is mastered. While requiring repeated visits, this technique is not complex and might, therefore, be within the boundaries of primary care (depending on the clinician's time, comfort, and interest and the availability of specialists to whom one could refer).

One major (and often unappreciated) objective of "sensate focus" in the treatment of erectile dysfunction is change in the communication pattern between partners so they could, with "permission" (i.e., encouragement), and with a minimum of tension and embarrassment, tell one another what is, and is not, pleasurable. (Rather than the communication exercise it is, sensate focus is sometimes mistakenly thought of as a way of allowing one to discover previously unappreciated physical feelings in particular body areas.) A second objective of "sensate focus" is to remove the demand for intercourse. Since the man does not "need" an erection for any purpose other than intercourse and intercourse is not to take place, theoretically the "pressure" on the man to "perform" will be removed and the worry (which is thought to inhibit his erection) will disappear, thus allowing his erection to develop unhindered.

> Rather than the communication exercise it is, sensate focus is sometimes mistakenly thought of as a way of allowing one to discover previously unappreciated physical feelings in particular body areas.

Two obstacles to sensate focus have been described[11] (p. 189). First, the passive process of sensate focus is contrary to the need of aging men for active and direct penile stimulation for an erection to develop. Second, the idea of performance anxiety is so popular that general knowledge of the concept has rendered its treatment less effective. Consequently, LoPiccolo coined the term *metaperformance anxiety* to explain why, on some occasions, "eliminating performance anxiety does not lead to erection during sensate focus body massage"[11] (p. 189).

> Functional men can become aroused on demand, whereas the same request in dysfunctional men results in interference with the arousal process.

Recently the role of "anxiety" in producing erectile troubles and the expected relief with its disappearance has been reexamined and reviewed from a research rather than clinical viewpoint.[22] Functional and dysfunctional men have been shown to respond differently to anxiety. The results of these studies are summarized as follows:

1. Functional men can become aroused on demand, whereas the same request in dysfunctional men results in interference with the arousal process (similar results were found in laboratory studies)
2. Functional men report their subjective arousal to be greater than dysfunctional men regardless of what occurs physically
3. (Particularly interesting from a therapeutic viewpoint) functional men report distraction to be an obstacle to sexual response, whereas this is neutral or actually helpful to dysfunctional men[16]

> Functional men report distraction to be an obstacle to sexual response, whereas this is neutral or actually helpful to dysfunctional men.[16]

The third theme concentrates on sexual "script" modification (i.e., changes to what actually occurs sexually between two people). The *fourth theme concentrates on relationship issues* such as intimacy, control, conflict resolution, and trust. The *fifth theme concentrates on the prevention of relapse.* Since the third, fourth, and fifth areas are often more within the interests, practice pattern, and skills of the sex therapist, they are not discussed at length here.

Little published information exists on the treatment of situational erectile dysfunction by methods usually reserved for occasions when the etiology is "organic, mixed, or undetermined" (see below in the chapter). Few quarrel with the concept of considering such an approach when psychologically-oriented methods have been unsuccessful. However, when medical techniques are used early in the course of treatment, the concept is more problematic. The rationale sometimes given is one of providing the man an opportunity to have a erection in worry free circumstances as a way of overcoming an undefined obstacle. The rationale continues that after the man engages in successful sexual experiences that require an erection he will be able to do so without extra support.

> A study of the use of intracavernosal injections in 15 men with "psychogenic impotence" did not convey a sense of optimism about the outcome of such an approach.[23] The authors concluded that performance anxiety was not alleviated, that dependence on injections for intercourse remained, and that the capacity for intimacy did not improve.

A study of the use of intracavernosal injections in 15 men with "psychogenic impotence" did not convey a sense of optimism about the outcome of such an approach.[23] The authors concluded that performance anxiety was not alleviated, that dependence on injections for intercourse remained, and that the capacity for intimacy did not improve. One can well imagine that the consequences (benefits and disappointments) of the use of such treatments for men with situational erectile difficulties become magnified when men who have these problems ask for, and are given, an oral medication such as sildenafil (see below in the chapter).

Few long-term follow-up studies have been conducted on the treatment of erectile dysfunction. Results for "primary" and "secondary" (i.e., acquired) erectile dysfunction were reported by Masters and Johnson as an "overall failure rate" (OFR) and were based on personal interviews conducted five years after the patients were originally treated[9] (p. 367). The OFR for "primary impotence" was 41%. This modest improvement supports the clinical experience of greater complexity in the treatment of this form of the erectile dysfunction syndrome. Furthermore, it suggests that insofar as "primary" impotence is concerned, a focus on performance anxiety without considering other factors will likely result in quite limited gains.

The OFR reported by Masters and Johnson for the "secondary" form was 31%.[9] Another follow-up study in the United States, carefully conducted after three years, found that of the 18 men presenting with "difficulty achieving or maintaining erection," ten maintained the improvement, four were the same, and three were worse.[24] The authors found that there was "significant improvement maintained across time in erectile capability during intercourse . . . . improved satisfaction in the sexual relationship . . . [and] . . . longer duration of foreplay." Hawton and his colleagues conducted a rigorous one to six year follow-up study in the United Kingdom and found that the "gains made during therapy by couples who presented with erectile dysfunction were reasonably well sustained."[25] Of the 18 couples who undertook treatment, 14 reported the problem resolved or mostly so at the end of therapy, and 11 reported the same at follow-up.

Indications for Referral for Consultation or Continuing Care by a Specialist

1. Since the "primary" form of situational erectile disorders is so often associated with complex individual diagnosable psychiatric conditions rather than interpersonal conflicts, referral to a mental health professional for individual treatment is usually the most reasonable course of action[19] (p. 245). If the health professional is not also a sex-specialist, it may be useful to consult with one before proceeding with the referral.

2. Solo men with the "secondary" form of situational erectile dysfunction (i.e., those without a partner, with an uncommitted partner, in a relationship that is filled with so much discord that they are unable to cooperate with each other, or who have been raised in a culture in which men are clearly in control and women entirely submissive) often require an amalgam of traditional psychotherapy and sex therapy. Such men are candidates for individual care with a sex-specialist who is also a mental health professional.

3. Couples in which the man has the "secondary" form of situational erectile dysfunction and who would benefit by a here-and-now focus on information and performance anxiety (previously described in the treatment of situational problems in this chapter) could be cared for in primary care. Couples who do not respond to this approach may require an additional focus on two of the other elements: "script" modification and attention to relationship conflicts. Given the time and experience involved in providing these other components, referral would be reasonable in these circumstances. If referral does take place, the health professional should be a sex-specialist who also has clinical experience in the mental health area.

4. Consultation with a sex-specialist is warrented when consideration is given to providing a form of treatment usually reserved for men with erectile dysfunction of "organic, mixed, or undetermined origin." The purpose would be to examine the possibility of integrating biological and psychologically oriented treatment methods.

Generalized Erectile Dysfunction: Organic, Mixed, or UnDetermined Origin

The assessment of generalized erectile disorders is summarized in Figure 11-4.

Description

> The key differentiating feature of the acquired and generalized form of erectile dysfunction is that the difficulty experienced by the man exists in all major circumstances when he would be expected to have an erection: with a partner, masturbation, and with sleep (including the time when he awakens in the morning).

The key differentiating feature of the acquired and generalized form of erectile dysfunction is that the difficulty experienced by the man exists in all major circumstances when he would be expected to have an erection: with a partner, masturbation, and with sleep (including the time when he awakens in the morning). In addition, he describes little or no difficulty with erectile function in the past. Typically in his 50s or older, his erection problems began in recent years. Sexual desire is usually present but, depending on the status of his health and the nature of any previous health troubles, there may have been problems with ejaculation or orgasm. Relationship conflict was not apparent except as a possible result of reluctance to seek help despite his partner's encouragement. Although unhappy, he is not clinically depressed.

A couple in their mid-60s were seen because of the man's erectile difficulties. They were married for seven years, both for the second time. Five years before, he held an executive position in a major computer software company but as a result of "downsizing" lost his job and subsequently retired. His wife had always been in good health but he had a "mild" heart attack about three years before. He felt well since then, stopped smoking, and was not taking any medications. On his last medical visit several months earlier, he talked with his physician about erection troubles, which had begun about one year before. Further history-taking revealed that the fullness of his erections during sexual activity with his wife (as well as in the morning and with masturbation—which occurred once every few months) had become consistently about 50% of what he had previously experienced. The last time he could recall having a full erection at any time was about one year earlier. He was referred to a urologist and after a thorough investigation he was told that the reason for his trouble was "organic." Intracavernosal injections were suggested. He was reluctant to pursue this option and wanted a second opinion from a sex therapist. This consultation primarily confirmed the opinion of the urologist and as a result he began injection treatment. He changed to sildenafil (Viagra) when this became available and after three months of use, he and his wife reported that they were pleased with the results.

Etiology/Risk Factors

Many medical disorders are identified as "organic causes" of erection difficulties (see Box 11-2), however, only a few seem to account for a great many cases where the etiology is known. Major etiological factors are discussed below.

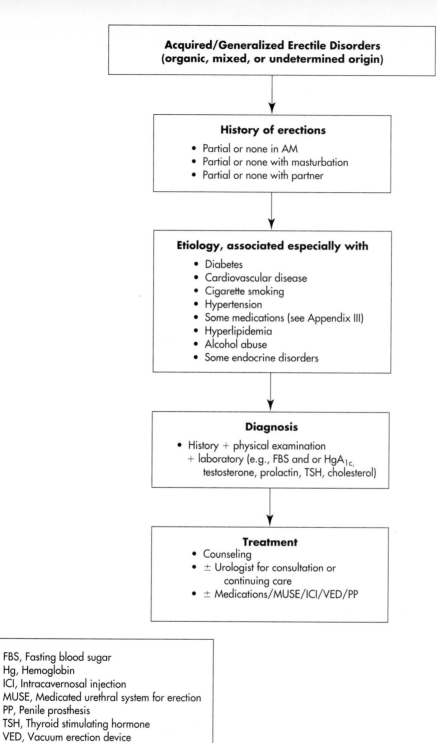

Figure 11-4 Assessment of acquired/generalized erectile dysfunction.

Box 11-2

Causes of Generalized Erectile Dysfunction

Organic Causes of Impotence*

Inflammatory
Urethritis
Prostatitis
Seminal vesiculitis
Cystitis
Urethral stricture

Mechanical
Congenital deformities
Peyronie's disease
Morbid obesity
Hydrocele
Phimosis
Malignancy

Postsurgical
Perineal prostatic biopsy
Prostatectomy (simple, radical)
Abdominal perineal resection
Aortoiliac surgery
External sphincterotomy

Occlusive Vascular
Atherosclerosis
Arteritis
Priapism
Thrombosis
Embolism

Traumatic
Penectomy
Ruptured urethra

Endurance Factors
Postmyocardial infarction
Pulmonary insufficiency
Anemias
Systemic illnesses (infection, nutritional)
Metabolic (renal and hepatic failure)
Sleep disorders

Neurogenic
Parkinson's disease
Temporal lobe lesions
Head injuries
Cord tumors/resection/injuries
Multiple sclerosis
Tabes dorsalis
Neuropathies
Spina bifida
Subacute combined degeneration
Amyotrophic lateral sclerosis

Chemicals
Hypnotics
Sedatives
Phenothiazines
Antidepressants
Antihypertensives
Antiparkinson agents

Endocrine
Diabetes
Pituitary disorders
Thyroid disorders
Adrenal disorders
Klinefelter's syndrome
Gonadal dysfunction

From Lakin MM: Diagnostic assessment of disorders of male sexual function. In Montague DK (ed): *Disorders of male sexual function*, Chicago/London/Boca Raton, 1988, Year Book Medical Publishers, Inc. Reprinted with permission.
*Modified from Smith AD: *Urologic Clinics of North America*. Philadelphia, WB Saunders, 1981, vol 8, no. 1, p. 83.

In the Massachusetts Male Aging Study, health status was ascertained by asking if diabetes, heart disease, and hypertension were present.[6] These three "were significantly associated with changes in the impotence probability pattern." After adjusting for age, 28% of men with treated diabetes, 39% of men with treated heart disease, and 15% of those with treated hypertension were described as having "complete impotence."

Diabetes

Estimates of the prevalence of erection problems in men with diabetes range from 27% to 71%.[26] As many as 50% of people with type 2 diabetes remain undiagnosed (about 8 million people in the United States), a serious situation since hyperglycemia in this condition causes microvascular disease and may contribute or cause macrovascular disease.[27] Erection problems may well be a manifestation of micro- and/or macrovascular disease. In the MMAS sample, "the age-adjusted probability of complete impotence was three times greater in subjects reporting treated diabetes than in those without diabetes."[6] In an attempt to clarify the connection between diabetes and erection problems and to eliminate the confounding effects of associated illness and medications, 40 men with diabetes (but free of other illness or drugs apart from antidiabetic medication) were compared to an equivalent group of age-matched healthy controls.[26] The men with diabetes were found to have a wide variety of sex-related difficulties, including:

> Forty men with diabetes with no other illnesses and taking no drugs other than antidiabetic medication were compared to the equivalent group of age-matched healthy controls.[26] The men with diabetes were found to have a variety of sex-related difficulties, including erectile function with attempts at intercourse, during sleep, and with masturbation; sexual desire; frequency of intercourse; premature ejaculation; and sexual satisfaction.

1. Erectile dsyfunction with attempts at intercourse, during sleep, and with masturbation
2. Sexual desire disorders
3. Diminished frequency of intercourse
4. Premature ejaculation
5. Diminished sexual satisfaction

In another study, *sexually functional* men with diabetes were shown to have significantly diminished Nocturnal Penile Tumescence (NPT) profiles when compared to a similar control group.[28]

Cardiovascular Disorders

The association between erectile difficulties and cardiovascular disorders is well studied. "Vascular disorders" include two groups: arterial (i.e., obstruction to the penile inflow tract) and veno-occlusive (i.e., the inability to trap blood in the corpus cavernosum).[29] The former has attracted particular attention.

The presence of four *arterial* risk factors (ARF) (diabetes, smoking, hyperlipidemia, and hypertension) was assessed in 440 "impotent" men.[30] The frequency of "organic impotence" occurred in 49% of men without any ARF, and 100% when there were three or four risk factors.

Cigarette Smoking

The link between cigarette smoking and arterial disease is well established. Smoking was found to be significantly more prevalent in men who were "impotent" compared to estimates of smoking among men in the general population.[31] In one study, two groups of men with and without penile arterial disease were compared, and the former was found to have smoked more pack-years.[32] In the MMAS, "complete impotence" was higher in current smokers (versus current nonsmokers) who were also treated for heart disease, hypertension, or arthritis, and, as well, in those taking cardiac drugs, antihypertensives, or vasodilators.[6] In subjects with treated heart disease the probability of "complete impotence" in the MMAS was 56% for current smokers compared to 21% for current nonsmokers. Likewise, treated hypertension together with smoking increased the probability of "complete impotence" to 20% of those who had both factors, as compared to 9% among hypertensive men who did not smoke. Apart from particular connections between smoking and other risk factors, "a general effect of current cigarette smoking was not noted."

> In the MMAS, "complete impotence" was higher in current smokers (versus current nonsmokers) who were also treated for heart disease, hypertension, or arthritis, and, as well, in those taking cardiac drugs, antihypertensives, or vasodilators.[6]

Hypertension

The relationship between "impotence" and "erection dysfunction" and hypertension was examined in a review of studies that were conducted in the 1970s and 1980s[33](p. 204). Impotence was found in 7% of men with normal blood pressure. Impotence was found in 17% to 23% of untreated men with hypertension and in 25% to 41% of men who were treated for hypertension. From these studies, the association between "impotence" and hypertension (apart from drugs used in its treatment) is clearly evident.

> Impotence was found in 7% of men with normal blood pressure. Impotence was found in 17% to 23% of untreated men with hypertension and in 25% to 41% of men treated for hypertension.[33]

Lipids

In the MMAS, a negative correlation was found between "impotence" and high density lipoprotein cholesterol, although this was not so with total serum cholesterol. "In the older men (age 56 to 70 years), the age-adjusted probability of 'moderate impotence' increased from 6.7% to 25% as high density lipoprotein cholesterol decreased from 90 to 30 mg./dl."[6]

Medications

A variety of drugs used presently and in the recent past have been shown to interfere with erectile function in men (see Appendix III). The increase in the number of new drugs that are currently being introduced for various human ailments and the increased speed with which they appear on the market make it likely that unanticipated side effects (including sexual side effects) of these agents will become apparent only *after* they have been used for a period of time. Physicians must therefore be constantly sensitive to the possibility of sexual side effects (including effects on the mechanism of erection) of newer drugs. The following comment was made about hypotensive agents but applies equally to other drugs as well: "Although . . . certain agents . . . . are likely to have sexual side effects [while] other agents . . . are unlikely to be associated with erectile dysfunction, it is important to stress that *any* agent may cause erectile difficulties in certain patients . . . there is

> The increase in the number of new drugs that are currently being introduced for various human ailments and the increased speed with which they appear on the market make it likely that unanticipated side effects (including sexual side effects) of these agents will become apparent only after they have been used for a period of time. Physicians must therefore be constantly sensitive to the possibility of sexual side effects (including effects on the mechanism of erection) of newer drugs.

[also] considerable individual variation in vulnerability of erectile function to different drugs. In other words, *the existing literature can only serve as a general guide to patient management"* (italics added)[34] (pp. 111-112).

In the MMAS study, "complete impotence" was found to be present significantly more often in men taking the following medications than in the sample as a whole (10%)[6]:

- Hypoglycemic agents (26%)
- Antihypertensives (14%)
- Vasodilators (36%)
- Cardiac drugs (28%)

This association was not found with lipid-lowering drugs.

Two groups of drugs (antihypertensives and medications used in psychiatry) have been particularly implicated in the development of erectile dysfunction[33] (pp. 197-337).

Issues learned from sexual side effect research on antihypertensive drugs (that apply to other substances as well) include the following items[32] (pp. 206-207):

- Possibility of late appearance (6 months or more)
- Lack of information about their effects on women
- Importance of assessing sexual symptoms of the underlying disease
- Need to include information from partners
- Usefulness of information about masturbation
- Need to assess alcohol use and abuse

> Issues learned from sexual side effect research on antihypertensive drugs include the possibility of their late appearance (6 months or more), the lack of information about their effects on women, the importance of assessing sexual symptoms of the underlying disease, the need to include information from partners, the usefulness of information about masturbation, and the need to assess alcohol use and abuse[32] (pp. 206-207).

Alcohol

"With just a few drinks, most men experience transient boosts in sex drive and sociability. With continued drinking, however, erection and ejaculation abilities systematically decrease in a dose-related fashion to a point of total dysfunction."[32] Although there are acute and chronic effects of alcohol on sexual function, comments here focus on the latter. Studies relating to chronic alcoholism and epidemiology, Nocturnal Penile Tumescence (NPT), hormonal and neurologic effects have been reviewed.[35]

An examination of clinical experience in the care of approximately 17,000 male alcoholics over 36 years revealed that 8% spontaneously described continued erectile problems after detoxification.[36] Years later, despite abstinence, 50% had not fully recovered their erectile function. The continuation of sexual desire in these men indicates that their erectile problems were unlikely to be simply a result of insufficient testosterone but rather more fundamental structural and functional body changes, including:

> An examination of clinical experience in the care of approximately 17,000 male alcoholics over 36 years revealed that 8% spontaneously described continued erectile problems *after* detoxification.[36] Years later, and despite abstinence, 50% had not fully recovered their erectile function.

- Effect on testosterone receptors
- Influence of estrogen
- Damage to organs in the body, including the central nervous system, testicles, and liver
- Existing diseases caused or made worse by alcohol abuse such as diabetes, heart disease, and peripheral neuropathy

In addition, two controlled studies on the effects of alcoholism on sexual function demonstrate that erectile dysfunction[37] and also desire problems[38] were more common in alcoholic men.

In an effort to assess the effect of alcohol use on NPT, 26 sober, healthy, sexually functional, and medication-free chronic alcoholics and controls were studied for two nights in a laboratory setting.[39] The subjects had fewer full penile tumescent episodes that were also shorter in duration. The authors speculated on the possible contribution of central processes to the effects of alcohol on erections.

The impact of chronic alcoholism on pituitary-gonadal function appears at both levels. Apart from liver disease, chronic alcoholic men show evidence of hypogonadism, abnormalities in spermatogenesis, and testicular atrophy.[40] Such men also demonstrate diminished androgens, elevated estrogens, and increased prolactin levels.

The neuropsychiatric effects of chronic alcoholism on sexual function may involve central and peripheral processes. Alcohol-induced peripheral neuropathy may result in both erectile and ejaculatory disorders. Schiavi outlined many of the psychological factors that may also be present such as preexisting personality problems, mood disorder, and feelings of inadequacy.[35] He concluded that "the reciprocal interaction between drug intake and psychological factors is so closely interwoven that it is impossible to identify the nature of this relation."

Endocrine Abnormalities

> Erectile dysfunction in all situations, including the lack of nocturnal erections, strongly suggests that a general medical condition or substance use is the cause.[5]

"Erectile dysfunction of exclusively endocrine origin is uncommon. . . . In most cases the primary effect of the endocrine abnormality is loss of sexual interest."[12] The authors of the MMAS study arrived at a similar conclusion.[6'] Of the 17 hormones measured in the MMAS, "only dehydroepiandrosterone showed a strong correlation with impotence." Specifically, no correlations were found between "impotence" and the following hormones:

- Testosterone (total or free)
- Sex hormone binding globulin (SHBG)
- Estrogens
- Prolactin
- Luteinizing hormone (LH)
- Follicle stimulating hormone (FSH)

When hormonal difficulties occur in the context of erectile dysfunction, the more common clinical abnormalities are those that involve the hypothalamus-pituitary-gonadal axis and include: hypo- and hypergonadotropic hypogonadism, hyperprolactinemia, and hypo- and hyperthyroidism.[41] (p. 85). The frequency of the association of endocrine and erectile problems depends on the age of the sample and the clinical context of the investigation (e.g., outpatient medical, urology, endocrine, or sex therapy clinics), as well as the nature of the sample.

When the particular association of erection problems and hyperprolactinemia (HPRL) was reviewed, the observation was made that this was "often the first, and for a long time the only symptom of HPRL, an important point because in many cases the cause is a pituitary tumor."[12]

Buvat and Lemaire reviewed large published series of endocrine abnormalities in cases of erectile dysfunction and when combining their own results with others found an 8% prevalence for low testosterone and 0.7% of prolactin levels greater than 35 ng./ml.[42]

Aging

See "Sexual-developmenl History: The Older Years" in Chapter 5.

Laboratory Investigation

When the history and physical examination (see the "General Considerations" section above in this chapter) leave doubt about the origin of a patient's erectile dysfunction, the clinician must also consider the use of laboratory tests.

The availability of orally administered treatments for erectile dysfunction (for example, sildenafil—see "Treatment" below in this chapter) that appear to be easy to use, often effective, and have minimal side-effects may well have profound effects on the process of evaluating erectile dysfunction. The initial use of these medications by a patient may, itself, become a test, and in so doing may replace some other investigatory procedures. Nothing, however, should replace a *careful clinical assessment* and "when there is suspicion of an organic factor, one should rely (as well) on a combination of investigations."[13]

Laboratory investigation of generalized erectile dysfunction chiefly entails examining three body systems:

- Endocrine
- Vascular
- Neurological

Several diagnostic tests involving these three systems have been developed. The criteria used in considering which diagnostic tests are appropriate for investigating generalized erectile dysfunction on a primary care basis are:

1. Usefulness
2. Low cost
3. Noninvasiveness
4. Low complexity
5. Availability

Endocrine Blood Tests

Endocrine and blood tests for diabetes are probably the *only* procedures that fulfill the criteria outlined immediately above. Despite agreement on the endocrine disorders most commonly associated with erection difficulties,". . . . there is disagreement on the specific tests to be employed or the interpretation thereof"[41] (p. 85). Many suggest the need to measure Testosterone (T) and Prolactin (PRL) in all men with erection difficulty (PRL can be abnormal when T is not). However, others promote a more specific policy. For example, Buvat and Lemaire suggest that *before* age 50, T should be determined only in cases of (accompanying) low sexual desire and abnormal physical examination but that *after* age 50 it should be measured in all men, and that PRL should be determined only in

> These authors also direct clinicians to repeat first results of abnormal prolactin and testosterone determinations because of their finding of normal second results in 40% of their cases.

cases of (accompanying) low sexual desire, gynecomastia, and/or testosterone less than 4 ng/ml.[42] These authors also direct clinicians to repeat first results of abnormal prolactin and testosterone determinations because of their finding of normal second results in 40% of their cases.

Apart from measuring total testosterone, this hormone also can be determined in the bioavailable form (BAT) and as free testosterone (FT). BAT consists of FT and the fraction that is bound to albumin[41] (p. 76).

Conflicting opinions exist over the need to also immediately test some or all of the following other factors without waiting for an abnormal T or PRL result:

- Follicle Stimulating Hormone (FSH)
- Luteinizing Hormone (LH)
- Sex Hormone Binding Globulin (SHBG)
- Thyroid function tests

Cost of testing and the nature of the clinical context are two elements resulting in differences of opinion. In the literature, it seems assumed that these other factors would be measured in the event of an abnormal T or PRL level.

Tests for Diabetes

Fasting blood sugar (FBS) or fasting plasma glucose (FPG) and/or glycosylated hemoglobin (HgA_{1C}) is widely used as a screening test for diabetes. A positive test indicates that a confirming diagnostic test is warranted.[43]

Vascular Tests

Since the penis is, basically, a vascular organ, vascular tests are often important elements in the evaluation of erectile difficulties, particularly when there is suspicion that vascular elements may contribute to the etiology. However, tests of penile vascular function are mostly invasive, costly, complex, difficult to interpret, and have limited availability. As such they are generally conducted by urologists and *not* recommended in primary care unless a physician has special training. Although vascular testing procedures may not be recommended for use in primary care, clinicians should be aware of their potential diagnostic benefits and limitations to determine the need for urological consultation.

> The most worrisome complication of ICI is that of prolonged erection. After six hours of continuous erection, there is insufficient blood supply to the erectile tissue. The corpora cavernosa must be drained to decrease the intracavernosal pressure and an adrenergic agonist administered, injected intracavernously.[29] In clinical practice, patients must be told to contact a physician long before six hours if their erection persists.

Assessment of the penile response to the intracavernous injection (ICI) of vasoactive agents has been found to be particularly useful in considering vascular function. While structural problems with cavernosal arteries may explain a negative response, anxiety can as well.[44] "A positive erectile response implies normal veno-occlusive function. Nonresponders bear a high probability of a vascular origin with a predominance of veno-occlusive insufficiency."[29]

From a procedural viewpoint, the most common substances used for intracavernosal injections are papaverine, papaverine-phentolamine mixture, or prostaglandin E1 (PGE_1). The most worrisome complication of ICI is that of prolonged erection. A comparative study of these three medications demonstrates that PGE_1 had the highest erection rate (75%) and lowest prolonged erection rate (i.e., requiring "interruption" [0.1%]).[45] After six hours of continuous erection, there is insufficient blood supply to the erectile tissue. In this situation, the corpora cavernosa need to be drained to decrease the intracavernosal pressure and an adrenergic agonist (e.g., 10 mg of adrenaline) injected intracavernosly.[29] *In clinical practice, patients must be told to contact their physician long before six hours if their erection persists.*

Pharmacopenile Duplex Ultrasonography (PPDU) provides "an estimate of penile arterial inflow and venous outflow . . . [and] . . . has become a first-line test to define vascular [erectile dysfunction]"[29] It allows for accurate location of penile arteries and measurement of the diameter of each artery and provides evidence of the thickness and pulsatility of arterial walls.[12] In addition to assessment of the state of the cavernosal arteries, PPDU can locate well-defined pathological conditions such as Peyronie's disease. The procedure for PPDU involves the creation of an erection through ICI (needed because the procedure is unreliable when a penis is in the flaccid state) and then simultaneously combining ultrasound color imaging of the arteries to the cavernosal bodies of the penis with an analysis of blood flow patterns.

Nonspecific Tests: Nocturnal Penile Tumescence (NPT)

Any discussion of erectile dysfunction assessment is incomplete without including NPT testing, since it is so widely used and so frequently included in the literature on this subject. NPT is based on the discovery that a period of sleep involves different stages and that one of those stages (REM) is associated with many body changes, including the development of erection in men (three or four times each night and occupying about 20% of total sleep time). It was assumed that erections that occur at night and those which occur during the day involve the same body mechanisms and that by comparing sleep and daytime erections, it would be possible to distinguish the psychological or organic nature of the etiology of erection dysfunction. Sleep erections are considered to be unaffected by waking psychosocial factors.

When used in-home, NPT testing fulfills many of the primary care criteria previously described insofar as it is inexpensive, not extraordinarily complex to use, noninvasive, and available. However, when done in a sleep laboratory, NPT is the opposite in that it is expensive, cumbersome, and frequently unavailable in many geographic areas. The chief doubt about NPT is its usefulness.

When used in such a way as to provide clearest interpretation, the test is performed in a sleep laboratory with measurement of other sleep parameters such as electroencephalograph (EEG), respiration, and electromyograph (EMG), and recordings are made on at least two nights. The purpose in monitoring other sleep parameters is the detection of interference with sleep or REM such as might happen with illness or medication, which might result in mistaken conclusions.

Because of the complexity, expense, and difficulties with availability associated with formal testing of NPT in a hospital setting, three in-home procedures have been developed[46] (p. 153):

1. The "stamp" test (a ring of stamps placed around the base of a man's penis)
2. Snap Gauge Band (one ring of a thin plastic material containing three others that break at three different levels of tension as a penis enlarges)
3. Portable NPT monitoring

"Stamp" test results are difficult to interpret because of such problems as false-positive findings due to accidental tearing of the stamps for reasons other than an erection, false-negative results due to slippage, and lack of standardization. Snap Gauge has similarly been found to be of limited value. Both the stamp test and Snap Guage provide information about changes in circumference only, nothing about rigidity or stiffness (a vital issue in the assessment of erectile capacity for intercourse), and no data concerning the number or duration of tumescent episodes each night.

Portable monitors (e.g., Rigiscan) measure rigidity as well as the number and duration of NPT episodes. Measurement of rigidity has for some time been regularly included in NPT testing (now sometimes called NPTR with the "R" referring to rigidity). Reasons include the finding of substantial "interindividual differences in the increase of circumference associated with full erections and the recognition that maximal increases in shaft circumference did not indicate adequate rigidity."[47]

As inviting as these in-home methods of NPT testing might be, clinicians should be fully aware of their considerable limitations. It is suggested that this test "should be used only as screening tools in the context of a comprehensive medical and psychological evaluation"[46](p. 153).

Although the use of the Rigiscan at-home is certainly less troublesome and expensive than NPT in a sleep laboratory, opinions differ concerning its usefulness. "Apart from the lack of sleep data, it is impossible to know if such devices have been misused, manipulated, or otherwise mishandled by the patient. Deliberate faking of results cannot be excluded. . . ."[12]

Apart from issues of technology, patient reliability, and cost, the utility of NPT itself has been questioned. After many years, the importace of NPT in the process of evaluation of erectile dysfunction remains unclear. So, too, is the question about the equivalency of sleep and sexual erections. Confusion abounds in findings that show, for example, *abnormal* NPT results in *men who are not sexually dysfunctional* in circumstances such as aging,[47] depression,[48] and diabetes.[49] Conversely, *normal* NPT is reported in men with multiple sclerosis *who have daytime erectile difficulties.*[50]

Conclusions about the use of NPTR when used in the clinical evaluation of erectile dysfunction (in a sleep laboratory or at home) are summarized Box 11-3.

Treatment

"Whether psychological issues are co-determinates of the erectile problem or are reactive to it is immaterial. A man's emotional reaction to his erectile failure may be such that it serves to maintain the erectile problem even when the initial physiological causes are resolved . . . no patient, even those with a clear organic impairment of erectile capacity, can be considered inappropriate for psychological as well as relevant surgical or drug therapies for his sexual problem".[54] For these reasons, everything that was written immediately above about the treatment of situational erectile difficulties is also applicable to the acquired and generalized form.

Specific Treatments

Specific disorders and their sexual symptoms are often (not always) therapeutically responsive to specific treatments. Therapy for hyper- and hypogonadotropic hypogonadism and hyperprolactinemia have been reviewed elsewhere[41] (pp. 86-91). Details

---

Box 11-3

Nocturnal Penile Tumescence (NPT) Interpretation[45-47]

- Greatest benefit is to confirm a situational (psychogenic) erectile disorder
- Evidence of significant erectile activity during a single night may be sufficient to demonstrate the potential for normal functioning
- Repeated demonstration of insufficient rigidity in an otherwise normal male is not necessarily pathological
- Abnormal findings may coexist with normal daytime function in older men, men with diabetes, and nondepresssed men with a recent history of major depression
- May not be helpful in neurological disease in proving waking erectile capacity
- Should be conducted only in a sleep (versus home) laboratory when certain factors coexist (e.g., manual dexterity problems, dementia, malingering, medico-legal assessment, and sleep disorder)

---

concerning treatment will not be discussed here, since primary care health professionals likely seek consultation when encountering such a patient.

Other specific disorders and their sexual symptoms may not respond therapeutically to specific treatment methods. Diabetes is an example. Careful control of insulin-dependent and probably non-insulin-dependent diabetes mellitus will slow the onset and delay the progression of early vascular and neurologic complications, two body systems that have been particularly implicated in the etiology of erectile disorders in this disease.[55,56] Presumably, better control of diabetes would also delay the onset and slow the development of sexual dysfunctions, including erectile difficulties. When erectile dysfunction in specific disorders such as diabetes do not respond to specific treatment, nonspecific approaches can be used.

Nonspecific Treatments

Dramatic developments in the treatment of the acquired and generalized form of erectile dysfunction have been introduced in the past two decades in the form of intracavernosal injections, intraurethral medication, erections devices, and prostheses. As significant as these developments have been, they might well be overshadowed by the introduction of new oral therapies. The etiological and clinical heterogeneity of the acquired and generalized form of erection dysfunction will likely necessitate the continued use of several treatment approaches. Not everyone will benefit from the new oral therapies. For this reason, the oral therapies and many of the other currently used treatment approaches are discussed below.

Oral Therapies

Sildenafil (Viagra), is a new oral treatment that may be a critical advancement in the care of men with erectile difficulties (Box 11-4).

As a result of factors such as the ease of administration, sildenafil (and other orally administered substances currently being tested) will

> As a result of factors such as the ease of administration, sildenafil (and other orally administered substances currently being tested) will likely result in a substantial shift in the treatment of men with erectile difficulties away from specialists and toward physicians in primary care.

Box 11-4

Sildenafil (Viagra) Highlights[62, product monograph]

- MECHANISM OF ACTION: Sexual stimulation results in release of nitric oxide (NO); NO stimulates the production of cyclic guanosine monophosphate (cGMP), which relaxes smooth muscle and promotes the inflow of blood into the corpus cavernosum; phosphodiesterase type 5 (PDE5) is an enzyme that inhibits cGMP; sildenafil inhibits PDE5 (and therefore causes increased levels of cGMP)
- PLASMA CONCENTRATION LEVELS: Maximal within one hour after oral administration
- HALF-LIFE of 3 to 5 hours
- ADMINISTRATION: Taken on an "as needed" basis about one hour (0.5 to 4 hours) before sexual activity
- FREQUENCY OF USE: Maximum recommendation is once/day
- STARTING DOSE: Recommendation is 50 mg but can vary from 25 to 100 mg, depending on efficacy
- EFFICACY: Eighty percent of men with erectile dysfunction (ED) taking 50 mg will have sufficiently firm erections for intercourse
- ASSOCIATED SEXUAL STIMULATION: Necessary
- ETIOLOGY OF ED: Similar benefit regardless of etiology
- OTHER SEXUAL BENEFITS: Orgasmic function, intercourse satisfaction, and overall satisfaction but not for sexual desire
- PARTNERS: Verify erectile improvement and report significant enhancement of their satisfaction
- SIDE EFFECTS: Increase with increasing dose and include (at 50 mg): headache (21%), flushing (27%), dyspepsia (11%), rhinitis (3%), and visual disturbance (6%; change in the perception of color hue or brightness). No priapism reported
- CONTRAINDICATION: Potentiates hypotensive effects of organic nitrates. Therefore, not to be taken with organic nitrates in any form, including nitroglycerin

---

likely result in a substantial shift in the treatment of men with erectile difficulties away from specialists and toward physicians in primary care. Sildenafil demonstrated in initial trials to be well tolerated and "effective in improving erectile activity in patients with male erectile dysfunction for which there is no established organic cause."[57]

As described above (see "Mechanism of Erection" in this chapter), relaxation of smooth muscle is an essential aspect of the development of an erection. This relaxation is mediated by nitric oxide via cyclic guanosine monophosphate (cGMP).[59] Cyclic nucleotide phosphodiesterase (PDE) isozymes hydrolyse cGMP. It was reasoned that an inhibitor of PDE would therefore enhance the action of nitric oxide/cGMP on penile erectile activity. Sildenafil is such an inhibiting agent.[59] It is described as the first representative of a new class of agents: an enzyme inhibitor (type 5 cyclic guanosine monophosphate-specific phosphodiesterase isozyme) that results in the relaxation of corpus cavernosum smooth muscle cells and thereby enhances penile erection in response to sexual stimuli.[60]

An initial report on sildenafil involved 12 subjects and was conducted in two phases: (1) a single dose in a laboratory and (2) once-daily doses at home for seven days, 1 to 2 hours before sexual activity was likely to occur.[57] Both phases were placebo-controlled, double-blind, and involved a cross-over design. The first included use of the drug at three different doses and measured erectile response to visual sexual stimulation using subject-chosen explicit videos and magazines. In the second phase, subjects kept a diary and graded their erections. Results from the first phase demonstrated a significant difference in penile rigidity between all three doses of sildenafil and placebo, with the difference being more substantial as the dose increased. The in-home phase showed that higher quality erections occurred more often when men were on the drug. Adverse events were described as "mild and transient."

Another report on sildenafil was conducted on 250 patients with erectile dysfunction of "predominantly no known organic cause."[61] Patients previously were involved in an open dose study and were randomized to receive their optimum dose of the medication or placebo. They were asked to compare their erections in the present study to those they experienced in the open trial. Of those given sildenafil, 59% reported no change, and of those receiving placebo, 72% reported their erections as "much worse." The authors concluded that sildenafil must be continued for the erectile improvement to be maintained.

The most complete report on oral sildenafil (as of Spring 1998) was published in the New England Journal of Medicine (NEJM). It involved a total of 861 men with erectile dysfunction described as organic, psychogenic or mixed.[62] Two studies were conducted: (1) a dose-response study on 532 men treated with 25, 50, 100 mg or placebo and (2) a dose-escalation study involving 329 different men treated initially with 50 mg or placebo and subsequently with one half or twice the amount of the original dosage, depending on efficacy and tolerance. These studies were performed in a natural environment and therefore relied on the subjects' reports of efficacy.

In the first study (dose-response) in the NEJM report, increasing doses of sildenafil were associated with significantly increased "frequency of penetration" and maintenance of erections after entry ($p < 0.001$). Interestingly, the cause of the erection difficulty did not affect the outcome. In the second study (dose-escalation), improvement of the same two measures were significantly better for sildenafil compared to placebo ($p < 0.001$), as were several other measures, including "overall satisfaction." (However, in this same study, sexual desire scores were not different in the two groups). In the dose-response study, the frequency of erections sufficiently firm for intercourse to occur was 72%, 80%, and 85% for doses of 25 mg, 50 mg, and 100 mg, respectively (versus 50% for the placebo group; ($p < 0.001$). In the dose-escalation study, 69% of attempts at intercourse (versus 22% for the placebo group) were successful ($p < 0.001$).

> In a dose-response study, the frequency of erections sufficiently firm for intercourse to occur was 72%, 80%, and 85% for doses of 25 mg, 50 mg, and 100 mg, respectively (versus 50% for the placebo group; $p < 0.001$). In the dose-escalation study, 69% of attempts at intercourse (versus 22% for the placebo group) were successful ($p < 0.001$).

Yohimbine is one of the more widely used and studied oral agents used recently in the treatment of erectile dysfunction. It is an alkaloid derivative that is found in the bark of the yohimbine tree and has a long-standing reputation as an aphrodisiac.[63] Part of the attractiveness of yohimbine is the "benign side effect profile"[33] (p. 123). Pharmacologically, yohimbine is a preferential presynaptic alpha 2 antagonist. The dose ranges from 2 to 6 mg three times per day, and has shown to have a positive effect on sexual behavior in animals).[64] However, a review of the outcome of several studies of men with erectile dysfunction indicates that while yohimbine may have the capacity to affect sexual desire and performance in some subjects, "results have been far from conclusive [since] more than half of all patients studied thus far have shown little or no benefit from the drug."[63] A meta-analysis of studies of the effect of yohimbine in men with erection difficulties concluded the opposite, namely, that it was consistently helpful compared to placebo.[65] It may be that the heterogeneity of men with erection difficulties that is evident in many studies has disguised a beneficial effect of this substance in a particular subpopulation. One hypothesis suggests that men with a "nonorganic etiology" might derive a greater benefit than other men.[64]

Androgens often have been administered to men with erection difficulties, frequently without establishing the presence of an endocrinopathy. Studies of androgen treatment in erectile dysfunction that included hormonal assessments strongly suggest that it "is of little value in eugonadal males"[40] (p. 91). The hazards of androgen therapy in this situation have not always been considered. Given the fact that erectile dysfunction and prostate cancer become more evident with increasing age, clinicians need to be especially concerned about the potentially negative effect of androgens (even on a trial basis) on the prostate gland (see Etiology, "Endocrine Abnormalities" above in this chapter).

Intracavernosal Injections (ICI)

Injection of medications directly into one of the corpora cavernosa of a man's penis as a treatment of erectile dysfunction became an accepted and widely used treatment method in the 1980s. It would not be surprising to see this approach greatly diminish in popularity with the advent of an efficacious and safe oral medication.

Three substances are currently used for ICI:

- Papaverine hydrochloride
- Phentolamine mesylate
- Prostaglandin E_1 (PGE_1)

Papaverine has been used alone or in combination with phentolamine; PGE_1 has been used alone or together with papaverine and phentolamine as Trimix. One formulation of PGE_1 is alprostadil. The subject of ICI treatment is thoroughly reviewed elsewhere.[66,67] Dosages are generally titrated to the response of the patient. PGE_1 alone is the substance most commonly used by urologists and the dose is typically in the range of 1 to 40 μg.[67] Smaller doses of medications used in ICI are generally required in instances of neurogenic (and "psychogenic") erectile dysfunction.

ICI seems most efficacious in the context of a neurological deficit (e.g., spinal cord injury) and least helpful in men who have severe corporal veno-occlusive dysfunction and/or arterial insufficiency. Contraindications include poor manual dexterity, morbid obesity, and anticoagulant therapy.[67] Injection usually results in a partial erection within minutes and the addition of sexual stimulation usually increases the enlargement.[68] Patient's are taught the technique of injection (usually by a urologist or nurse-educator) and "observed while self-injecting so that the physician has an opportunity to advise and correct his technique." Patients then inject themselves at home.[67] One side effect, namely, prolonged erection (defined as more than four hours), requires immediate medical attention. The frequency of prolonged erection (priapism) and other side effects depends on the medication used. Side effects include the following:

- Fibrotic nodules (more with papaverine and/or phentolamine)
- Pain (about 10% to 34% with PGE_1 alone)
- Infection
- Bruising
- Liver function abnormalities
- Vasovagal episodes

Prolonged erections appear to more common with papaverine alone (10% of patients) than PGE_1 alone (2% of patients). The incidence of priapism seems to be less with the mixture of papaverine-phentolamine-PGE_1.[67] Priapism rates for home injections are considerably less (0.3%) than in-office trial injections. When priapism occurs, emergency intervention is required, and most cases resulting from papaverine and/or phentolamine respond to aspiration alone, or in combination with intracorporal installation of a diluted alpha-adrenergic receptor agonist such as epinephrine (limited to less than 15 μg at intervals of more than five minutes to avoid systemic side effects).[69]

Fibrotic plaques are reported to be less common with PGE_1 than with papaverine and/or phentolamine, and there have been no reports of liver disease with either of these substances or with PGE_1 despite abnormalities on liver function testing.[67] Pain during injection is commonly reported by men using PGE_1 (75% in one study) but pain is infrequent with papaverine and/or phentolamine.[67]

The impact of ICI on patients and their partners was studied and beneficial changes were described in each, particularly in the areas of self-esteem, sexual desire, frequency, and satisfaction.[66,67]

Although ICI is considered safe and reliable, many patients do not continue using it in the short-run for several reasons, including[67]:

1. The feeling that it was unnatural
2. Concerns about side effects
3. Lack of a regular partner
4. Fear of being belittled by the partner

In addition to immediate issues, there is a surprisingly high (50%) drop out rate at 12 month follow-up. Reasons given include loss of efficacy and loss of interest. The high drop out rate suggests the need for a careful initial evaluation of the motivation of the patient and partner and willingness to accept ICI on the part of both.

Transurethral Alprostadil

Alprostadil is a synthetic compound identical to PGE_1. A transurethral method of delivering this medication was developed as an alternative to intracavernosal injections. With medicated urethral system for erection (MUSE), a proprietary drug delivery system, the medication is put into a tiny pellet and deposited into the end of the urethra with an applicator. A man urinates before insertion of the applicator to lubricate his urethra.

Route of administration of any medication may result in different side effects even though the substance might be the same. In the form of intracavernosal injections, alprostadil enters directly into the corpus cavernosum of the penis. When given transurethrally, the medication is absorbed from the urethral mucosa, enters the body's blood stream, and then is returned to the penis.

In a double-blind and placebo-controlled study, 1511 men aged 27 to 88 with "chronic erectile dysfunction from various organic causes" were treated with transurethral alprostadil.[70] To determine maximal penile response, subjects were given the opportunity to use up to four alternative doses of the drug: 125, 250, 500, or 1000 µg. The 996 men who responded in a clinic setting were then randomly assigned to the selected dose or placebo. Eighty-eight percent of the men completed the three month course of treatment. Significantly more men in the alprostadil group (65%) reported having intercourse at least once and the medication was significantly more effective than placebo regardless of age or the cause of the erectile dysfunction.

The most common side effect of transurethral alprostadil was penile pain (reported by 33% of the men) but was considered mild and resulted in only 20% of the men leaving the study.[70] Other side effects include mild urethral trauma (5%), dizziness (2%), and urinary tract infections ("rare").

Transurethral alprostadil is particularly advantageous in primary care. For the physician the procedure is greatly simplified (compared to ICI) in that the medication is self-administered and does not require an in-office training procedure. From the patient's perspective, the process is less complex to learn and to use at home and free of the potentially serious side effects of priapism and fibrosis associated with ICI.

Vacuum Erection Devices

Vacuum erection devices (VEDs) are also called vacuum constriction, and external vacuum, devices (information available through Imagyn Technologies at 1-800-344-9688). Like intracavernosal injections, the use of VEDs may diminish considerably with the advent of a safe and effective oral treatment for erectile dysfunction. However, for the foreseeable future, VEDs are likely to remain in the armamentarium of health professionals who treat men with erectile dysfunction. The need is exemplified, for example, in men for whom a physical approach is recommended but who strongly prefer not to use any kind of drugs for an ailment that could be treated in a nonpharmacological manner. The subject of VEDs is reviewed in detail elsewhere.[66]

When first introduced in the early 1980s, "the concept [of VEDs] seemed difficult for physicians to accept. In an era of high technology, perhaps the low technology and simplicity of vacuum devices are disarming and provoke rejection"[66] (p. 297). Precisely because they are "low tech," safe, and efficacious, VEDs are likely to remain of particular interest to primary care clinicians.

The mechanism of action is fundamentally the same for the various VEDs that exist. Procedures are as follows:

- A cylinder is placed over a man's flaccid penis and pressed firmly against his body to create an airtight seal
- Air is pumped out of the cylinder to create a vacuum
- Blood is, in the process, drawn into his penis
- After an erection exists, a tension band is transferred from the VED to the base of the man's penis
- A vacuum release valve is then opened and the cylinder is removed

VED-induced erections are passively created by suction and venous stasis that results from constriction, in contrast to erections produced naturally (and by ICI), which are actively created by neurotransmitters and relaxation of corpora smooth muscle. Several studies demonstrate that 90% of men who have "organic," "mixed," and "psychogenic" erection dysfunction and use this system are able to have sufficiently firm erections for the purpose of intercourse.[66]

The most common side effects reported with VEDs are hematoma and petechiae (8% to 50%).[66] These are generally not considered serious and resolve without medical intervention. Other side effects include the following:

- Pain
- Numbness of the penis
- Pulling of scrotal tissue into the cylinder
- Blocked and painful ejaculation

Patient acceptance is estimated at 80% to 95%. The reasons for discontinuing the use of a VED include the following:

- Mechanical difficulty
- Failure to produce an adequate erection
- Feeling that the device is cumbersome
- A sense that the erection is artificial

There are three contraindications: men with Peyronie's Disease, concurrent blood dyscrasia or use of anticoagulants, and poor manual dexterity (which can be overcome by the use of a battery operated device).

Table 11-1 summarizes comparisons between VEDs and ICI. Since they are both equally efficacious and have a positive effect on patients, "the critical discriminations need to be made on the basis of cost, potential side effects, patient acceptance, and aesthetic preferences of the man or couple"[66] (p. 304).

Penile Prostheses

The use of prostheses (or implants) in the treatment of men with erectile dysfunction is generally considered "a last resort," since surgery involves the destruction of structures which are otherwise normally involved in the erectile process. The irreversibility of prosthesis implantation limits its use given the rapid progress in the development of more benign approaches to the treatment of this disorder. The subject of prostheses has been thoroughly reviewed elsewhere.[71]

> The irreversibility of prosthesis implantation limits its use given the rapid progress in the development of more benign approaches to the treatment of this disorder.

Implants have been used since the early 1950s and now exist in a variety of forms: semirigid silicone only; semirigid, silicone interior; and inflatable.[71] "Most operating rooms stock one type of semirigid device and the inflatable prosthesis used most often by the implanting surgeons" (p. 270). Some factors that influence the choice of device include: cost, availability, esthetics, and manual dexterity (to use the inflatable type) (p. 271).

In a follow-up examination on the satisfaction of patients (n = 52) and their partners (n = 22), which involved interviewing the two people separately and had a response rate of 72%, the kind of device implanted made little difference to the men.

Table 11-1   Comparison of Self-injection and External Vacuum Devices

FACTOR	SELF-INJECTION	EXTERNAL VACUUM DEVICES
Efficacy		
Neurogenic	Good response	Good response
Vasculogenic	Poor-good response	Good response
Idiopathic	Good response	Good response
Psychogenic	Adequate response	Adequate-good response
Psychological benefits	Positive effect	Positive effect
Patient acceptance	40%-50%	80%-95%
Cost	$75/monthly; $900/yearly	$200-$400 total outlay
Side effects	Prolonged erection	Hematoma, bruising
	Fibrotic nodules	Numbness
	Hepatotoxicity	Blocked/painful ejaculation
	Bruising	Pulling in scrotal tissue
	Pain	Fainting
	Vasovagal episodes	
	Infection	
Concealability	Easily concealed	Not easily concealed
Prolonged intercourse	Possible	Limited to 30 minutes
Frequency of Intercourse	Limited to twice weekly	No limitation
Conception	No limitation	Possible blocked ejaculation

From Althof SE, Turner LA: Self-injection therapy and external vacuum devices in the treatment of erectile dysfunction: methods and outcome. In Rosen RC, Leiblum SR (editors): *Erectile disorders: assessment and treatment*, New York, 1992, The Guilford Press. Reprinted with permission.

However, the patient's partner preferred inflatable implants.[72] All except four had intercourse more than "infrequently." Almost 80% of the men said they would undergo the operation again but only 60% of the partners said that they had no hesitations.

The goal of treatment with penile prostheses can vary greatly and depends to a large extent on the perspective of the discipline of the person stating an opinion. Some urologists focus specifically on the issue of erection, whereas mental health professionals and sex therapists concentrate more broadly on sexual satisfaction of the two partners. One follow-up study did not resolve the conflict (but leaned more toward the view of sex therapists), since it demonstrated that the greatest benefit is the sense of "restored manhood." "The feeling of being *capable* of coitus, was reported by many of the men in the study as a prime benefit of surgery" (italics added)[71] (p. 273). Screening issues have been identified to detect patients for whom penile prosthesis implantation is planned but who might benefit also from preventive counseling.[73] These include the following factors:

- Concern about the importance of penile size in sexual activity
- Disinterest in foreplay

- Low sexual desire in either partner
- Premature ejaculation
- Untreated vaginal atrophy in the woman

Indications for Referral for Consultation or Continuing Care by a Specialist

The treatment of solo men, or couples, in which the man has an acquired and generalized form of erectile dysfunction requires attention to both physical and psychological etiological issues. The more the etiologies are known, the more specific will be the treatment, as well as the kind of health professional needed to provide the necessary form of care. Referral for medical specialist *consultation* may be useful in, for example, the following specific and defined circumstances:

- Endocrine disorders
- Diabetes
- Cardiovascular disorders (including hypertension)
- Major depression

Referral to a urologist for continuing care might be beneficial in instances of "venous leak."

When complex, expensive, or physically invasive diagnostic procedures are necessary to clarify the etiology, consultation with a urologist who is knowledgeable about erectile disorders is required. Buvat reminded clinicians of " . . . Cochran's aphorism: 'before doing a test, decide what to do if it is (a) positive and (b) negative. If both answers are the same, don't do the test."[12]

When the etiology is unknown (or the etiology known but not responsive to specific therapy), treatment is nonspecific. The advent of safe and effective oral therapies will likely result in many more men with erectile dysfunction being identified and cared for on a primary care basis than at present. However, liberal use should be made of other health professionals (especially urologists and sex therapists) when cases are treatment-resistant (for the purpose of consultation and possible implementation of other nonspecific treatment approaches).

Summary

Impotence is a term that is widely used and accepted but falls short of being helpful for two reasons: (1) confusion, since several conditions are grouped in the same category and (2) even more confusion, since the disorders have nothing to do with power (the origin of the word "potency").

The prevalence of erectile disorders is 40% of men at age 40 and 66% at age 70. The resources needed to treat this widespread problem are substantial and will become even more substantial as the aging population increases.

In the same way that different cardiac disorders manifest in similar ways despite having several origins, so do erectile disorders. While the chief manifestation of an erectile disorder is a soft penis rather than a hard one, the pattern of erection function matters when considering etiology ("psychogenic" and "organic") and treatment. An erectile problem that is generalized (exists in all situations: with a partner, in the morning, and with masturbation) suggests a different etiological and treatment direction than one that is situational (erections are unimpaired in some situations). Likewise, it matters if erection problems have always existed, since the man has been sexually involved with others (lifelong) or developed more recently (acquired).

Causes of erectile disorders (often more than one) include the following:

- Medical disorders (endocrine, cardiovascular, neurological)
- Drugs
- Elevated blood lipids
- Cigarette smoking
- Psychiatric disorders
- Relationship problems
- Anxiety

In any investigation of an erectile disorder, history-taking is essential, a physical examination is necessary (although the yield is low), and laboratory tests are required if the pattern of erectile dysfunction even hints at being generalized.

Treatment of erectile disorders are sometimes specific to the etiology (e.g., replacing a hormone that exists in insufficient amounts) and sometimes nonspecific, for example, oral medications (sildenafil [Viagra], psychotherapy, or intracavernosal injections. Counseling intervention ranges from being central (sex therapy) to being an adjunct (e.g., information about the use of vacuum erection devices).

The prevalence of erectile disorders makes primary care health professionals central to the care of men (and couples) with this disorder. Their task will likely be made easier by the introduction of safe and effective oral therapies. However, even with the advent of new forms of care there still will be treatment-resistant patients and couples, and in those instances, liberal use should be made of other approaches and specialists.

POSTSCRIPT

When a patient takes no action after treatment suggestions are made for erectile difficulties, clinicians should not necessarily be surprised or discouraged.

A 57-year-old divorced computer analyst was seen because of long-standing (about ten years) erectile difficulties that appear when alone in masturbation and on the occasional times he is sexually active with a partner. He experienced a myocardial infarction four years before the referral. He lived alone for 25 years after a marriage that lasted three years. The longest relationship he had with a woman since then (he was not romantically or sexually interested in men) was four months and that was about 20 years before. Since then he had a few dates but none in the previous ten years because he felt that women would expect him to do what he felt was not possible, that is, to sexually "perform." Discontented with the suggestions made at the end of a thorough assessment, he insisted on special diagnostic vascular procedures about which he had read. He was unwilling to consider oral medications, intracavernosal injections, or VEDs and was angry about the suggestion of psychiatric care as part of a treatment "package." He did not appear again after two visits and canceled his last appointment.

A survey of men assessed for erectile problems in a urology clinic found that two years later over half had not followed up on recommendations.[74] Sexual and nonsexual reasons may have existed. A strong desire for return of erectile capability may not be durable after the discovery that treatment entails significant psychological and/or physical effort and discomfort. In addition, some men are quite resistant to the notion that the explanation for problems with the function of their genitalia may, in fact, lie elsewhere (e.g., the problems may be an expression of intimacy difficulties [see Appendix II]).

REFERENCES

1. Rosen RC, Leiblum SR: Erectile disorders: an overview of historical trends and clinical perspectives. In Rosen RC, Leiblum SR (editors): *Erectile disorders: assessment and treatment,* New York, 1992, Guildford Press, pp. 3-26.
2. Elliott ML: The use of "impotence" and "frigidity": why has "impotence" survived, *J Sex Marital Ther* 11:51-56, 1985.
3. Impotence. NIH Consensus Statement 10:1-31, 1992
4. Lue TF, Tanagho EA: Functional anatomy and mechanism of penile erection. In Tanagho EA, Lue TF, McClure RD (editors): *Contemporary management of impotence and infertility.* Baltimore,1988, Williams & Wilkins.
5. *Diagnostic and Statistical Manual of Mental Disorders, ed 4, Primary Care Version,* Washington, 1995, American Psychiatric Association.
6. Feldman HA et al: Impotence and its medical and psychosocial correlates: results of the Massachusetts male aging study, *J Urology* 151:54-61,1994.
7. Rosen RC, Leiblum SR: Erectile disorders: an overview of historical trends and clinical perspectives. In Rosen RC, Leiblum SR (editors): *Erectile disorders: assessment and treatment,* 1992, The Guilford Press, pp. 3-26.
8. Spector IP, Carey MP: Incidence and prevalence of the sexual dysfunctions, *Arch Sex Behav* 19:389-408, 1990.
9. Masters WH, Johnson VE: *Human sexual inadequacy,* 1970, Little, Brown and Company.
10. Althof SE, Seftel AD: The evaluation and management of erectile dysfunction, *Psych Clin N Am* 18:171,1995.
11. LoPiccolo J: Postmodern sex therapy for erectile failure. In Rosen RC, Leiblum SR (editors): *Erectile disorders: assessment and management,* New York, 1992, The Guilford Press, pp. 171-197.
12. Buvat J et al: Recent developments in the clinical assessment and diagnosis of erectile dysfunction, *Ann Rev Sex Res* 1:265-308,1990.
13. O'Leary MP et al: A brief male sexual function inventory for urology, *Urol* 46:697-706, 1995.
14. Schover LR, Jensen SB: *Sexuality and chronic illness: a comprehensive approach,* New York, 1988, The Guilford Press.
15. Slag MF et al: Impotence in medical clinic outpatients, *JAMA* 249:1736-1740, 1983.
16. Rosen RC, Leiblum SR, Spector IP: Psychologically based treatment for male erectile disorder: a cognitive-interpersonal model, *J Sex Marital Ther* 20:67-85, 1994.
17. Levine SB: Intrapsychic and interpersonal aspects of impotence: psychogenic erectile dysfunction. In Rosen RC, Leiblum SR (editors): *Erectile disorders: assessment and treatment,* 1992, The Guilford Press, pp. 198-225.
18. Masters WH, Johnson VE: *Human sexual response,* Boston, 1966, Little, Brown and Company.
19. Althof SE: Psychogenic impotence: treatment of men and couples. In Leiblum SR, Rosen RC (editors): *Principles and Practice of Sex Therapy: Update for the 1990s,* ed 2, New York, 1989, The Guilford Press, pp. 237-265.
20. Zilbergeld B: *The new male sexuality,* New York, 1992, Bantam Books.

21. Goldman A, Carroll JL: Educational intervention as an adjunct to treatment of erectile dysfunction in older couples, *J Sex Marital Ther* 16:127-141,1990

22. Cranston-Cuebas MA, Barlow DH: Cognitive and effective contributions to sexual functioning, *Ann Rev Sex Res* 1:119-161, 1990.

23. Turner LA et al: Self-injection of papaverine and phentolamine in the treatment of psychogenic impotence, *J Sex Marital Ther* 15(3):163-176, 1989.

24. De Amicis LA et al: Clinical follow-up of couples treated for sexual dysfunction, *Arch Sex Behav* 14:467-489, 1985.

25. Hawton K et al: Long-term outcome of sex therapy, *Behav Res Ther* 24:665-675, 1986.

26. Schiavi RC et al: Diabetes mellitus and male sexual function, *Diabetologia* 36:745-751, 1993.

27. Report of the expert committee on the diagnosis and classification of diabetes mellitus, *Diabetes Care* 20:1183-1197, 1997.

28. Nofzinger EA et al: Results of nocturnal penile tumescence studies are abnormal in sexually functional diabetic men, *Arch Internal Med* 152:114-118, 1992.

29. Meulemann EJ, Diemont WL: Investigation of erectile dysfunction: diagnostic testing for vascular factors in erectile dysfunction, *Urol Clin N Am* 22:803-819, 1995.

30. Virag R, Bouilly P, Frydman D: Is impotence an arterial disorder? *Lancet* 8422:181-184, 1985.

31. Condra M et al: Prevalence and significance of tobacco smoking in impotence, *Urol* 27:495-498, 1986.

32. Rosen MP et al: Cigarette smoking: an independent risk factor for atherosclerosis in the hypogastric-cavernosus arterial bed of men with arteriogenic impotence, *J Urol* 145:759-763, 1991.

33. Crenshaw TL, Goldberg JP: *Sexual pharmacology: drugs that affect sexual function*, New York, 1996, W.W. Norton & Company, Inc.

34. Segraves RT, Segraves KB: Aging and drug effects on male sexuality. In Rosen RC, Leiblum SR (editors): *Erectile disorders: assessment and treatment*, New York, 1992, The Guilford Press, pp. 96-138.

35. Schiavi RC: Chronic alcoholism and male sexual dysfunction, *J Sex Marital Ther* 16:23-33, 1990.

36. Lemere F, Smith JW: Alcohol-induced sexual impotence, *Am J Psychiatry* 130:212-213, 1973.

37. Whalley LJ: Sexual adjustment of male alcoholics, *Acta Psychiatr Scand* 58:281-298, 1978.

38. Jensen SB: Sexual function and dysfunction in younger married alcoholics: a comparative study, *Acta Psychiatr Scand* 69:543-549, 1984.

39. Snyder S, Karacan I: Effects of chronic alcoholism on nocturnal penile tumescence, *Psychosom Med* 43:423-429, 1981.

40. Bannister P, Lowowsky MS: Ethanol and hypogonadism, *Alcohol Alcoholism* 22:213-217, 1987.

41. Davidson JM, Rosen RC: Hormonal determinents of erectile function. In Rosen RC, Leiblum SR (editors): *Erectile disorders: assessment and treatment*, New York, 1992, The Guilford Press, pp. 72-95.

42. Buvat J, Lemaire A: Endocrine screening in 1,022 men with erectile dysfunction: clinical significance and cost-effective strategy, *J Urol* 158:1764-1767, 1997.

43. WHO Expert Committee on Diabetes Mellitus: *World Health Organization Technical Report Series 646*, Geneva, 1980 World Health Organization.

44. Buvat J et al: Is intracavernous injection of papaverine a reliable screening test for vascular impotence? *J Urol* 135:476-478, 1986.

45. Porst H: Diagnotic use and side-effects of vasoactive drugs—a report on over 2100 patients with erectile failure, *Int J Impotence Res* 2(2):222-223,1990.

46. Schiavi RC: Laboratory methods for evaluating erectile dysfunction. In Rosen RC, Leiblum SR (editors): *Erectile disorders: assessment and treatment*. New York,1992, The Guilford Press, pp. 141-170.

47. Schiavi RC et al: Healthy aging and male sexual function, *Am J Psychiatry* 147:766-771, 1990.

48. Nofzinger EA et al: Sexual function in depressed men, *Arch Gen Psychiatry* 50:24-30, 1993.

49. Nofzinger EA et al: Results of nocturnal penile tumescence studies are abnormal in sexually functional diabetic men, *Arch Intern Med* 152:114-118, 1992.

50. Kirkeby HJ et al. Erectile dysfunction in multiple sclerosis, *Neurology* 38,1366-1371, 1988.

51. Kirkeby HJ, Andersen AJ, Poulsen EU: Nocturnal penile tumescence and rigidity: translation of data obtained from normal males, *Int J Impotence Res* 1:115-125, 1989.

52. Levine LA, Carroll RA: Nocturnal penile tumescence and rigidity in men without complaints of erectile dysfunction using a new quantitative analysis software, *J Urol* 152:1103-1107, 1994.

53. Levine LA, Lenting EL: Use of nocturnal penile tumescence and rigidity in the evaluation of male erectile dysfunction, *Urol Clin N Am* 22:775-788, 1995.

54. Schreiner-Engel P: Therapy of psychogenic erectile disorders, *Sex Disability* 4:115-122, 1981.

55. The Diabetes Control and Complications Trial Research Group. The effect of intensive treatment of diabetes on the development and progression of long-term complications in insulin-dependent diabetes mellitus, *N Engl J Med* 329:977-986, 1993.

56. McCullough DK et al: The prevalence of diabetic impotence, *Diabetologia* 18:279-283,1990.

57. Boolell M et al: Sildenafil, a novel effective oral therapy for male erectile dysfunction, *Brit J Urology* 78:257-261, 1996.

58. Lue T: Editorial Comment, *J Urol* 157:2021, 1997.

59. Boolell M et al: Sildenafil: an orally active type 5 cyclic GMP-specific phosphodiesterase inhibitor for the treatment of penile erectile dysfunction, *Int J Impotence Res* 8:47-52, 1996.

60. Wicker P: Phosphodiesterase inhibitors and male erectile dysfunction. Presented at the 1997 Annual Meeting of the Society for Sex Therapy and Research, Chicago, 1997.

61. Virag R et al: (Pfizer Central Reseach, UK): Sildenafil (Viagra), a new oral treatment for erectile dysfunction (editor): an 8 week double-blind, placebo-controlled parallel group study. Presented at the VII World Meeting of the International Society for Impotence Research, San Francisco, 1996.

62. Goldstein I et al: Oral sildenafil in the treatment of xerectile dysfunction, *N Engl J Med* 338:1397-1404, 1998.

63. Rosen RC, Ashton AK: Prosexual drugs: empirical status of the "new aphrodesiacs," *Arch Sex Behav* 22:521-543, 1993.

64. Mann K et al: Effects of Yohimbine on sexual experiences and nocturnal penile tumescence and rigidity in erectile dysfunction, *Arch Sex Behav* 25:1-16, 1996.

65. Carey MP, Johnson BT: Effectiveness of Yohimbine in the treatment of erectile disorder: four meta-analytic integrations, *Arch Sex Behav* 25:341-360, 1996.

66. Althof SE, Turner LA: Self-injection therapy and external vacuum devices in the treatment of erectile dysfunction. In Rosen RC, Leiblum SR (editors): *Erectile disorders: assessment and treatment*, New York, 1992, The Guilford Press, pp. 283-309.

67. Fallon B: Intracavernous injection therapy for male erectile dysfunction, *Urol Clin N Am* 22:833-845, 1995.

68. Donatucci CF, Lue TF: The combined intracavernous injection and stimulation test: diagnostic accuracy, *J Urol* 148:61-62, 1992.

69. Lue TF et al: Priapism: a refined approach to diagnosis and treatment, *J Urol* 166:104-108, 1986.

70. Padman-Nathan H: Treatment of men with erectile dysfunction with transurethral alprostadil, *N Eng J Med* 336:1-7,1997.

71. Melman A, Tiefer L: Surgery for erectile disorders: operative procedures and psychological issues. In Rosen RC, Lieblum SR (editors): *Erectile disorders: assessment and treatment*. New York, 1992, The Guilford Press, pp. 255-282.

72. Pederson B et al: Evaluation of patients and partners 1 to 4 years after penile prosthesis surgery, *J Urol* 139:956-958, 1988.

73. Schover LR: Sex therapy for the penile prosthesis recipient. *Urol Clin N Am* 16:91-98, 1989.

74. Tiefer L, Melman A: Adherence to recommendations and improvement over time in men with erectile dysfunction, *Arch Sex Behav* 16:301-308, 1987.

CHAPTER 12

ORGASMIC DIFFICULTIES IN WOMEN

Although not as prominent a sexual problem as it once was, failure to achieve orgasm continues to be a major complaint of many women. . . . the manner, method, and ease of orgasmic attainment has received wide publicity, and the woman who does not regularly achieve orgasm feels deficient, deprived, and often depressed.

LIEBLUM AND ROSEN, 1989[1]

PROLOGUE

In a study of written descriptions of orgasms obtained from 24 men and 24 women, pronouns were deleted and the accounts given to 70 health professionals who were "blinded" men and women.[5] The latter were unable to distinguish the descriptions on the basis of gender.

Clinical experience suggests that the meaning of orgasm to men and women is not always the same. Men tend to focus attention on their own and their partner's orgasm. Many women also put great weight on the intimacy and closeness that accompanies a sexual experience.

Why are orgasm troubles in women considered separately from phenomena that are known by the same name in men? Is there a difference between the two? When considering only the subjective sensation of an orgasm, probably not. Masters & Johnson,[2] Kaplan,[3] and DSM-IV[4] do not separate men and women. Perhaps even more tellingly, in a study of written descriptions of orgasms obtained from 24 men and 24 women, pronouns were deleted and the accounts given to 70 health professionals who were "blinded" men and women.[5] The latter were unable to distinguish the descriptions on the basis of gender.

What about the equivalency of orgasm and the word "sex?" For many, the answer is that they are not the same. A patient may be better served if a clinician goes beyond a consideration of orgasms only and thinks also about sexual *satisfaction*.[6] Clinical experience suggests that the meaning of orgasm to men and women is not always the same. Men tend to focus attention on their own and their partner's orgasms. Many women also put great weight on the intimacy and closeness that accompanies a sexual experience.

THE PROBLEM

A 27-year-old single woman was concerned about never having an orgasm. Since her late teens, sexual experiences were a regular and satisfying part of three long-term and several brief relationships with men. Despite her usual high level of sexual desire and arousal and the absence of discomfort with intercourse, as well as her obvious pleasure with sexual activity, partners often wondered why she was not experiencing orgasm. They questioned if they were somehow not "doing something right" and generally gave the impression that she was missing out on a universal and gratifying sexual experience. She wondered if something was wrong with her sexual response. She felt that her partners must be knowledgeable about such issues, since they had the wherewithal to compare her to other women with whom they had had sexual experiences (one was actually explicit in saying so). Over the years, she read books and articles in women's magazines suggesting masturbation as a way of learning to become orgasmic but many attempts at self-stimulation proved unsuccessful. Psychotherapy was directed at focusing on her sexual pleasure rather than whether or not she experienced an orgasm. She was still not orgasmic one year later but the level of arousal that she experienced with sexual activity had markedly increased. She described herself as much more sexually content.

TERMINOLOGY

"Climax" is often used as a synonym for orgasm. On a colloquial level, the word "come" has become the verbal equivalent of orgasm (for women and men), and some women use the more euphemistic words "peak" or "satisfaction."

DEFINITION

Orgasm in a man is not difficult to detect, since it is usually accompanied by ejaculation. The process is more subjective in women, although Masters and Johnson[2] (pp. 128-137) described psychophysiological and measurable phenomena associated with female orgasm such as vaginal contractions. They also described (p.5) three patterns in the sexual response cycle experienced by women. While two patterns reached the level of orgasm, one (designated pattern "B" [see Figure 3-2 in Chapter 3]), reached sustained plateau level response without orgasm apparently occurring. Since their first book, *Human Sexual Response,* described "normal" sexual anatomy and physiology, the implication was thus left that the three patterns of female sexual response were all "normal" and so, too, was a high level of female sexual response without orgasm. Unfortunately, there was no commentary accompanying the description of pattern "B" so the frequency (as well as associated changes in physiology, thoughts, and feelings) of these women remains a mystery.

CLASSIFICATION

Female Orgasmic Disorder is defined in DSM-IV-PC[7] (p. 117) in the same terminology as for the male: "Persistent or recurrent delay in, or absence of, orgasm following a normal sexual excitement phase. This can be present in all situations, or only in specific settings, and causes marked distress or interpersonal difficulty. This diagnosis is not appropriate if the difficulty in reaching orgasm is due to sexual stimulation that is not adequate in focus, intensity, and duration." Additional clinical information is provided: "In diagnosing Orgasmic Disorder, the clinician should also take into account the person's age and sexual experience. Once a female learns how to reach orgasm, it is uncommon for her to lose that capacity, unless poor sexual communication, relationship conflict, a traumatic experience (e.g., rape), a Mood Disorder, or a general medical condition intervenes. . . ."

Two common clinical presentations of orgasmic dysfunction in women are: (1) lifelong and generalized (also called primary, pre-orgasmia, anorgasmia, and lifelong global) and (2) lifelong and situational (also called situational and secondary). (The term *secondary* can also refer to women who not only experience orgasm through masturbation but who do not experience orgasm "through any type of partner stimulation [and] who define their limited repertoire of stimulation techniques leading to orgasm as problematic").[8] A third form of orgasmic dysfunction is that which is acquired and generalized.

Clinicians commonly hear a concern from a woman that she is experiencing orgasm with masturbation (perhaps easily, and either alone or with partner touch) but not during penile-vaginal intercourse. Masters and Johnson viewed the absence of orgasm specifically during penile-vaginal intercourse (while present otherwise), to be a disorder requiring treatment[9] (pp. 240-241). Many women objected to this idea, since it seemed to echo a previously held idea that orgasms experienced apart from intercourse

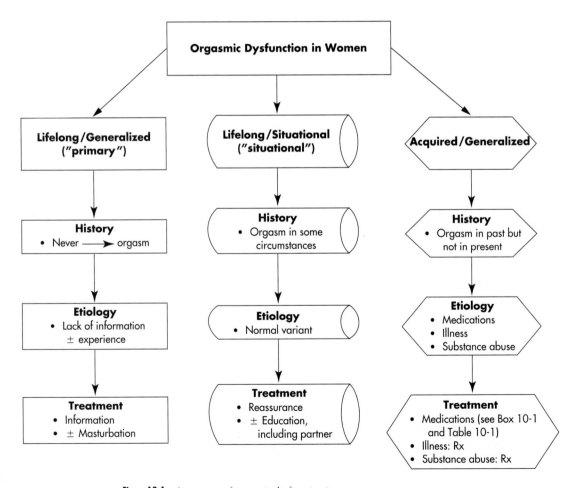

Figure 12-1   Assessment of orgasmic dysfunction in women.

were considered "immature" in contrast to the "mature" orgasms with intercourse. The accumulation of epidemiological information about patterns of orgasmic response in women suggests that orgasm during intercourse is not universal. In fact, one survey found that the *majority* of respondents in partner-related sexual activity usually came to orgasm outside of penile-vaginal intercourse.[10] This new information resulted in a change in the view of health professionals treating women with orgasm concerns to one of thinking that this pattern may not represent pathology but "may constitute a normal variation of female sexuality"[3] (p. 398).

The assessment of orgasmic dysfunction in women is outlined in Figure 12-1.

DESCRIPTION

Lifelong and Generalized ("*primary*")

In the past, many women who reported a lifelong and generalized history of orgasmic dysfunction were considered to be otherwise physically and psychologically healthy. A woman with lifelong and generalized orgasm would describe the following symptoms:

1. Unlike other women she knew, she never had an orgasm
2. She enjoyed sexual experiences with a partner for the closeness but never felt much sexual enjoyment
3. She never tried masturbation
4. She read little or nothing about sex and orgasm
5. She talked to virtually no one about these subjects

Today, women who are concerned about the absence of orgasm often report:

1. A high level of sexual response when with a partner and feeling close to "something"
2. Having read about sexual matters and orgasm
3. Talking to partners about orgasm
4. Having "tried" to masturbate but finding that it "didn't work" (and possibly also used a "toy" such as a vibrator)

Reports of masturbation attempts in the past require more detailed questioning, since they vary from meager (a few opportunities for brief periods) to considerable (many times involving great effort and lengthy duration).

A recently married 26-year-old woman talked to her family doctor about her sexual response. Specifically, she said that while she generally enjoyed sexual experiences with men, she never had an orgasm by any means whatsoever. She read in books and women's magazines about masturbation as a way of experiencing orgasm, little reservation about this approach, and tried it but found it to be sexually frustrating. When asked how many times she tried and for how long, she related that she tried about six times during a two-month period about two years before, and for about five minutes on each occasion. She stopped trying when she experienced little change in her sexual feelings. She also reported that when male sexual partners stimulated her clitoris, she generally found this irritating and eventually asked them to stop.

The patient's doctor used the opportunity of her periodic pelvic examination and pap smear to explain aspects of female genital anatomy and physiology, about which the patient was not well informed. This was done during the examination by placing the patient in a semi-reclining position while she held a mirror that reflected her genitalia, so that she could more easily understand the doctor's explanation.

After the examination, the patient was encouraged to buy and read a self-help book about women and orgasm and to masturbate at home several times each week for a much longer period of time (at least 15 to 30 minutes) before she stopped. When she returned as scheduled three weeks later, the patient reported the following:

- That she purchased and read the recommended book
- That she experimented with self-stimulation as suggested
- That she experienced a high level of arousal in the process

She was encouraged to continue, and to direct her husband in stimulating her as she might do when alone. Three weeks after that visit, she reported having orgasms regularly when alone since shortly after the previous visit. She also described being less shy with her husband, more candid in her directions, and reaching a much higher level of arousal with him. She was confident that orgasm during sexual activity with her husband would eventually occur.

Lifelong and Situational ("situational")

Women who are situationally nonorgasmic on a lifelong basis usually report that with masturbation they have no difficulty coming to orgasm. (Some may, alternatively, describe infrequent orgasms with a partner.) Some may be orgasmic with partner-related sexual practices other than intercourse and, in general, describe sexual experiences as quite pleasurable. A lack of orgasm usually extends over a lifetime of sexual encounters for the woman (although it is not unusual to hear that orgasm during intercourse occurred once or a few times in the past). Sometimes this pattern of response is presented as a sexual concern. With greater depth of questioning, the woman often says that orgasms with intercourse would be her preference if they could easily happen. However, she states that she feels quite satisfied if she can come to orgasm in some form or another when with her partner, (e.g., with oral stimulation) and that the notion that this must occur specifically with intercourse derives more from the wishes of her partner rather than herself.

Acquired and Generalized

In the acquired and generalized form, the woman reports the recent loss of the ability to come to orgasm by any means whatsoever with a partner or when alone, or alternatively, a recent change in her sexual response pattern such that orgasm occurs only after an unusually lengthy process.

A 39-year-old woman was seen because she recently became nonorgasmic. She was in a harmonious lesbian relationship for the past 10 years. The quantity of sexual activity was considerably greater initially but diminished over the years, largely because of a discrepancy in sexual desire between the two (the patient's partner was less interested). Sexual events were qualitatively uncomplicated. In the past, both were easily orgasmic and the patient masturbated to orgasm several times each week (an experience that she highly valued) between sexual times with her partner. She (the patient) had mild episodes of depression in the past that were treated with psychotherapy. However, more recently, she had a more severe episode and she accepted the inclusion of antidepressant medication (an SSRI) in her treatment. Within a week, she noticed that coming to orgasm with masturbation was becoming more difficult, and shortly after she found that achieving orgasm became impossible by any means (despite continued desire and a high level of arousal). Even though she felt improvement in her mood, the medication was changed because of the sexual side effect. When she became orgasmic once again, however, her symptoms of depression worsened. It proved difficult to find a medication that was effective in treating her mood problems without also causing a loss of orgasm. The benefit of the antidepressant was so substantial that she chose abandoning her orgasms for what she expected to be a limited period of time.

EPIDEMIOLOGY

In response to a question in the Laumann et al. study ("In the last 12 months, has there ever been a period of several months or more when you were unable to come to a climax?") 24% of women respondents said "yes".[11] This was the second most common sexual dysfunction reported by women (the first was "lacked interest in sex"). Orgasm difficulties in women were more often associated (p. 371) with the following:

> In response to a question in the Laumann et al, study ("In the last 12 months, has there ever been a period of several months or more when you were unable to come to a climax?") 24% of women respondents said "yes".[11] This was the second most common sexual dysfunction reported by women.

1. Less education (30% of those who had "less than HS")
2. Low income (27% of those who were "poor")
3. Impaired health (33% of those who were in "fair" health)
4. Personal unhappiness (40% of those who were "unhappy most times")
5. Younger age (less than 40 years old)
6. Marital status (highest [29%] in divorced women)
7. Race (highest [29%] in black women)
8. Religion (highest [29%] in women who reported "none")

Information on subclassification can be gained from a review of community based research on the epidemiology of orgasmic dysfunction in women.[12] Various studies show that 5% to 20% of women have never, or infrequently, experienced orgasm. In the language of DSM-IV-PC, such women would be classified as having the lifelong and generalized form of orgasmic dysfunction.[7] There is inadequate data on the frequency of the situational, and acquired and generalized forms.

In a review of the frequency of orgasmic problems in women as the presenting problem in sex therapy clinics, there was a reported range in several studies from 18 to 76%[13] (p. 42). Variations probably relate to the year the particular study was conducted (several are from the 1970s and early 1980s) and the focus of the clinic from which the particular report emerged.

ETIOLOGY

Most of the comments about the etiology of orgasmic dysfunction in women are general and have not been made in relation to any particular subtype. After reviewing the literature on physiological, sociological, psychological and interpersonal, and cultural factors that might influence orgasm in women, Morokoff concluded that ". . . one association is clearly uncontested: Birth later in the century is related to higher frequency of orgasm[14] (p. 156). Whatever cultural changes in attitude toward female sexuality are at work, it seems possible that women who are better educated, have higher social standing, and/or do not have rigid religious morals have been more easily influenced."

Gebhardt related the experience of orgasm to the extent of happiness of a woman in her relationship. He found that a certain group of women (35% to 41%) reached "coital orgasm" regardless of the degree of contentment.[15] Since the percentage was appreciably higher (59%) in women from "very happy" marriages, he concluded that there were also women who were quite sensitive to the state of their relationship and who would not experience orgasm unless the quality of this alliance was at a high level.

While the importance of psychological issues in the possible causes of orgasmic dysfunction remain unclear from a research perspective, they are difficult to ignore clinically.

A 27-year-old woman, recently separated after a five year marriage, was referred because of never having been orgasmic. In her previous sexual encounters, she was usually interested, had no difficulty becoming vaginally wet, and did not experience pain with attempts at intercourse. She described many of the physiological phenomena associated with a high level of arousal and felt herself "close," at which point "something would happen." Her arousal level and her feeling of sexual desire would drop precipitously. The same pattern existed with other partners before her marriage, as well as with masturbation.

She wondered about sexual abuse during her childhood but had no memory of any such experience. However, she also described a family-of-origin where her father was uncommunicative, unaffectionate, and critical. As an adult, she found relationships with men difficult, particularly in the areas of trust and control. She felt that her distrusting attitude toward men derived directly from her family and, moreover, was underlined by her discovery of a relationship between her husband and another woman.

After one year of psychotherapy, she had a better understanding of the origins of her attitudes toward men and how they shaped her life in the present. She also felt more sexually responsive for longer periods than had been the case in the past, although to her chagrin, she remained nonorgasmic. However, she was optimistic that this situation might change.

Orgasmic dysfunction that is acquired and generalized can result from various medications, illnesses, and abused substances. However, as compared to impaired ejaculation/orgasm in men, there seems to be considerably less specific information in the literature on the effects of these phenomena on orgasm in women (see "Delayed Ejaculation/Orgasm" in Chapter 10). Segraves comments that women may be less likely to report orgasmic difficulty than men, since they often are more prepared to attribute the problem to an interpersonal conflict than a biological explanation.[16] Although his statement was made in relation to antidepressant medications, it is equally valid in other situations as well, and hence it is necessary to ask specific questions when determining the presence of side effects.

> Women may be less likely to report orgasmic difficulty than men, since they often are more prepared to attribute the problem to an interpersonal conflict than a biological one.[16]

Some medications used in psychiatry, to control high blood pressure and other ailments seen in medical practice have a particular predilection for interfering with the orgasm part of the sex response cycle (see Appendix III).[17] Psychiatric drugs that have a specific effect on orgasm in women have been reviewed.[16,18,19] Antidepressants (tricyclics, MAOIs, and SSRIs), antipsychotics (some phenothiazines), and antianxiety drugs (some benzodiazepines) are reported as causing anorgasmia in women. In a recent (1997), comprehensive, and family-practice-oriented report on the sexual side effects of medications, Finger and his colleagues provided information on *all* such effects (not only those related to one part of the sex response cycle), specified the nature of the problems encountered, commented on their relative frequency, and included gender-specific observations (see Appendix III).[20] Some of their notations are relevant to the issue of orgasmic dysfunction in women.

Some medical disorders result in symptoms that affect orgasmic response for men and women. Specific observations on diabetes[21] and multiple sclerosis (MS) in women[22] are reported. One study on sexual problems in women with MS refers to "difficulties" in achieving orgasm. The authors of another study[23] on the same subject found that when a patient had genital sensory disturbance, the kind of sexual practice that occurred became significant when considering whether or not the patient came to orgasm. Three sexual practices were described:

- Intercourse, least effective
- Oral stimulation, intermediate
- Manual stimulation, most effective

Studies of the effects on alcohol use on sexual expression in women are confusing. In a study of the effects of acute intoxication on a group of 18 university women subjects,[24] alcohol was shown to result in a progressively greater depressant effect on orgasmic response as blood levels increased. Specifically, alcohol was associated with longer latency to orgasm and diminished intensity of the feeling but, paradoxically, greater sexual arousal and pleasure associated with orgasm.

In an attempt to obtain more information on the effects of alcohol on the sexual activity of nonalcoholic women, a prospective study involving daily logs of alcohol intake and sexual activity was conducted on 69 subjects.[25] Three groups were defined:

- No alcohol
- Moderate intake
- Heavy consumption

The only significant finding was that female-initiated sexual activity occurred twice as often *without* alcohol (versus with alcohol). No significant effects were found on sexual arousal, pleasure, or orgasm. These findings indicate errors in retrospective accounts on the stimulative effects of alcohol use on sexual expression in women.

INVESTIGATION

History

History-taking provides core information. Issues to inquire about and questions to ask include:

1. Duration (see Chapter 4, "lifelong versus acquired")

Suggested Question: "HOW LONG HAS THIS (NOT COMING TO ORGASM) BEEN A CONCERN TO YOU?"

(Comment: asking about a non-experience is admittedly rather awkward).

2. Partner-related sexual experiences other than intercourse (see Chapter 4, "generalized versus situational")

Suggested Question: "DOES YOUR HUSBAND (PARTNER) TOUCH YOUR GENITAL AREA WITH HIS FINGERS OR HIS MOUTH DURING LOVE MAKING (OR SEXUAL) TIMES TOGETHER?"

Additional Question: "HAVE YOU EVER COME TO ORGASM THAT WAY?"

3. Masturbation experience (see Chapter 4, "generalized versus situational")

Suggested Question: "HAVE YOU HAD EXPERIENCE WITH STIMULATING YOURSELF OR MASTURBATING?"

Additional Question if the Answer is Yes: "HAVE YOU EVER COME TO ORGASM WITH SELF-STIMULATION OR MASTURBATION?"

Additional Question: "HAVE YOU EVER USED A VIBRATOR?"

Additional Question if the Answer is Yes: "DID YOU COME TO ORGASM WHEN YOU DID?"

4. Level of arousal (see Chapter 4, "description")

Suggested Question to a Woman who has not Experienced an Orgasm: "IF YOUR COMPARE YOUR SEXUAL EXCITEMENT TO CLIMBING A MOUNTAIN AND ORGASM IS THE PEAK, WHAT HEIGHT DO YOU ACHIEVE WHEN THE TWO OF YOU MAKE LOVE?"

Additional Question if Husband (or partner) Touches Woman with Hands or Mouth: "WHAT ABOUT WHEN YOUR HUSBAND (PARTNER) TOUCHES YOU WITH HIS HANDS OR MOUTH?"

Additional Question if the Patient has Experience with Masturbation or Use of a Vibrator: "WHAT ABOUT WHEN YOU WERE MASTURBATING (OR USING A VIBRATOR)?"

Additional Question if Woman has been Orgasmic: "COULD YOU DESCRIBE WHAT AN ORGASM FEELS LIKE PHYSICALLY?" "PSYCHOLOGICALLY?"

5. Psychological accompaniment (see Chapter 4, "patient and partner's reaction to problem")

Suggested Question: "WHAT ARE YOU THINKING ABOUT WHEN YOU HOPE FOR AN ORGASM AND IT DOESN'T OCCUR?"

Additional Suggested Question: "WHAT DOES YOUR HUSBAND (PARTNER) SAY AT SUCH TIMES?"

Physical Examination

The physical examination is usually unproductive diagnostically in an apparently healthy woman but can be important when conducted for educational purposes.

Laboratory Examinations

No specific laboratory examinations appear useful in an apparently healthy woman.

TREATMENT

Lifelong and Generalized

"Directed Masturbation" is the preferred treatment method and, in principle, involves education, self-exploration and body awareness, and encouraging the patient to masturbate to first experience an orgasm by herself before expecting it to happen when sexually active with a partner.[26] The objective of this approach is for the woman to initially become comfortable with the experience of orgasm when alone, with the hope that she will subsequently feel equally comfortable when experiencing an orgasm during partner-related sexual activities such as intercourse or oral stimulation. Alternatively, or in addition, she could teach her partner to stimulate her in the same manner as she learned to stimulate herself. Several studies have show this approach to be beneficial and even superior to other treatment procedures.[27,28]

Orgasm initially experienced through masturbation was helpful to a great many middle-class women in the 1970s and 1980s who were born in North America and continues to be widely used as a treatment procedure. However, since the "sexual revolution" in the 1970s, the availability of books on the sexuality of women, sexual information in women's magazines, and the appearance and discussion of explicit sexual issues in movies, videos, and the Internet have provided women (and men) with a substantial amount of sexual information. The resulting change in self-acceptance and self-awareness has greatly affected all aspects of the sexuality of women including knowledge about body function generally and orgasm specifically. As a consequence, most adult women are better informed about their body function in a sexual sense than their counterparts in the 1970s and early 1980s. However, patients who have sexual concerns sometimes avoid reading the information available and may need encouragement to do so. Primary care clinicians are in a particularly advantageous position to provide such assistance. Provision of information and encouragement might be especially valuable to certain groups of women such as teens and adults who immigrated to North America from countries where gender roles are rigid and women are clearly subservient to men (especially in relation to sexual practices).

When supplying information and promoting the directed masturbation approach, one method is to proceed step-by-step through the process of learning to masturbate to the point of orgasm. If the major etiological factors are, indeed, lack of sexual knowledge and experience, the number of visits required and the extent of health professional involvement may be minimal and therefore easily within the pattern of practice in primary care. A less time-consuming approach is to suggest to the patient that she read and use one of the readily available self-help soft-cover books describing women's sexual response in general[10] and masturbation techniques in particular.[29,30] In a study that has particular applicability to primary care, a 15-session treatment program was compared to a four-visit program.[31] Both were found to be equally effective in helping the woman come to orgasm with masturbation, and the authors concluded that " . . . therapist contact time can be reduced without loss of effectiveness" and that lifelong and generalized orgasmic dysfunction can be viewed as a "skill deficit." One of the self-help books[29] also has an accompanying videotape that many women find useful (available through Focus International, 1-800-843-0305).

> In a study that has particular applicability to primary care, a 15-session treatment program was compared to a four-visit program.[31] Both were equally effective in helping the woman come to orgasm with masturbation, and the authors concluded that . . . "therapist contact time can be reduced without loss of effectiveness" and that lifelong and generalized orgasmic dysfunction can be viewed as a "skill deficit."

Many women are currently knowledgeable about some sexual aspects of female body function. However, many are unaware of and curious about the details of female genital anatomy (understandably, because the vulva is ordinarily hidden from view and comparisons between girls are therefore not made in earlier developmental years, as often happens with boys in school shower rooms). Many women thus welcome the reassuring opportunity to compare themselves anatomically to others through the use of a self-help book with color photographs showing the panorama of vulvar shapes.[32]

Vibrators, fantasy, and Kegel's exercises have been suggested as adjuncts to directed masturbation, particularly when ordinary techniques do not achieve the objective of the woman coming to orgasm. On the basis of clinical experience, use of a vibrator can be helpful, since the intensity of the stimulation can not be matched by other methods. Some professionals are concerned about the development of dependency on a vibrator[3] (pp. 388-389); others are not[28]. Vibrators are easily available at pharmacies, department stores, and "sex" shops. No single type is judged superior. Information about vibrators is available in a specific self-help book on this subject.[33] Physicians can arrange for vibrators to be "dispensed" by a specific pharmacy to minimize patient embarrassment.

Books and films that encourage the use of erotic fantasy during sexual activity may also be useful as an adjunct. In a study of "reasonably normal married women," the occurrence of sexual fantasy during intercourse was found to be common and one conclusion derived was that it "could be used adaptively to enhance sexual interest".[34] In another study, women with a sexual desire disorder were found to have significantly fewer sexual fantasies than controls who described a "satisfactory sexual adjustment".[35] From these and other investigations, it is thought that women with desire disorders and other sexual dysfunctions might derive benefit from creating fantasies if they did not experience such phenomena in the ordinary course of sexual events. Books describing sexual fantasies in women can be used as a method of assisting women in learning to fantasize. An example of such a book is *Herotica 2*.[36]

In relation to the sexually arousing effects of films on women, one study showed that the subjective experience of arousal appeared to be greater in women-made films as compared to those made by men, although the genital response to both was described as substantial.[37]

Some clinicians also promote the use of "Kegel's exercises".[38] Kegel was a urologist who taught women who were experiencing stress incontinence to strengthen their pubococcygeus muscle by repeatedly contracting their perivaginal muscles. In the process of doing this, some women reported an increase in their perception of genital sensations and in the frequency of orgasm. Hence the notion was developed that such exercises be used adjunctively in the treatment of orgasmic dysfunction. In nondysfunctional women (and consistent with Kegel's original observations), Kegel's exercises have shown to increase subjective ratings and physiological measures of arousal.[39] However, in women with orgasmic dysfunction, such exercises have not proven to be helpful with the lifelong and generalized form or the situational form (the latter despite an increase in pubococcygeal strength).[40] Whatever beneficial effects exist may derive from an increased focus of attention of the patient on her genitalia.

LoPiccolo and Stock report that of approximately 150 women treated with directed masturbation, "about 95%" were able to reach orgasm through masturbation.[8] "Around 85%" were also able to come to orgasm with the direct stimulation of a sexual partner. "About 40%" of these women were able to also experience orgasms via penile-vaginal intercourse.

Lifelong and Situational

In accordance with the concept that orgasm with a partner (e.g., with touch but not with the thrusting movements of intercourse) is a normal variation in the sex response cycle experienced by women, most clinicians who treat people with sexual difficulties approach this concern by "normalizing," and providing information and reassurance to the patient. One aspect of this reassurance is to help the patient place the issue of how an orgasm occurs in perspective. Doing so might involve

In accordance with the concept that orgasm with a partner (e.g., with touch not including intercourse) is a normal variation in the sex response cycle experienced by women, most clinicians who treat people with sexual difficulties approach this concern by "normalizing," and providing information and reassurance to the patient.

clarification of the notion that, while pleasure is one of the desired "outcomes" of sexual activity and pleasure and orgasm are connected, if the woman is left feeling inadequate because orgasm does not occur with a specific sexual practice, this feeling could substantially interfere with her sexual pleasure.

A 35-year-old married woman was referred because she was anorgasmic. She was seen alone because she was taking a summer course in a city that was not where she ordinarily lived. Her family remained at home. In the course of history-taking, it quickly became apparent that she regularly and easily experienced orgasm with touch (her own or her husband's) but not during intercourse, a situation that she and her husband thought to be abnormal. Information was given to her about the variability of orgasm experiences in different women, and reading matter on this subject was suggested. When she returned several weeks later for a second (and final) visit, she summarized the interval as follows:

1. She talked with her husband on the telephone on the evening after the first visit
2. She indicated that her own concerns had greatly diminished
3. She reassured her husband about her normality
4. The couple concluded that they did not have any sexual difficulties

---

Verbal reassurance about the normality of not experiencing orgasm during intercourse is powerfully assisted by also referring the patient to published information on this subject. For example, the Hite Report concerning sexuality in women declared that about two thirds of the 3,000 women who were surveyed reported that although they were usually orgasmic, they did not have an orgasm when penile-vaginal intercourse was occurring.[10]

One method used to treat the concern about not experiencing orgasm during intercourse is to provide information about "the bridge maneuver"[41] (p. 87-93). This approach initially involves the patient (with fingers or vibrator) or her partner bringing her to orgasm by direct clitoral stimulation, and the partner then entering her vagina while orgasm is taking place. Subsequently, vaginal entry occurs just before orgasm which, theoretically, would be provoked by penile stimulation alone.

A 37-year-old woman, married for 12 years, described a concern that she never had orgasms during intercourse. Her husband accompanied her to the appointment but remained in the background. In response to questions, he indicated that he was supportive of what she wanted but at the same time was quite content with their present sexual experiences.

She was regularly and easily orgasmic alone with masturbation and, as well, when her husband stimulated her clitoris with his fingers or orally. She was not reassured when given information indicating that her sexual and orgasmic response pattern was within the range of normal. However, she did not want to give up her objective of orgasm during intercourse.

The approach used was to provide information about the "bridge maneuver" to the patient and her husband, and to see them again in several weeks. During the follow-up visit, both partners reported the following:

1. Having tried the technique twice without any change
2. Less concern on her part about how she would experience orgasm
3. Both felt better about their relationship, since they talked more about nonsexual issues

---

Male partners tend to be more involved than was the case in this story. In addition to their current partner, women with orgasmic difficulties have often been questioned in the past about the sexual response of other partners. Male partners often imply that 'having an orgasm during intercourse is important to my sexual pleasure and so it must be for you too. If you are not having the same kind of experience as I am, you must not be enjoying yourself. Something is wrong with this situation'. In addition, there is an unvoiced (although sometimes voiced) concern by the man that he is doing "something wrong" and is therefore a "lousy lover." The man in this situation often seems to have difficulty accepting his partner's reassurance. However, the same reassurance given to the man from a health professional authority seems to be quite powerful. Thus it is important to see both partners together.

Acquired and Generalized

Clarifying the possible etiological role of medications, illness, or substance abuse is essential if this is not already apparent to the patient. Medications that interfere with orgasm are outlined in Appendix III. Strategies for managing delayed ejaculation/orgasm resulting from medication use were reviewed in Chapter 10 (see "Delayed Ejaculation/Orgasm, Box 10-1, and Table 10-1). These same treatment approaches apply to men and women.

INDICATIONS FOR REFERRAL FOR CONSULTATION OR CONTINUING CARE BY A SPECIALIST

1. Lifelong and Generalized: for the woman who experiences this syndrome but who is also sexually uneducated and inexperienced a directed masturbation treatment program with appropriate reading materials should be implemented. For the woman who is sexually educated and experienced, the approach is not so clear. If she is focused on orgasm rather than her feelings of pleasure and does not respond readily to reassurance about the likely positive outcome, referral to a sex specialist might be helpful.
2. Lifelong and Situational: most patients respond positively to an approach that normalizes their experience while at the same time not minimizing their concern. It may be essential to direct this message to the partner as well. A patient who does not want to accept this pattern as a normal variant should be referred to a sex therapist.

3. Acquired and Generalized: when orgasms were a feature of a woman's sexual response in the past but cease to be so in the present, a search for some biological explanation should be made. A physician needs to be involved if the primary care professional is not an MD. When a medication is found to interfere with orgasm, the clinician should make use of the information in Box 10-1 and Table 10-1 in Chapter 10. Illnesses and substance abuse should be specifically treated, since the sexual phenomena are usually symptoms rather than disorders. Clinicians must always consider the possibility that disrupted sexual function could be the presenting symptom of a disorder rather than, for example, the side effect of a medication.

SUMMARY

Orgasmic dysfunction is the second most common problem among women in the general population (24%) but appears as less of a clinical complaint then it did a decade or two ago. When a concern does surface, it can take one of three forms:

1. Lifelong and generalized (primary): the woman never had an orgasm by any means (5% to 10% of women)
2. Lifelong and situational: the woman is orgasmic by one means (e.g., masturbation) but not by other means (e.g., intercourse) (very common)
3. Acquired and generalized: the woman has lost the capacity that she once had to come to orgasm (infrequent in a healthy population).

History-taking is essential in the investigation of the complaint of orgasmic dysfunction (physical and laboratory examinations are distinctly less helpful [other than for educational and reassurance purposes]) in an apparently healthy woman. The lifelong and generalized form is usually a result of lack of awareness of sexual issues affecting women and is responsive to educational input and initial experience of orgasm through masturbation. The concept of the generalized and situational form as a problem requiring treatment has changed substantially so that today this pattern is considered a "normal" variant of female orgasmic response. Women with this concern are generally responsive to reassurance although this often involves the partner as well. The acquired and generalized form usually results from medication side effects, symptoms of illness, or direct effects of abused substances. When a side effect of medications is responsible (see Appendix III), several treatment approaches (see Box 10-1 and Table 10-1 in Chapter 10) can be employed. Only in the occasional instance does specialized care seem necessary for any of the three forms described.

REFERENCES

1. Leiblum SR, Rosen RC: Orgasmic disorders in women (introduction). In Leiblum SR, Rosen RC (editors): *Principles and practice of sex therapy: update for the 1990s*, New York, 1989, The Guilford Press, pp. 51-88.
2. Masters WH, Johnson VE: *Human sexual response*, Boston, 1966, Little, Brown and Company.
3. Kaplan HS: *The new sex therapy: active treatment of sexual dysfunctions*, New York, 1974, Brunner/Mazel, Inc.

4. *Diagnostic and statistical manual of mental disorders*, ed 4, Washington, 1994, American Psychiatric Association.

5. Vance EB, Wagner NN: Written descriptions of orgasm: a study of sex differences, *Arch Sex Behav* 5:87-98, 1976.

6. Jayne C: A two-dimensional model of female sexual response, *J Sex Marital Ther* 7:3-30, 1981.

7. *Diagnostic and Statistical Manual of Mental Disorders*, ed 4, *Primary Care Version*, 1995, Washington, American Psychiatric Association.

8. LoPiccolo J, Stock WE: Treatment of sexual dysfunction, *J Consult Clin Psychol* 54:158-167, 1986.

9. Masters WH, Johnson VE: *Human sexual inadequacy*, Boston, 1970, Little, Brown and Company.

10. Hite S: *The Hite report: a nationwide study on female sexuality*, New York, 1976, Macmillan.

11. Laumann EO et al: *The social organization of sexuality: sexual practices in the United States*, Chicago, 1994, The University of Chicago Press, pp. 35-73.

12. Spector IP, Carey MP: Incidence and prevalence of the sexual dysfunctions, *Arch Sex Behav* 19:389-408, 1990.

13. Wincze JP, Carey MP: *Sexual dysfunction: a guide for assessment and treatment*, New York, 1991, The Guilford Press.

14. Morokoff PJ: Determinants of female orgasm. In LoPiccolo J, LoPiccolo L (editors): *Handbook of sex therapy*, New York, 1978, Plenum Press, pp. 147-165.

15. Gebhard PH: Factors in marital orgasm, *Journal of Social Issues* 22:88-95, 1966.

16. Segraves RT: Overview of sexual dysfunction complicating the treatment of depression, *J Clin Psychiatry Monograph* 10:4-19, 1992.

17. Crenshaw TL, Goldberg JP: *Sexual pharmacology: drugs that affect sexual function*, New York, 1996, W.W. Norton & Company.

18. Segraves RT: Psychiatric drugs and inhibited female orgasm, *J Sex Marital Ther* 14:202-207, 1988.

19. Shen WW, Sata LS: Inhibited female orgasm resulting from psychotropic drugs: a five-year, updated clinical review, *J Reprod Med* 35:11-14, 1990.

20. Finger WW, Lund M, Slagle MA: Medications that may contribute to sexual disorders: a guide to assessment and treatment in family practice, *J Fam Prac* 44:33-43, 1997.

21. Zemel P: Sexual dysfunction in the diabetic patient with hypertension, *Am J Cardiol* 61:27H-33H, 1988.

22. Lundberg PO: Sexual dysfunction in female patients with multiple sclerosis, *Int Rehab Med* 3:32-34, 1980.

23. Hulter BM, Lundberg PO: Sexual function in women with advanced multiple sclerosis, *J Neurol Neurosurg Psychiatry* 59:83-86, 1995.

24. Malatesta VJ et al: Acute alcohol intoxication and female orgasmic response, *J Sex Res* 18:1-17, 1982.

25. Harvey SM, Beckman LJ: Alcohol consumption, female sexual behavior, and contraceptive use, *J Stud Alc* 47:327-332, 1986.

26. LoPiccolo J, Lobitz WC: The role of masturbation in the treatment of orgasmic dysfunction, *Arch Sex Behav* 2:163-171, 1972.

27. Kohlenberg RJ: Directed masturbation and the treatment of primary orgasmic dysfunction, *Arch Sex Behav* 3:349-356, 1974.

28. Riley AJ, Riley EJ: A controlled study to evaluate directed masturbation in the management of primary orgasmic failure in women, *Br J Psychiatry* 133:404-409, 1978.

29. Heiman JR, LoPiccolo J: *Becoming orgasmic: a sexual and personal growth program for women*, editor revised and expanded, New York, 1976, Prentice Hall Press.

30. Barbach LG : *For yourself: the fulfillment of female sexuality*, New York, 1975, Anchor Books.

31. Morokoff PJ, LoPiccolo, J: A comparative evaluation of minimal therapist contact and 15-session treatment for female orgasmic dysfunction, *J Consult Clin Psychol* 54:294-300, 1986.

32. Blank, J: *Femalia*, San Francisco, 1993, Down There Press.

33. Blank, J: *Good Vibrations: the complete guide to vibrators*, San Francisco, 1989, Down There Press.

34. Hariton BE, Singer JL: Women's sexual fantasies during sexual intercourse: normative and theoretical implications, *J Consult Clin Psychol* 42:313-322, 1974.

35. Nutter DE, Condron MK: Sexual fantasy and activity patterns of females with inhibited sexual desire versus normal controls, *J Sex Marital Ther* 9:276-282, 1983.

36. Bright S, Blank J: *Herotica 2: a collection of women's erotic fiction*, New York, 1991, Down There Press.

37. Laan E et al: Women's sexual and emotional responses to male- and female-produced erotica, *Arch Sex Behav* 23:153-169, 1994.

38. Kegel AH: Sexual functions of the pubococcygeus muscle, *West J Surg Obstet Gynecol* 60:521-524, 1952.

39. Messe MR, Geer JH: Voluntary vaginal musculature contractions as an enhancer of sexual arousal, *Arch Sex Behav* 14:13-28, 1985.

40. Chambless DL et al: Effect of pubococcygeal exercise on coital orgasm in women, *J Consult Clin Psychol* 52:114-118, 1984.

41. Kaplan HS: *The illustrated manual of sex therapy*, ed 2, New York, 1987, Brunner/Mazel, Inc.

CHAPTER 13

INTERCOURSE DIFFICULTIES IN WOMEN: PAIN, DISCOMFORT, AND FEAR

Female dyspareunia . . . may be one of the earliest recognized sexual dysfunctions . . . the most common . . . possibly the most underreported . . . and the sexual dysfunction most linked to physiological pathology. Perhaps one of the reasons why the literature . . . is filled with absolutes is because of one further distinction - it is clearly the most underinvestigated . . .

MEANA AND BINIK, 1994[1]

THE PROBLEM

A 32-year-old nurse was seen in consultation with her 35-year-old husband. They were married seven years and had two children. Their sexual experiences had always been pleasurable and free of problems until two years ago. Immediately after the birth of their second child, she experienced persistent pain whenever intercourse was attempted. The pain was located at the entrance to her vagina and became evident only with entry. Before her vaginal pain began, the frequency of intercourse was several times each week but now was reduced to once or twice each month. She and her husband remained sexually interested and sexual activity (excluding, by agreement, attempts at intercourse) occurred several times each week.

The use of tampons had never been a source of difficulty for her but she stopped using them after her last childbirth. Vaginal examinations by her doctor were uncomfortable in the past but now they were associated with great pain. At her request her husband stopped inserting his finger into her vagina during sexual experiences. On examination by a gynecologist, there was vaginal spasm at the introitus and mild reddening in the 4 to 9 o'clock area of the vestibule. The cotton swab test (see Figure 13-2 and `Physical Examination' below in this Chapter) showed exquisite tenderness in this same region, indicating a diagnosis of vulvar vestibulitis.

Anesthetic ointment relieved her pain temporarily but also diminished pleasurable feelings. Vaginal dilators helped relieve the vaginal spasm so that when intercourse occurred it was less painful. Surgery was discussed with her and while she and her husband viewed this as a possible option, they preferred to wait until other approaches were exhausted.

A 23-year-old school teacher was seen with her husband of eight months because intercourse was attempted on many occasions but had never actually occurred (either during her marriage or before). She reported experiencing vaginal discomfort when intercourse was attempted. Both were born of families that emigrated from Asia and had known each other since childhood. The marriage was born of a love relationship rather than having been arranged but they nevertheless refrained from including intercourse in their sexual activities before their wedding because of family, religious, and cultural proscriptions. Both families were applying not-so-subtle pressure on the couple to have children. No one else knew of their inability to have intercourse. She was terrified of pain and expected to experience pain with anything entering her vagina (or going out, hence also her fear of childbirth). Her dread of pain with intercourse was so strong that she cried out when he neared her vulva (a reaction that made him progressively less enthused about making any attempt at vaginal entry).

In an initial inspection-oriented pelvic examination, the patient was in a semi-reclining position and watched the procedure with a handheld mirror. Cotton swab test was negative. When on a subsequent occasion the end of the physician's finger was introduced into the patient's vagina, the physician could feel a ring of surrounding muscle. The diagnosis of vaginismus was made and the patient and her husband began a treatment program. About four months later, intercourse occurred successfully on many occasions, and when last seen she was pregnant.

TERMINOLOGY

Terminology problems have more to do with health professionals than with patients or the lay public. *Vulvodynia* is a general term recommended by the International Society for the Study of Vulvar Disease (ISSVD) to describe any chronic discomfort or pain in the vulvar region regardless of etiology and not necessarily related to sexual activity.[2] *Dyspareunia* is more specific in describing pain associated with sexual intercourse. Dyspareunia could be felt at the point of vaginal entry, associated with the back and forth movements of intercourse, or deep within the patient's vagina. Insofar as pain with intercourse is discussed, this chapter concerns itself principally with the first.

However, patients may complain of vaginal "discomfort," rather than pain, when intercourse occurs. Whether such discomfort always represents mild pain, does so sometimes, or is something else altogether is unclear. The multiplicity of problems that are inherent in the present use of the word "dyspareunia" were outlined by Meana and Binik and include issues such as unclear definition, disagreement over the inclusion or exclusion of certain disorders (such as vaginismus and post-menopausal vaginal dryness), confusion about the role of physical and psychological factors in the etiology, and the meaning of not finding abnormalities on pelvic examination.[1] Another source of confusion can be found in the use of the word *vaginismus*, which in the literature describes (1) a physical sign accompanying various casuses of painful intercourse and (2) a specific disorder. (In this Chapter, the words "vaginal spasm" will be used to describe the former, and "vaginismus" will refer to the latter).

Vulvar vestibulitis (VVS) is a specific diagnostic term that is defined and discussed below in this chapter.

CLASSIFICATION

While the heading "Sexual Pain Disorders" was not carried over from DSM-IV[3] to DSM-IV-PC[4], both classification systems continue a tradition of asking clinicians to think of two disorders (dyspareunia and vaginismus), and to do so in an either/or fashion. The criteria for both are summarized in the PC version respectively as follows: "recurrent or persistent genital pain . . . before, during, or after sexual intercourse, causing marked distress or interpersonal difficulty" (p. 117) and "recurrent or persistent involuntary spasm of the musculature of the outer third of the vagina that interferes with sexual intercourse, causing marked distress or interpersonal difficulty" (p. 118).[4]

CLASSIFICATION PROBLEMS: DISTINGUISHING DYSPAREUNIA AND VAGINISMUS

In relation to the problem of pain, discomfort, and/or fear of intercourse in women, DSM-IV-PC[4] definitions and accompanying clinical information often conflict with clinical experience and result in confusion when trying to distinguish dyspareunia and vaginismus. The two often occur together. For example, when intercourse is attempted in the context of vaginismus, patients usually complain of pain (although *fear* of pain may be much more prominent). Likewise, when persistent painful intercourse occurs for reasons other than vaginismus, it is clinically commonplace to see associated vaginal spasm. In such instances, vaginal spasm seemingly functions as a symptomatic and defensive (usually involuntary) reaction of the woman to protect herself against anticipated pain.

SUBCLASSIFICATION: DESCRIPTIONS

Theoretically, the subclassification of disorders that cause fear, discomfort, or pain-related difficulties with intercourse in women involve the assessment of whether the problem is lifelong or acquired, situational or generalized. In clinical practice, the first two patterns described below are most commonly seen; the third probably occurs frequently in the community but is uncommonly presented to health professionals. The assessment of pain, discomfort, or fear associated with attempts at intercourse in women is outlined in Figure 13-1.

Lifelong and Generalized

When hearing that pain or fear associated with attempts at intercourse have always existed, the history is often that of an unconsummated marriage. Not only has a man's penis never entered her vagina, but the same story is also heard concerning her own, or her partner's fingers, tampons or a physician's fingers or speculum. Alternatively, vaginal entry of a current or previous partner's penis may have taken place but pain persisted through much of the experience of intercourse. Prior to intercourse attempts (e.g., in the premarital period when a woman resolutely decides against having intercourse before marriage), she often found herself sexually interested, wet, and possibly orgasmic. While this response may have continued in the short run (e.g., after marriage), the pattern may have altered in the long run as a result of pain and fear connected to present attempts at penile entry. In such a situation, women typically feel

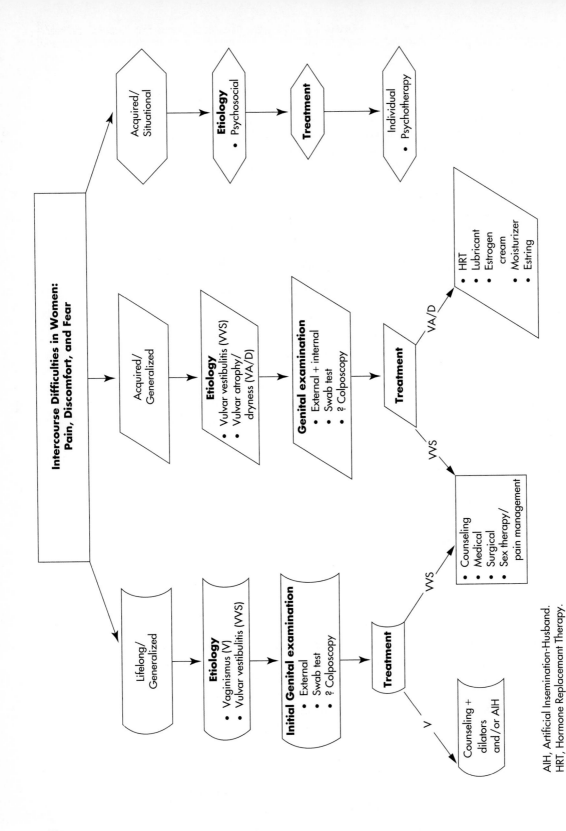

Figure 13-1 Assessment of intercourse difficulties in women: pain, discomfort, and fear.

AIH, Artificial Insemination-Husband.
HRT, Hormone Replacement Therapy.

self-deprecatory, saying that they feel "abnormal" as women and as a marital and sexual partner. In a frenzy of ambivalence, she may have explicitly suggested to her partner that he "find himself someone else" while simultaneously fearful that he will do exactly that. The agony of feeling unable to become pregnant through intercourse is often the final straw that drives her to the humiliating admission that help is necessary to accomplish what television, magazines, and billboards shout is a common event for the rest of mankind.

A 22-year-old woman saw her family doctor because she had married three weeks before but was unable to have intercourse despite numerous attempts. It was evident that she was fearful of vaginal entry but it was not evident whether she also experienced pain when intercourse was attempted. She and her husband were sexually active with one another in the three years of their courtship but decided for religious reasons that intercourse should be included only after they married. Their sexual practices did not include vaginal insertion of his fingers, and, as well, she never had intercourse with a previous sexual partner, did not like the idea of tampons, and never had a vaginal examination from a physician. Neither she nor her husband described any other difficulties with their sexual function.

A pelvic examination was scheduled for the following day when the physician could allocate a greater amount of time. The external vulvar examination revealed no structural pathology and a negative swab test. The physician then explained her diagnostic impression of vaginismus and aspects of the anatomy and physiology of the patient's vagina, reassured the patient that there were no apparent structural problems impeding intercourse, described the importance of control by the patient in relation to vaginal insertion, and encouraged the patient to insert her own and then the doctor's finger part-way into her vagina. With patience and encouragement from the doctor, finger insertion took place. The patient was enormously pleased and felt a sense of accomplishment. She was encouraged to guide her husband's penis into her vagina in the same manner as her own finger. When seen one week later, the patient related that intercourse occurred on three occasions, the last two times without any difficulty.

A 38-year-old woman was seen alone because of a lifelong inability to have intercourse. Her first marriage was annulled after five years, primarily because of "nonconsummation." She had pleasurable sexual experiences since her separation ten years before but she always managed to avoid attempts at intercourse. Over the years, she was unwilling to accept suggestions made by her family physician (aware of the problem because of the impossibility of vaginal examinations) for referral to a sex therapist. Presently, she was in the midst of a serious relationship and was contemplating marriage. However, she was also fearful of the implications of her inability to engage in intercourse. Her partner was accepting of this limitation but at the same time was encouraging her to obtain medical care.

A vaginal examination, conducted by a consultant, resulted in a negative swab test, and it was possible to only partially insert a single finger because of enormous fear of pain and severe muscular tightness at the vaginal entrance. A suspected diagnosis of vaginismus was confirmed. She remained unwilling to consult a sex therapist and insisted on not involving her partner in the treatment program, explaining that she had this problem long before their relationship began. She was unable to insert the smallest dilator and felt pessimistic about the benefit of this approach. When last seen she had remarried and was sexually active without intercourse.

Acquired and Generalized

In this syndrome, the most commonly heard story concerning vaginal pain with intercourse is that the woman had no prior difficulty. Typically, her previous sexual enthusiasm, ease of arousal, and orgasm contrasts sharply with her present reticence. The current experience of pain tends to be associated with anything entering her vagina (penis, fingers, a vaginal speculum), and the discomfort is particularly located at the vaginal entrance and especially in the "horseshoe" 4 to 8 o'clock area. The intercourse pain is described as "tearing" and occurs with initial vaginal entry but is sometimes characterized as burning and connected more with the friction of continuous coital movement. Discomfort may continue for several hours after the sexual experience.

A 27-year-old woman, married four years, was seen by her family physician because of pain associated with intercourse. She related that before the past two years, she only rarely experienced pain during intercourse and it lasted only a matter of seconds and was relieved by change in position. Her sexual interest was equal to that of her husband and other male partners before she married, she had no difficulty becoming vaginally wet when interested, and would easily come to orgasm. Since the past two years, all of this had changed. Pain associated with vaginal entry had become gradually more common and increasingly severe and as a result she found herself only marginally interested in sexual activities, often used an artificial lubricant because of insufficient vaginal lubrication, and only occasionally would come to orgasm. She described the pain as in the 6 o'clock area of her introitus, burning in character, and somewhat relieved by the cessation of intercourse, although the discomfort after would necessitate her sitting in a bath to obtain some lessening of the feeling of irritation.

On examination, the swab test was positive in many locations and a diagnosis of vulvar vestibulitis (VVS) was made. With an initial focus on her diminished sexual desire, psychologically oriented treatment was begun. Counseling also focused on helping her and her husband explore other sexual practices other than intercourse. Intercourse occurred periodically and was eventually experienced with little or no discomfort on her part. Despite improvement on many levels, her lack of sexual enthusiasm did not change and more aggressive treatment of her VVS at that time was not something she thought desirable.

Acquired and Situational

In contrast to the lifelong form, the history reveals intercourse without difficulty in the past, and in contrast to the generalized form, only vaginal entry of a man's penis in the present results in discomfort (rather than tampons, fingers, and speculum). Other features of the syndrome may include the following:

- Variability in appearance of the pain, age of patient (youth), sexual inexperience
- The presence of psychosocial explanatory factors
- The lack of pathological findings with pelvic examination

None of these features are pathognomonic.

A 19-year-old single woman was concerned that since about six months ago, intercourse was associated with pain—a facet of her sexual experiences that had never occurred before in previous relationships. Although dyspareunia was frequent now, it was also quite irregular. Her relationship with her boyfriend of ten months was frequently stormy, and on two occasions they decided to stop dating. She was still unsure about continuing the relationship and had not told him of her sexual discomfort. She had no difficulty using tampons now or in the past during her menstrual periods, and likewise, experienced no problems with pelvic examinations by a physician. The pain that she experienced was not localized, would arise only with vaginal entry, and disappeared when his penis left her vagina. Pelvic examination revealed no structural pathology and the swab test was negative. When seen three months later, she had begun a relationship with another man with whom she was in love and found that her dyspareunia had disappeared.

EPIDEMIOLOGY

In the general population study conducted by Laumann and his colleagues, respondents were asked the following question: "During the last 12 months, has there ever been a period of several months or more when you experienced physical pain during intercourse?"[5] (p.371) Overall, this was answered with a "yes" by 14% of the women (in contrast to 3% of the men). The age group in which this was most commonly reported was 18 to 24 (22%) and was least commonly reported in those over 50 (7% to 9%). As with other sexual problems, pain with intercourse was positively correlated with the respondent's health status (p. 373) (9% of women who's health status was "excellent" compared to 23% of those in "fair" health). There was also a positive correlation with "happiness" (p. 374) in that pain with intercourse was reported by 12% of those who were "extremely happy" versus 28% of those who were "unhappy most times." While intercourse pain is obviously common among women in the general population, vaginismus as a specific disorder seems unusual. Subtypes of pain associated with intercourse, and the subject of unconsummated marriages, were not addressed in the Laumann[5] or Kinsey[6,7] studies.

> When asked the question: "During the last 12 months has there ever been a period of several months or more when you experienced physical pain with intercourse?"[5] 14% of the women answered "yes."

Meana et al. completed a descriptive study of a nonclinical sample of 112 women recruited by newspaper advertisement and ranging in age from 19 to 65[8] with pain relating to intercourse. Subjects underwent thorough psychological and gynecological examinations. The subjects were eventually grouped under four diagnostic subheadings:

- The largest (46%) were diagnosed as having vulvar vestibulitis
- The next largest (24%) had no dyspareunia-related physical findings
- The third (17%) was "mixed" (described by the authors as a "catch-all")
- The fourth (13%) was the vulvar/vaginal atrophy group

Apart from community studies, Goetsch provided information on the prevalence of dyspareunia and vulvar vestibulitis in an unreplicated study of a general gynecology practice.[9] All patients (n = 10) seen by her in a six month period were questioned and their examination included a swab test. Twenty percent described symptoms of pain and all except three had a positive swab test. Thirty-one patients (15% of the entire group) were diagnosed as having vulvar vestibulitis. Affected patients were typically premenopausal.

Information about the epidemiology of vulvar/vaginal atrophy (typically found in postmenopausal women) and its consequences was assessed in a general population study conducted in Sweden on a random sample of 5990 women ranging in age from 46 to 62 (five birth cohorts).[10] Subjects were sent a questionnaire (response rate 76%) that included questions on various climacteric symptoms. Vaginal dryness was reported by 21% overall and showed a linear increase (4% to 34%) in each cohort. In spite of lubrication difficulty, approximately 60% had a "regular sex-life" and only 8% of the entire sample reported that vaginal dryness was the reason for the absence of sexual activity (although 32% of the 62-year-old women said so).[11] It is instructive to note that in another study which involved the transition to menopause, one third of premenopausal women reported vaginal dryness, thus indicating that factors other than hormones can have a major influence on vaginal lubrication.[12] In addition, a study of 48 postmenopausal women that included psychophysiological measurements supported the notion that vaginal dryness in postmenopausal women might well be related to nonhormonal sexual arousal problems.[13]

In a review of the incidence and prevalence of sexual dysfunctions in "sex clinics," vaginismus was found to vary from 12% to 17% "of the females presenting with problems in sexual dysfunction clinics . . . reflecting a rather stable rate."[14] In the same review, dyspareunia rates were estimated at 3% to 5% but the authors wondered if this complaint was more often made to family physicians and gynecologists than sex therapists. Support for this was given by the Laumann data[5], and, as well, a survey of physicians[15] who reported that "dyspareunia, or painful intercourse" was the sixth most common sexual problem seen out of a list of 20 items.

ETIOLOGY

Entry dyspareunia that lasts for a short period of time (days to weeks) is probably common and may result from vaginal irritation as a consequence of infection or allergy. Although there are many explanations for more persistent entry dyspareunia,[16] three problems probably account for most cases of pain, discomfort, or fear of intercourse in women:

- Vulvar vestibulitis
- Postmenopausal vulvar/vaginal atrophy and consequent vaginal dryness
- Vaginismus

Vulvar Vestibulitis

Friedrich[17] coined the term *vulvar vestibulitis* (VVS) and described three criteria for the diagnosis:

1. Severe pain on vestibular touch or attempted vaginal entry
2. Tenderness to pressure localized within the vulvar vestibule
3. Physical findings confined to vestibular erythema of varying degrees

> Three problems probably account for most cases of pain, discomfort, or fear of intercourse in women:
>
> - Vulvar vestibulitis
> - Postmenopausal vulvar/vaginal atrophy and consequent vaginal dryness
> - Vaginismus

Women with VVS are typically in their 20s and 30s and of Caucasian origin. Goetsch (see Epidemiology above) provided details of her 31 subjects (plus seven who were diagnosed with VVS before the beginning of her six month study).[9] The median length of the complaint was 8.5 years and half of the respondents first noted pain with tampon use rather than with sexual intercourse. Half of the women *always* had pain dating from the first attempt at intercourse (often designated as "primary"). A significant subgroup (21%) experienced dyspareunia in the postpartum period, and delivery by cesarean section made no difference in its appearance.

The etiology of VVS is unknown, giving rise to several theories.[17-19] Infectious agents have received much attention. Some observers note a high rate of repeated vaginal and/or urinary tract infections (such as candidiasis). Human papillomavirus (HPV) is also suspected. A majority of Goetsch's patients had no known association with HPV. However, "unusually large doses of fluorouracil cream . . . had caused severe chemical burns in two patients and evolved into the most severe cases of vestibulitis seen in the survey."[9] "The only infectious agent found to directly cause or worsen vestibulitis was group B streptococcus" in two patients.[9] Eighty percent of patients in the Goetsch study who always had pain and who had sisters knew of a female relative with dyspareunia or intolerance of tampons. There was no such association in those whose pain began later. Investigators into the psychological status of patients with dyspareunia generally found evidence of more symptoms than no-pain matched controls.[8] However, no differences were found when those who specifically had VVS were separated from other subtypes.

Goetsch concluded that swab testing demonstrated a continuum from those who were positive but had no clinical pain to those who were dysfunctional.[9] Likewise, she indicated that when pain was present, it was "minor for many, and accommodation was aided even by getting an explanation of the problem."[9] Last, she noted that many had sensitivity that *predated* sexual exposure.

> Goetsch concluded that swab testing demonstrated a continuum from those who were positive but had no clinical pain to those who were dysfunctional.[9] Likewise, she indicated that when pain was present, it was "minor for many, and accommodation was aided even by getting an explanation of the problem."[9]

Postmenopausal Vulvar/Vaginal Atrophy

Vaginal lubrication largely depends on estrogen stimulation of the vaginal mucosa and, therefore, vaginal dryness is usually considered to be associated with the diminution of estrogen that accompanies menopause. Atrophic alterations occur to the vaginal epithelium in the absence of estrogen and are associated with increased vaginal pH, decreased vaginal fluid, and decreased vaginal blood flow.[20] Exogenous estrogens appear to reverse these changes. However, a woman's level of sexual activity (including masturbation) and her circulating androgens have also been demonstrated to influence the extent of vaginal atrophy.[21] While vaginal atrophy and dryness is often reported as uncomfortable, the extent to which actual pain is experienced during intercourse is unclear.

> While vaginal atrophy and dryness is often reported as uncomfortable, the extent to which actual pain is experienced during intercourse is unclear.

Vaginismus

Vaginismus represents an involuntary spasm of the muscles surrounding the outer third of the vagina, resulting in narrowing of the vaginal entrance and inability or difficulty in allowing vaginal entry in the waking state. The sex-related result of vaginismus is the inability to engage in intercourse (either at all or without significant discomfort). The history is usually lifelong (that is, since the patient tried to put anything into her vagina) but not all such lifelong histories represent this disorder. A similar story may be given in some instances of vulvar vestibulitis (see Vulvar Vestibulitis above).[9] Patients give various explanations for vaginismus including[22]:

1. Thinking sexual activity to be sinful or offensive
2. Fear of pregnancy or childbirth
3. Lack of anatomical awareness
4. Homoerotic feelings
5. Dislike of semen
6. Aversion to a man's penis or men in general

> When patients were asked for possible causes of vaginismus, they placed pain and fear of intimacy high on the list.

Some specialists view such phenomena as symptoms rather than causes.[23] As counterintuitive as it might seem, a history of genital trauma or sexual violence in the histories of women with vaginismus is unusual.[24] When patients were asked their opinions about possible causes, they placed fear of pain and fear of intimacy high on the list.[25] Patients may describe pain with intercourse attempts but *fear* of vaginal entry rather than the actual experience of pain may be the principal factor that interferes with intercourse. Other sexual difficulties (e.g., a desire disorder) may be present in the patient and may have antedated awareness of intercourse trouble.

> Patients may describe pain with intercourse attempts but *fear* of vaginal entry rather than the actual experience of pain may be the principal factor that interferes with intercourse.

INVESTIGATION

History

History is only one element, albeit an essential one, in defining fear, discomfort, or pain in women associated with intercourse attempts, and in many instances, helping to delineate the cause. Issues to inquire about and suggested questions include:

1. Duration (see Chapter 4, "lifelong versus acquired")

Suggested Question: "HOW LONG HAS THIS BEEN A PROBLEM FOR YOU?"

Alternative Suggested Question if Intercourse Occurred in the Past: "**HAVE YOU EVEN BEEN ABLE TO HAVE INTERCOURSE WITHOUT EXPERIENCING PAIN?**"

2. Intravaginal experience in the past (see Chapter 4, "generalized versus situational")

Suggested Question: "**WHAT HAS BEEN YOUR EXPERIENCE WITH TAMPONS?**"

Suggested Question: "**WHAT HAS BEEN YOUR EXPERIENCE WITH INSERTING YOUR OWN FINGER INTO YOUR VAGINA?**"

Suggested Question: "**WHAT HAS BEEN YOUR EXPERIENCE WITH A SEXUAL PARTNER INSERTING A FINGER INTO YOUR VAGINA?**"

Suggested Question: "**WHAT HAS BEEN YOUR EXPERIENCE WITH DOCTORS PERFORMING A PELVIC EXAMINATION AND USING FINGERS OR A SPECULUM?**"

Suggested Question: **WHAT HAS BEEN YOUR EXPERIENCE WITH WEARING TIGHT CLOTHES SUCH AS JEANS?**

3. Intravaginal experience in the present (see Chapter 4, "generalized versus situational")

Suggested Question: "**WHAT IS IT LIKE FOR YOU NOW WHEN A SEXUAL PARTNER ATTEMPTS TO INSERT HIS PENIS (OR HIS FINGER) INTO YOUR VAGINA?**"

Additional Suggested Question: "**DOES IT MATTER IF YOU ARE WITH A DIFFERENT SEXUAL PARTNER?**"

4. Location of the pain (see Chapter 4, "description")

Suggested Question if Intercourse Occurs: "**WHERE DO YOU ACTUALLY FEEL THE PAIN? AT THE ENTRANCE? WITHIN YOUR VAGINA DURING INTERCOURSE? OR DEEP INSIDE?**"

Additional Suggested Question for Entry Pain: "**IF YOU WERE TO COMPARE THE OPENING TO YOUR VAGINA TO A CLOCK, AT WHICH POINT ON THE CLOCK DO YOU FEEL PAIN?**"

Additional Suggested Question to Determine if Pain is Associated with Thrusting: "**IS THE PAIN FELT ON THE INSIDE OF YOUR VAGINA AS HE IS MOVING IN AND OUT?**"

Additional Suggested Question to Determine if the Pain is Deep: "**WHEN HE INSERTS HIS PENIS DEEPLY, DOES IT FEEL AS THOUGH HE IS POKING SOMETHING?**"

5. Character of the pain (see Chapter 4, "description")

Suggested Question: **"SOMETIMES A PERSON EXPERIENCES FEAR OF INTER-COURSE MORE THAN ACTUAL PAIN. DOES THIS EVER HAPPEN TO YOU?"**

Additional Suggested Question if Intercourse Occurs: **"WHAT DOES THE PAIN FEEL LIKE? FOR EXAMPLE, DOES IT FEEL AS THOUGH IT IS TEARING OR BURNING?"**

6. Factors that result in improvement or worsening (see Chapter 4, "description")

Suggested Question: **"IS THERE ANYTHING THAT MAKES THE PAIN BETTER?"**

Additional Suggested Question: **"IS THERE ANYTHING THAT MAKES THE PAIN WORSE?"**

Additional Suggested Question if Intercourse Occurs: **"WHAT DOES IT FEEL LIKE WHEN HE EJACULATES?"**

Physical Examination

> Any complaint of persistent pain associated with vaginal entry requires a complete physical examination, which need not take place on the first visit or be completed on one occasion.

> Considerably more time (and patience) is usually required for a pelvic examination involving persistent pain associated with vaginal entry than is required in a more "ordinary" pelvic examintion.

Any complaint of persistent pain associated with vaginal entry requires a complete physical examination, which need not take place on the first visit or be completed on one occasion. For example, in the context of vaginismus, a vaginal examination might well be terrifying to the patient and, as well, impair the physician-patient relationship. A speculum examination under such circumstances may have even more severe consequences. Rafla described a case in which a vaginal examination in the context of vaginismus resulted in physical injury and a blood loss of 1000 ml.[26] Considerably more time (and patience) is usually required than in a more "ordinary" pelvic examination (see "Physical Examination" in Chapter 6).

When the patient's history is one where intercourse has never occurred because attempts resulted in pain, discomfort, or fear, it is reasonable to engage in a preparatory process before an actual intravaginal examination.[27] The patient touches herself as close to the introitus as possible, daily, in private, and for five to ten minutes. While this is taking place, she is asked to imagine herself being examined, view her genitalia with a mirror, and is shown how to insert her own fingertip around the anterior vaginal wall using diagrams or models. This preparation is meant to convey to the patient that she will be in control of the examination when it does occur.

The actual pelvic examination in such a patient begins with an inspection of the external genitalia. In the syndrome of vulvar vestibulitis, inspection may reveal varying degrees of erythema of the vestibular mucosa.[17] On this first occasion, there is no necessary reason to extend the examination beyond inspection and explanation. However, if the patient permits, the examiner can also gently probe the vestibular openings to major and minor gland ducts (the "swab test") with a sterile water-moistened cotton-tipped applicator, to exclude the possibility of vulvar vestibulitis (Figure 13-2). (The

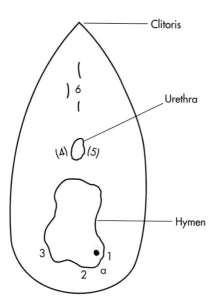

Figure 13-2 Swab test sites: a comparative site for reference (a) and six sequential test sites (from Goetsch MF: Vulvar vestibulitis: prevalence and historic features in a general gynecologic practice population, *Am J Obstet Gynecol* 164:1609-1616, 1991.)

vestibule is bordered medially by the hymenal ring, laterally by Hart's line, anteriorly by the frenulum of the clitoris, and posteriorly by the fourchette. The area contains opening of major [Bartholin's, Skene's, and periurethral] and minor vestibular glands.)[28]

When the swab test is positive, colposcopy might be "helpful in identifying discrete lesions, which [are] often difficult to see without aceto-white staining and magnification".[18]

When the swab test is negative, examination of the interior of the vagina might then take place. One method of allowing the patient control over this part of the examination is to have her hold the physician's wrist while she slowly introduces one of the examiner's fingers into her vagina. This process may extend over several visits. Speculum and bimanual examination of the patient with a history of lifelong vaginismus should be delayed (barring some urgent reason) until a later time when vaginal entry is no longer associated with pain, discomfort, or fear.

> Speculum and bimanual examination of the patient with a history of lifelong vaginismus should be delayed (barring some urgent reason) until a later time when vaginal entry is no longer associated with pain, discomfort, or fear.

Valins provided a vivid and poignant first-person account of the pelvic/vaginal examination of a woman with vaginismus with a description of how her gynecologist approached the examination[29] (pp. 203-210).

Laboratory Examination

When vaginal infection is considered, several tests can be done to eliminate the possible presence of various pathogens. In addition, biopsy of the vulvar epithelium on a patient with suspected vulvar vestibulitis often shows evidence of chronic inflammation. However, the *normal* histology of this area has not been well described. In a comparison of tissues obtained by punch biopsy done on women with VVS and normal controls, both showed evidence of inflammation, thereby casting doubt on the value of finding evidence of inflammation on histological examination of vulvar epithelial tissue.[30]

TREATMENT

Lifelong and Generalized

Most women who have the lifelong and generalized form of vaginal pain or fear to the extent that intercourse has never occurred will likely be diagnosed as having vaginismus (although some will have primary vulvar vestibulitis [see below]). Drenth suggest that when considering the treatment of vaginismus, couples should separate the issues of wanting to overcome the intercourse difficulty from wanting to become pregnant, decide which is of higher priority, and focus on that goal.[31] In any instance, primary care treatment may be sufficient.

Both partners should be involved in treatment, although the apparent passivity of many husbands of women with vaginismus (noted by many authors) may contribute to his relatively small contribution.[32] (p. 34). On an impressionistic basis, many women with vaginismus seem to have difficulty talking about their thoughts and feelings, which in turn makes insight-oriented psychotherapy with them difficult. With couples where the man is passive and the woman unexpressive, visits are often brief and the focus is on progress using dilators and other functional aspects of their care.

> When overcoming the fear or pain associated with attempts at intercourse is the principal objective, couples are initially advised to stop any form of vaginal insertion even if the circumstances seem favorable. (Emphasis on thoughts are crucial, since it is the anticipation that leads to worry.)

When the diagnosis is vaginismus and pregnancy is the principal objective, Drenth suggests artificial insemination using (1) the husband's semen (AIH) and (2) the insemination procedure performed by the couple themselves.[33] When overcoming the fear/pain associated with attempts at intercourse is the principal objective, couples are initially advised to stop attempting to insert the man's penis into the woman's vagina (or anything else such as his finger), and even to not consider any form of vaginal entry even if the circumstances seem favorable. (Emphasis on thoughts are crucial, since it is the anticipation that leads to worry.) At the same time, they are encouraged to continue enjoying the sexual activities other than intercourse that previously occurred.

> The word "dilator" is a misnomer when used in the treatment of vaginismus since dilatation does not occur and in any case is not the purpose of the procedure. The problem is not with the structure of the muscle surrounding the vaginal opening but rather with its function.

After the diagnosis of vaginismus is confirmed and VVS excluded, as well as insufficient knowledge of sex-related anatomy and physiology, vaginal dilator use could be considered. (Flesh-colored, silicone dilator sets of four are available at 1-800-621-1278 through Milex Products, 5915 Northwest Highway, Chicago, ILL 60631). Although recommended decades ago for this same purpose, vaginal dilators have become a therapeutic mainstay since they were suggested by Masters and Johnson in 1970.[34] The word "dilator" is a misnomer when used in the treatment of vaginismus since dilatation does not occur and in any case is not the purpose of the procedure. The problem is not with the structure of the muscle surrounding the vaginal opening but rather with its function. A "dilator" works rather as an "accommodator" in providing an opportunity for the woman to become used to having something in her vagina without fear or pain, and entirely in her control.

Supervision of dilator use through the progressively larger sizes in a set can be readily undertaken in a primary care setting. Insertion of dilators should occur daily for the longest period of time that the patient can manage, and when she is alone so that the process remains entirely under her control (rather than at the urging of her partner). The largest dilator in the set that does not also cause discomfort should initially be used. Liberal amounts of over-the-counter water-soluble jelly (e.g., K-Y Jelly) should be applied to the dilator. Progression to the next size should only take place when there is complete absence of discomfort with the size currently used. Eventually, when she is comfortable with a size that approximates her partner's erect penis, she should be instructed to insert his penis almost as if it were another dilator. Since intromission by the woman is accomplished relatively easily when she is in the superior position, the couple should practice using that position before penile insertion is actually attempted.

If this appears to be a mechanical approach, it probably is a correct perception, but only from the health professional's viewpoint. Much more than mechanical manipulations are taking place from the couple's perspective. While hope extends backward to the time the physician's finger was first inserted into the patient's vagina, only her actual experience of painless penile insertion represents concrete evidence of change. Paradoxically though, patients tend to be more subdued when describing the first occasion of intromission than is the treating health professional. The explanation might be an absence of confidence that the remainder of the therapeutic tasks can be successfully completed. However, it is well to remember at this point that penile insertion may not be immediately translated into feelings of pleasure for either person. This depends on the extent of sexual freedom that the couple enjoyed before. Some couples absorb the newly found sexual skills quickly and zealously. In other instances, pleasure for the women may take place in an evolutionary way, extending over a period of time and in the context of the confidence that is linked with not having to think about the placement of body parts. Confidence in that circumstance tends to occur with repeated successful experiences.

Most observers use intercourse (consummation) as the sole criterion for success in the treatment of vaginismus. Masters and Johnson describe excellent treatment results (100%) in their five-year follow-up.[34] Van de Wiel et al. conducted a meta-analysis on treatment results involving 20 surveys and 17 case studies published between 1960 and 1990.[35] They conclude that several treatment approaches appear to be equally effective (except surgery, which was not a subject of a published report) and that the average rate of success was about 80%. Some describe a more modest outcome. Drenth et al. reports on a questionnaire survey of 57 patients (response rate 86%) diagnosed with "primary vaginismus."[33] Consummation occurred in 54% overall. In couples who wanted to become pregnant, consummation occurred in 74% compared to 33% who sought treatment only for the intercourse difficulty. Problems encountered in the treatment of vaginismus[31] include the following:

1. Lack of clarity around therapeutic aims
2. Intimacy difficulties on the part of the woman and consequent unwillingness to involve her partner
3. The emergence of other fears

Desire for a child may be a stronger motivating factor for the treatment of vaginismus than desire for intercourse. The survey by Drenth et al. also provided information on obstetrical issues.[33] Almost one half (25) of the patients became pregnant (10 as a result of artificial insemination and 15 through intercourse). Patients who chose self-insemination did so for reasons that include the pressure of time (resulting from a delay in seeking treatment) or slow therapeutic progress. The authors felt that insemination by a physician represented "unnecessary medicalization" and, furthermore, might unduly influence any ambivalence toward pregnancy experienced by the couple.

When self-insemination (also known as home insemination or AIH [artificial insemination by husband] is undertaken, it, may be helpful for a physician to provide technical advice to the couple and to review methods of ovulation detection. Briefly, the insemination process is as follows*: The man ejaculates [volume of ejaculate is usually in the range of 2 to 6 cc] into a clean, dry, plastic or glass container such as a urine collection bottle from a medical laboratory. Regular condoms are undesirable for collecting semen because they may contain a spermicidal agent. The semen is kept at body temperature for about 10 minutes (the sample is then more liquid) and then is drawn, with minimal accompanying air, into a narrow syringe (as small as 1 cc in instances of severe vaginismus but perhaps as large as 10 to 12 cc). The syringe is inserted as deep into the woman's vagina as possible and the semen is deposited by pushing on the plunger. During this process, the woman's hips should be slightly elevated with a pillow and she should remain in this position for about 20 to 30 minutes. The same process can be repeated in about 24 hours.

Drenth et al. also reported on 26 deliveries and found that assisted deliveries were 10% higher in patients with vaginismus than in their clinic population.[33] Reasons included the presence of vaginismus and the (older) age of the mother. However, they concluded that having vaginismus does not, in itself, require special precautions during labor and delivery. They also observed that: however counterintuitive the notion might be, childbirth does not automatically result in pain- and fear-free intercourse. "Obviously, a pushing out movement is experienced quite differently from a pushing-in movement."[33]

Acquired and Generalized

As outlined above (see Etiology in this chapter), vulvar vestibulitis and vulvar/vaginal atrophy probably account for the majority of patients seen with the acquired and generalized form of dyspareunia. When such disorders are resistant to definitive treatment within the health care system, active involvement of the patient in her own care may

---

*Personal communication, Stacu Elliott, M.D., Co-director, Vancouver Sperm Retrieval Clinic, VHHSC, 1998.

be necessary and beneficial. Membership in the National Vulvodynia Association (NVA) may prove useful, especially since the organization produces an informative and patient-oriented newsletter. (The NVA can be reached through its Web site [see Appendix IV], by telephone at [301] 299-0775, or by mail at P.O. Box 4491, Silver Spring, MD 20914-4491)

Vulvar Vestibulitis (VVS)

Bergeron and her colleagues[19] reviewed the treatment of VVS and grouped the existing studies into three categories:

- Surgical intervention
- Medical management
- Cognitive-behavioral/pain management therapy

Surgical interventions consist of vestibulectomy and laser therapy. Vestibulectomy has been the most investigated VVS treatment and the one reported as having the best outcome. Laser treatment is described as controversial and sometimes associated with negative consequences. Surgery is usually undertaken after the failure of medial management. The surgical procedure is typically described as a modified perineoplasty, which is performed as day surgery under general anesthesia. Surgical success usually has been measured through a one-time self-report rating of pain with intercourse, and rates vary from 43% to 100%, with the majority more than 60%.[19]

Schover et al. reports an improved outcome when surgery is combined with sexual counseling.[18] They describe an eight-month follow-up study on the evaluation and treatment of a group of 45 women with VVS. All were treated by conservative local excision of the vulvar lesions. One of the factors that indicated a better outcome included willingness to engage in initial psychological evaluation and brief post-operative sexual counseling. Of 32 such patients, 50% reported that they were much improved. Other positive predictors were higher socioeconomic status and localized (versus diffuse) areas of pain. The authors hypothesize that women who could accept that their dyspareunia and vulvar pain was multifactorial in origin took an active role in rehabilitative efforts after surgery, and, as a result experienced a better outcome. They hypothesize that patients who could not do so might be poor surgical candidates.

Medical management of VVS typically involves the use of topical ointments (including anesthetics, antifungals, and antibiotics), systemic medications, and other treatments such as interferon.[19] Topical anesthetics are of limited value, since their effect is short-term and allergic reactions may occur. Nonscented lubricants are also of short-term value but do not have adverse effects. Other topical ointments (antibiotics, antifungals, antiviral, and corticosteroid creams) are considered to be ineffective but have not been carefully studied. Acyclovir (oral), capsaicin (topical), and calcium citrate tablets have been reported to be beneficial to some patients. Alpha interferon is not recommended if colposcopy or biopsy lesions do not show evidence of HPV changes.

Pain management of VVS has consisted of biofeedback, behavior and sex therapy, cold application, and acupuncture.[19] Some patients have found benefit from each of these four approaches. Since vaginal spasm (often referred to as vaginismus in the literature) is often found during the pelvic examination of a patient with VVS, some have found the inclusion of vaginal dilators to be a treatment adjunct.[36]

Bergeron et al. compared treatment results for 78 patients with VVS who were randomly assigned to surgery (vestibulectomy), biofeedback, or sex therapy/pain management.[37] Measurements were made pre- and post-treatment and at six-month follow-up. Self-reported coital pain was significantly improved in all groups from before and after treatment and from before to 6 month follow-up. However, the vestibulectomy group was significantly better than the sex therapy/pain management group post-treatment. All groups improved significantly when the frequency of intercourse was compared post-treatment to 6 months later. In summary, patients from all three groups reported significantly more subjective improvement from post-treatment to 6 month follow-up. However, the vestibulectomy group was significantly better than the sex therapy/pain control group.

> Patients from three groups (vestibulectomy, biofeedback, and sex therapy/pain management) reported significantly more subjective improvement from post treatment to 6 month follow-up. However, the vestibulectomy group was significantly better than the sex therapy/pain control group.

Vulvar/Vaginal Atrophy

Estrogen replacement therapy generally reverses the vaginal changes associated with menopause. However, restoration of vaginal tissue function may require up to 18 to 24 months. The long duration may explain the reason for continued vaginal dryness and dyspareunia (if the woman is sexually active) in spite of hormonal and cytologic return to premenopausal values.[38] However, only a distinct minority of postmenopausal women use hormone replacement therapy (HRT). Reasons include the following:

- Personal preference
- Adverse side effects
- It is contraindicated

In addition, some women find that even with HRT, there is little urogenital benefit. Thus local (vaginal) forms of treatment have been developed to counter vaginal dryness in women who are not on HRT or who need supplemental therapy for urogenital symptoms.

Vaginal creams containing estrogen represent one example of a local form of treatment. Since estrogen is absorbed from the vaginal mucosa, a fact that may limit its acceptability in some patients, attempts have also been made to find nonhormonal agents, or, alternatively, to minimize the absorption of estrogen.

The estradiol vaginal ring represents a second local treatment option for vaginal dryness and other urogenital consequences of estrogen loss. The development of the ring is based on the notion that compared to the amount of estrogen necessary to reverse vasomotor symptoms (50 mg/day), the amount of estrogen necessary to alleviate urogenital atrophy is much smaller (7 to 10 µg/day).[39] The ring delivers a low dose of 17 β-estradiol directly to the urogenital tissues and has a low level of systemic absorption. Bachmann reviewed the results of 11 clinical trials with the estradiol vaginal ring.[40] She found that it reversed urogenital atrophy, induced minimal stimulation of the endometrial lining, had few adverse side effects, and that a single ring was efficacious for three months of continuous use. Of the 946 postmenopausal women with treatments up to 96 weeks, "there were cytological, physiological, physician rating and patient reporting of either elimination or amelioration of urogenital atrophy signs and symptoms."[40] She concluded that" the risk/benefit ratio has a clear pref-

> "The ring provides a safe and effective method of pharmacological therapy for women who require treatment for symptoms of urogenital aging."[40]

erence to benefit with risks being very low. Therefore, the ring provides a safe and effective method of pharmacological therapy for women who require treatment for symptoms of urogenital aging."[40]

A vaginal moisturizer is a third local treatment option. "Replens" is a nonhormonal nonsystemic vaginal moisturizing gel that has a low pH, appears to bind to vaginal tissue, and is applied three times per week. Replens is based on a polymer (called polycarbophil), which becomes saturated with water, diffuses into vaginal epithelial cells, and then is sloughed off with epithelial cell turnover.[41] This substance has been studied in nonhuman primates[41] and humans.[42-44] In two open-label studies of women, Replens was compared to a locally applied estrogen cream and found to be safe and effective.[42,43] In one of the studies, both therapies exhibited statistically significant increases in vaginal moisture, vaginal fluid volume, and vaginal elasticity with a return of the premenopausal pH state. Replens has also been compared to a water-soluble lubricating placebo in a double-blind study of women with a history of breast cancer and similarly found to be effective.[44]

A fourth local treatment form that has been used for many years is an over-the-counter lubricating gel (e.g., K-Y Jelly).

Acquired and Situational

Little is known about this syndrome except from patients who describe the problem of vaginal discomfort with intercourse in the past, and who have watched it disappear with the advent of a new relationship. On the assumption that the difficulty relates to *inter*personal or *intra*personal psychosocial conflicts, the most reasonable therapeutic course of action is (1) reassurance to the woman about the integrity of her genitalia and (2) psychotherapy, either individual or couple-related depending on the circumstances.

INDICATIONS FOR REFERRAL FOR CONSULTATION OR CONTINUING CARE BY A SPECIALIST

1. The evaluation of persistent pain associated with intercourse should always include a physical/pelvic examination. Thus, medical consultation should always be included when a patient with dyspareunia has been evaluated only by a non-medical health professional.

2. Lifelong vaginismus can often be successfully treated by primary care health professionals regardless if the goal is sexual or reproductive. Consultation with a physician should take place if the treating health professional is not a MD to eliminate the possible coexistence of VVS. When artificial insemination (AIH) is desired, the couple should be referred to a physician for advice and possible assistance. When treatment that is aimed at overcoming vaginismus becomes problematic, the couple should be referred to a sex therapist for continuing care.

3. Primary (lifelong) VVS may be amenable to explanation and brief sexual counseling within primary care. Consultation with a gynecologist for the purpose of confirming the diagnosis may be helpful. The time and skills of a sex therapist

may be particularly useful when intercourse has never occurred in the past because of discomfort, and for patients who are otherwise experiencing significant sexual difficulty.

4. Secondary (acquired) VVS varies in the degree of pain experienced. The greater the extent of pain and sexual complications, the more a primary care professional would want to engage the assistance of other health professionals such as gynecologists and sex therapists.

5. When dyspareunia in a postmenopausal woman persists despite adequate vaginal lubrication, consultation with a sexual medicine specialist would be desirable to consider the possibility of other contributing factors.

SUMMARY

Penile-vaginal intercourse is sometimes accompanied in women by persistent pain, discomfort, or fear. Pain can exist at the point of entry, or deep in the vagina. This chapter is concerned with the former. *Vulvodynia* is a term that encompasses vulvar pain regardless of etiology, whereas *dyspareunia* is specific to pain that occurs with intercourse. DSM-IV suggests that "dyspareunia" and "vaginismus" should be separated. However, if a clinician considers that "vaginismus" as described in the literature includes both the disorder as well as vaginal spasm occurring in the context of several vaginal disorders, then in fact, vaginismus and dyspareunia often occur together and separation becomes clinically difficult.

In community studies, about 15% of women say they have experienced pain with intercourse for a few months during the last year. When dyspareunia is lifelong and generalized, the causes are usually vaginismus (the disorder) or vulvar vestibulitis (VVS). When acquired and generalized, the etiology is usually VVS (the most common cause in premenopausal women) or vulvar/vaginal atrophy with associated vaginal dryness (the most common cause in postmenopausal women). When acquired and situational, the genesis of dyspareunia is most often related to interpersonal or intrapersonal difficulties.

The assessment of persistent vaginal pain involves a history and a physical/pelvic examination. The latter should include a swab test whenever vulvar vestibulitis is considered. In cases where vaginal entry has never occurred or where there is severe introital pain, the pelvic examination may require more than one visit and a lengthy period of time to complete.

Early or mild instances of vaginismus may respond to education and supportive counseling. Treatment of patients who are not helped by such an approach depends heavily on the use of dilators and the support of the patient's partner and health care clinician. Sometimes the couple is primarily interested in reproduction rather than solving the intercourse problem. In such an instance, assisting in the process of artificial insemination using the husband's sperm (AIH) may be most productive.

Vulvar vestibulitis is sometimes amenable to explanation, but in other instances it may be difficult to treat. Several medical, surgical, and sex therapy/cognitive-behavior therapy methods have been suggested. Surgery (vestibulectomy) has received the most attention in the VVS treatment literature and studies indicate this form of treatment to provide the best results.

At least five approaches can be used in the treatment of women with dyspareunia resulting from vulvar/vaginal atrophy and associated vaginal dryness: oral hormone replacement therapy (HRT), estrogen cream, the estradiol vaginal ring (Estring), a nonhormonal vaginal moisturizer ("Replens") and nonhormonal and nonscented lubricants.

REFERENCES

1. Meana M, Binik YM: Painful coitus: a review of female dyspareunia, *J Nerv Ment Dis* 182:264-272,1994.
2. Paavonen J: Diagnosis and treatment of vulvodynia, *Ann Med* 27:175-81, 1995.
3. *Diagnostic and statistical manual of mental disorders, ed 4,* Washington, 1994, American Psychiatric Association.
4. *Diagnostic and statistical manual of mental disorders, ed 4, Primary Care Version,* Washington, 1995, American Psychiatric Association.
5. Laumann EO et al: *The social organization of sexuality: sexual practices in the United States,* Chicago, 1994, The University of Chicago Press.
6. Kinsey AC, Pomeroy WB, Martin CE: *Sexual behavior in the human male,* Philadelphia and London, 1949, W.B.Saunders.
7. Kinsey AC et al: *Sexual behavior in the human female,* Philadelphia and London, 1953, W.B.Saunders.
8. Meana M et al: Dyspareunia: sexual dysfunction or pain syndrome?, *J Nerv Ment Dis* 185:561-569, 1997.
9. Goetsch MF: Vulvar vestibulitis: prevalence and historic features in a general gynecologic practice, *Am J Obstet Gynecol* 164:1609-1616, 1991.
10. Stadberg E, Mattsson L-A, Milson I: The prevalence and severity of climacteric symptoms and the use of different treatment regimens in a Swedish population, *Acta Obstet Gynecol Scand* 76:442-448, 1997.
11. Stadberg E, Mattsson L-A, Milson I: Womens attitudes and knowledge and the climacteric period and its treatment. A Swedish population-based study, *Maturitas* 27:109-116, 1997.
12. Larson B, Collins A, Landgren A-M: Urogenital and vasomotor symptoms in relation to menopausal status and the use of hormone replacement therapy (HRT) in healthy women during the transition to menopause, *Maturitas* 28: 99-105, 1997.
13. Laan E, van Lunsen RHW: Hormones and sexuality in postmenopausal women: a psychophysiological study, *J Psychosom Obstet Gynecol* 18:126-33, 1997.
14. Spector IP, Carey MP: Incidence and prevalence of the sexual dysfunctions, *Arch Sex Behav* 19:389-408, 1990.
15. Burnap DW, Golden JS: Sexual problems in medical practice, *J Med Educ* 47:673-680, 1967.
16. Abarbanel AR: Diagnosis and treatment of coital discomfort. In LoPiccolo J, LoPiccolo L (editors): *Handbook of sex therapy,* New York, 1978, Plenum Press.
17. Friedrich EG: Vulvar vestibulitis syndrome, *J Reprod Med* 32:110-4,1987.
18. Schover LR, Youngs DD, Cannata R: Psychosexual aspects of the evaluation and management of vulvar vestibulitis, *Am J Obstet Gynecol* 167:630-636, 1992.
19. Bergeron S et al: Vulvar vestibulitis syndrome: a critical review, *Clin J Pain* 13:27-42, 1997.
20. Semmens J, Wagner G: Estrogen deprivation and vaginal function in postmenopausal women, *JAMA* 248:445-448, 1982.
21. Leiblum SR et al: Vaginal atrophy in the postmenopausal woman: the importance of sexual activity and hormones, *JAMA* 249:2195-2198, 1983.
22. Blazer JA: Married virgins: a study of unconsummated marriages, *J Mar Fam* 26: 213-214, 1964.

23. Dawkins S, Taylor R: Non-consummation of marriage: a survey of seventy cases, *Lancet* ii:1029-1033,1961.
24. Barnes J: Primary vaginismus (part 2): aetiological factors, *Irish Med J* 79:62-65, 1986.
25. Ward E, Ogden J: Experiencing vaginismus: sufferers' beliefs about causes and effects, *Sexual Marital Ther* 9:33-45, 1994
26. Rafla N: Vaginismus and vaginal tears, *Am J Obstet Gynecol* 158:1043, 1988.
27. Basson R: Lifelong vaginismus: a clinical study of 60 consecutive cases, *Soc Obstet Gynecol Can* 18:551-561, 1996.
28. Marinoff SC, Turner MLC: Vulvar vestibulitis syndrome: an overview, *Am J Obstet Gynecol* 165:1228-33, 1991.
29. Valins L: *When a woman's body says no to sex: understanding and overcoming vaginismus,* New York, 1992, Viking Penguin.
30. Lundqvist EN et al: Is vulvar vestibulitis an inflammatory condition? A comparison of histological findings in affected and healthy women, *Acta Derm Venereol (Stockh)* 77:319-322, 1997.
31. Drenth JJ: Vaginismus and the desire for a child, *J Psychosom Obstet Gynecol* 9:125-137, 1988.
32. Friedman LJ: *Virgin wives: a study of unconsummated marriages,* London, 1962, Tavistock Publications.
33. Drenth JJ et al: Connections between primary vaginismus and procreation: some observations from clinical practice, *J Obstet Gynecol* 17:195-201, 1996.
34. Masters WH, Johnson VE: *Human sexual inadequacy,* Boston, 1970, Little, Brown and Company.
35. Van de Wiel HBM et al:Treatment of vaginismus: a review of concepts and treatment modalities, *J Psychosom Obstet Gynecol* 11:1-18, 1990.
36. Abramov L, Wolman I, David MP: Vaginismus: an important factor in the evaluation and management of vulvar vestibulitis syndrome, *Gynecol Obstet Invest* 38:194-197, 1994.
37. Bergeron S et al: *A randomized controlled comparison of vestibulectomy, electromyographic biofeedback, and group sex therapy/pain management in the treatment of dyspareunia resulting from vulvar vestibulitis.* Paper presented at the meeting of the Society for Sex Therapy and Research, Fort Lauderdale, March, 1998.
38. Semmens JP et al: Effect of estrogen therapy on vaginal physiology during menopause, *Obstet Gynecol* 66:15-18, 1985.
39. Heimer G, Samsioe G: Effects of vaginally delivered estrogens, *Acta Obstet Gynecol Scand* 163(Suppl):1-2, 1996.
40. Bachmann G: The estradiol vaginal ring: a study of existing clinical data, *Maturitas* 22(Suppl):S21-S29, 1995.
41. Hubbard GB et al: Evaluation of a vaginal moisturizer in baboons with decreasing ovarian function, *Lab Anim Sci* 47:36-39, 1997.
42. Nachtigall LE: Comparative study: Replens versus local estrogen in menopausal women, *Fertil Steril* 61:178-180, 1994.
43. Bygdeman M, Swahn ML: Replens versus dienoestrol cream in the symptomatic treatment of vaginal atrophy in postmenopausal women, *Maturitas* 23:259-263, 1996.
44. Loprinzi CL et al: Phase III randomized double-blind study to evaluate the efficacy of a polycarbophil-based vaginal moisturizer in women with breast cancer, *J Clin Oncol* 15:969-973, 1997.

Appendix I

First Assessment Interview With A Heterosexual Couple

(The following is a compilation of several taped and edited interviews with different patients, together with comments on what was said by me and why. Names and other identifying information have been changed for confidentiality purposes.)

Comment: The couple is greeted in the waiting room. Introductions and handshakes are exchanged and they are then ushered into my office.

WLM: Let me first explain what I'd like to do. I'd like to meet with you together today, separately on another occasion, and then together again after that. Each visit will be for about one hour. The purpose of these first few visits is to get a clear understanding about why you're here, what sort of help you're looking for, and what I might do to be of some assistance to you. It usually takes more than one visit to accomplish all of that. Do you have any questions about what we're going to be doing?

Comment: I explain as much as possible about the process beforehand on the telephone (I make my own appointments) so that there are no surprises such as the unexpected presence of a student. However, repeating the information in the office is also essential. People often do not fully absorb an explanation the first time it is given. Also, a question may have arisen since the telephone conversation.

Patients: No.

WLM: I received some information from your family doctor. I know that you're here because of sexual concerns, but before talking about that subject, I'd like to get to know both of you a little better. Perhaps each of you could tell me something about yourself such as your age, your living circumstances, and how you spend your days.

Comment: I always acknowledge the existence of a sexual problem at the beginning of an interview before going on to ask about "identifying information" (see Chapter 6). As I learned from experience, people wonder why questions are being asked about issues that, seemingly, have nothing to do with sexual matters. Also, I strongly believe in the value of a few minutes spent on "neutral" subjects at the beginning of a first interview to allow patients to "settle in" to new surroundings and adjust to the idea of talking with a stranger to whom they are about to reveal very private information. This allows people a few moments to decide whether I seem to be trustworthy or not.

Woman: (They look at each other) You go first.

Man: No, you.

Woman: Well, I'm 32 and working as a school teacher. I've been doing that for seven years. We've been married for three years but knew each other on and off for about twelve.

WLM: Does anyone live with the two of you?

Woman: Just our cat.

WLM: (Directed to the man) What about yourself?

Man: I'm 32 and work for the telephone company installing phones.

WLM: (To the woman) May I ask why you made an appointment before, cancelled it, and then changed your mind about wanting to be here?

Comment: I feel it necessary to discuss issues that could potentially hinder the interview process and to do so as early as possible to minimize that interference. When someone is ambivalent about being in my office (apart from the expected and virtually universal nervousness and embarrassment), I like, if possible, to resolve that before talking about any specific sexual problems.

Woman: When your secretary said that you wanted to see both of us . . . it's my problem . . . I spoke to my family doctor again after I spoke with you . . . She said both of us should go. So, I spoke to my husband and he agreed to come.

WLM: Well, how do you feel now about him being here today?

Comment: It is not unusual for both partners to be unhappy about an initial conjoint visit but for different reasons. In this case she was prepared to shoulder complete responsibility for the existence of their trouble and its solution. In some instances, the other person arrives with a grumbling attitude about having to attend a visit and is prepared to do so only as someone giving information about the partner, rather than as an equal participant.

When either situation exists, it can seriously clash with the interviewing process. Usually, talking about this potential interference and explaining the benefits of having both of them there is enough for both people to be considerably more accommodating.

Woman: I still think it's my problem. I had it before we met.

WLM: (to the man) What do you think about being here today?

Man: No problem. It makes sense to me for both of us to be here.

Comment: His wife may well have thought that he was not sincere in telling her about his willingness to join her in the treatment process. His positive answer to a third party becomes important for her to hear.

WLM: (to the man) As I mentioned to your wife on the phone, my own opinion is that quite a bit of information can be obtained from talking to one person alone, but in terms of changing things, it's usually best if both partners are here. From my viewpoint, I'm very pleased that you're here.

Let me continue where we left off before. Is this the first marriage for both of you?

Woman: Yes.

WLM: Healthwise, how are the two of you doing? Do you have any major health troubles?

Comment: Ordinarily, I avoid asking someone two questions at the same time. When this happens, patients don't know which to answer. If it is more advantageous to answer one over the other, the person doing the answering will usually take the path of least resistance (as President Kennedy discovered in the Cuban Missile Crisis). The interviewer may be the loser (and, of course, ultimately, the patient). My only excuse in this instance was that the first question was more of a preamble to the second rather than an actual question. It would have been better phrased as a statement than a question.

This question is essential because some medical disorders can seriously interrupt sexual functioning.

Woman: I have an ulcer.

WLM: Tell me about that.

Woman: The pain started about two years ago. I had an X-ray but it didn't show anything. I took some medication . . . I don't remember the name . . . until about six months ago. It's much better now.

Man: My health is OK.

WLM: Do either of you take medications on a regular basis?

Woman: Nothing.

Man: Nothing.

WLM: Street drugs?

Woman: Neither of us has used any for years and even then just an occasional joint.

WLM: What about tobacco? Do either of you smoke?

Woman: We used to but stopped before we met.

WLM: Alcohol? What is usual for both of you?

Man: Only at parties. Hardly ever at home.

WLM: I understand that you do not have children. Has this been by choice or is there some other reason?

Woman: That's part of the reason we're here. We'd like to start a family.

WLM: Let me just ask you one more question before we talk about the reasons for the two of you being here. Have either of you had any kind of counseling in the past for sexual difficulties or any other problems?

Woman: No one apart from our family doctor and my gynecologist. I'm very selective about whom I talk to. I just can't go and talk to anyone about it.

WLM: You said something before about wanting to start a family and that was part of the reason for coming here. Could you explain that further?

Comment: Some medications can interrupt sexual functioning also; therefore this, too, is a necessary question.

Comment: The same can be said of street drugs.

Comment: The use of tobacco can have deleterious effects on relationships and on some aspects of sexual function.

Comment: Alcohol, as well, can have very serious effects on relationships and sexual function.

Comment: I have found this to be the most nonjudgmental way I can obtain this extremely sensitive information. The question is entirely descriptive and simply asks for explanation rather than justification. I prefer to avoid sounding like a reproachful relative.

Comment: My motivation in asking about experiences with other health professionals is not to be critical of others but rather to find out what approaches have been used in the past, and what has and has not been helpful. I would not be of much assistance to a patient if I simply repeated treatment methods used before without knowing why they were unsuccessful.

Comment: I did not need to ask them what the main problem was since she offered this spontaneously. As it was, I interrupted her somewhat by my previous question, something I am ordinarily loath to do. Patients do not easily explain the major reasons for coming to see me without my first asking. If someone does, I usually listen and don't ask questions until they finish talking.

Woman: Well, a lot of the problem is dealing with sexuality. We thought we could come and talk to you and that you might be able to help us. I have a habit of blocking things out that are unpleasant . . . I put things off . . . my family doctor thinks I'm nervous and tense about everything. . .and that maybe that has something to do with getting . . . you know . . . pregnant. We've . . . um . . . never done it . . . you know . . . intercourse. The gynecologist suggested an operation to make it easier but my family doctor said we should have counseling before considering that. We love each other very deeply but unfortunately this one area has been a problem.

WLM: Is it OK if I ask you some questions about intercourse?

Comment: Ordinarily in interviewing, it would be reasonable to ask an open-ended question at this point, for example, "Tell me more about the difficulty you have had with intercourse". In fact, I usually do so but I am never surprised when I receive a vaguely worded answer. I know by experience that patients find it onerous enough to indicate what the general area of the problem is, much less give details. She was hesitant about telling me and undoubtedly was embarrassed. An open-ended question at this juncture often meets with the type of reply that says "What is it that you want to know?" or "Ask me some specific questions." When this happens, I simply go on to ask direct questions about the specifics. In this particular instance, I used the "permission" format of asking the initial question. I did this for reasons explained in Chapters 2 and 3.

Woman: Yes.

WLM: Has there ever been a time when the two of you tried to have intercourse?

Woman: Yes. We've tried it quite a few times but it's always been painful for me and . . . um . . . my husband's so caring and understanding . . . he knows the way I am . . . he never forced it.

WLM: When was the first time the two of you tried?

Comment: I deliberately phrased it as the "two of you" so as not to force her into revealing information about sexual experiences with other partners, recently or in the past, that she may not have discussed previously with her husband. I wanted to know if the problem of not having intercourse was lifelong or acquired (see Chapter 4). With both partners together, I could find this out only in the context of this relationship (see Chapter 6).

Woman: Well, it was before we were married. I couldn't tell you exactly when . . . it was so long ago.

WLM: Has he ever actually entered your vagina, even part-way?

Woman: I really don't know. I mean . . . it's hard for me to know.

WLM: (to the man) can you shed some light on that question?

Man: Not really. I couldn't add anything to what she's said.

WLM: (to the woman) I'd like to ask you some questions about your experience with other things that might commonly be inserted into a woman's vagina. For example, have you ever used tampons?

Woman: No. I remember once I tried to use something that a doctor gave me for a yeast infection . . . it was to be inserted there and I couldn't.

WLM: A suppository?

Woman: Some sort of . . . there was this thing . . . I think it was a big pill actually . . . I told her I couldn't . . . she gave me something else . . . a cream or something. I think that's the only time I ever tried . . . I'm really squeamish . . . I don't like touching or looking down there.

WLM: Sometimes, for one reason or another, a woman might insert her own finger into her vagina. Have you ever had that experience?

Comment: This is an example of the statement/ question technique described in Chapter 2. It combines information as a preamble, with a question that follows.

Woman: No. My family doctor suggested that I try to stretch myself . . . I should have told her right then and there that I couldn't do it.

WLM: (to the man) Sometimes, a sexual partner might insert a finger into the woman's vagina as part of a couple's sexual activity. Has this ever been part of your experience together?

Comment: I was conscious of the fact that most of the discussion so far had been between myself and the woman, and that I needed to incorporate him in the conversation to a greater degree. From the viewpoint of being an observer of the communication pattern of the couple, it had (up to now) been enormously informative to me to see that she controlled the information flow and that he was passive.

Man: I wanted to but she won't ever let me. She used to jump when I went near that area so I don't do that anymore.

WLM: (to the woman) How have you felt about that?

Woman: It's sore enough when the doctor does it . . . she's the only one who's ever done that.

WLM: Tell me more about that.

Woman: I nearly jumped off the table.

WLM: When's the first time a doctor examined you?

Woman: The doctor that I've got now.

WLM: When did that occur?

Woman: When I was referred here.

WLM: When your doctor examined you, do you know if she put one finger inside or two?

Woman: I don't know.

WLM: Doctors often use what's called a speculum. It's made of metal or plastic and opens up inside a woman's vagina. Has your doctor ever inserted a speculum into your vagina?

Woman: I think she tried once and it didn't . . . it was too sore . . . is that for . . . like a Pap Test?

WLM: Yes. That's one of the reasons.

Woman: She couldn't go . . . or I couldn't go through with it and she said that would be OK until after I saw you.

Comment: My questions about tampons, suppositories, fingers, and doctor examinations were all asked in an attempt to establish whether the problem was generalized or situational (see Chapter 4). Except for the possibility of intercourse with other partners (which I did not want to ask about with her husband present), it seemed at this point that the problem was generalized.

WLM: Let me interrupt what we're doing and ask you how you're doing so far in talking here today?

Comment: I frequently stop the first interview midway and ask patients about the interview process and how it's affecting them. In so doing, I acknowledge that it is not easy for anyone to talk about this subject, since few people are used to doing so and it may feel strange to talk, in particular, with someone who is neither a family member nor a friend. I indicate that some discomfort is natural and even to be expected. After the process is discussed, I also talk about gender imbalances in the office (that is, the fact that there are two men and one woman) and invite patients (especially the woman) to mention any concerns they might have about this. It is rare that anyone ever does but simply raising the issue indicates sensitivity to the subject on my part and obviates worries that someone might have had before the visit. I always add, as well, that if this becomes a concern in the future, someone should let me know.

Woman: Good. It's not as bad as I thought it would be.

Man: It's OK.

WLM: Let me go back and ask you some other questions about your sexual experiences. I want to ask you about the location of the pain when your husband tried to put his penis inside. If you were to compare the opening of your vagina to the face of a clock, where did you feel the pain? Was it in any one location or was it all around the clock?

Comment: I attempt to obtain a partial description of the pain she initially was concerned about by asking about the location (see Chapters 4 and 13).

Woman: It was all around . . . I don't . . . a lot of it's in my head too.

WLM: What do you mean?

Woman: Well, with me being the way I am about pain . . . just something telling me this is going to hurt before it even . . . you know . . .

WLM: Do you mean that it's kind of frightening?

Comment: I try as much as possible to avoid leading questions. In this situation, I was trying to help her find the word she seemed to be looking for.

Woman: Yes. A lot has to do with that too.

WLM: It sounds like you're saying you might not even get to the point of experiencing pain?

Woman: I might have already told myself it's going to hurt.

WLM: I'd like to ask you one more question about the pain. Do you feel it only when he tries to enter or at other times too like when you are wearing tight jeans?

Woman: Only when he tried to go inside.

WLM: (to the man) I'd like to ask you some questions about the kinds of sexual experiences you and your wife might have together apart from attempts at have intercourse. Often when couples have intercourse troubles, they engage in other kinds of sexual activities such as, for example, holding each other, touching, and possibly bringing one another to orgasm outside of intercourse. Do the two of you have sexual experiences together apart from trying to have intercourse?

Man: Yes.

WLM: How often might that occur? I realize that it might vary from one time period to another.

Man: It does vary. Usually a few times a week.

WLM: Who's idea is that usually?

Man: She usually instigates it. I instigate it too but . . .

Woman: He's very laid-back (laugh). Maybe I shouldn't use that word! He is the type of person who appears very calm and is not what you call aggressive.

Comment: I avoid the word "sex", and talk instead about "sexual experiences" or "sexual activities." The word "sex" is often used by patients as a synonym for "intercourse," a method of speaking that I deliberately attempt to change. The point I wish to make for patients is that "sex" is much more than intercourse. To underline that concept, I might say that few quarrel with the idea that "sex" includes, for example, two individuals stimulating one another outside of intercourse to the point of orgasm. From the perspective of the interviewer, it is of great importance to discover all that is sexual in the life of an individual or couple, quite apart from intercourse.

Comment: Questions about the frequency of intercourse or other sexual activities, are, indeed, hard to answer, since sexual experiences tend to cluster in time, rather than occur at evenly spaced intervals.

Comment: Sexual jokes told by an interviewer are quite inappropriate in an interview situation. However, humor sometimes arises out of words that patients use. A sincere laugh helps lighten the atmosphere without diminishing the importance of the subject being discussed. The vital distinction is laughing "with", rather than "at."

While I particularly wanted to find out about their sexual desire levels, I was satisfied for the moment to obtain information about the subject of initiation. Desire and initiation are not identical. A person might be interested but not initiate sexual overtures. Likewise, a person can initiate a sexual encounter but not necessarily be interested.

WLM: How affectionate are the two of you with one another?

Comment: An interviewer must find out about intercourse and non-intercourse related sexual activities and also about the extent of affectionate exchanges such as hugs and kisses, between partners (see Chapter 4). The presence or absence of affectionate gestures may have great meaning, now in the history of the couple.

Woman: When we watch TV in the den or pass one another, we are always touching each other. He puts his arm around me and I will have my leg across his when he is sitting. So it's not as if we avoid one another. We are very loving toward each other and agree on everything and we don't raise our voices. It's the problem in the sexual area that is stressful for us.

WLM: (to the woman) I understand. (to the man) Let me go back and ask you some other questions about your sexual function. Do you have any problems with your erections.

Comment: At this point, I return to my task of defining the problem (see Chapter 4) after having obtained some information about sexual activities that do not continue on to intercourse, and exchanges of affection.

Man: No.

WLM: Does it sometimes happen that your wife stimulates your penis to the point where you'd ejaculate?

Man: That's what usually happens.

WLM: Any problems with your ejaculation?

Man: No.

WLM: (to the woman) Any problem with your own level of sexual interest or desire?

Woman: At some times. Most of the time I'd like to as long as he stays away from . . . you know.

WLM: Generally, when women feel a sense of desire, they also often experience some vaginal wetness or moisture as well. Does that happen with you?

Woman: Yes.

WLM: What about coming to orgasm? Has that been part of your experience?

Woman: Uh-huh.

WLM: Can I ask you some questions about that?

Woman: OK.

WLM: Is that something that happens just occasionally or frequently or most of the time?

Woman: I'd say most of the time nowadays.

WLM: How does that usually happen?

Woman: Well . . . uh . . . he . . . we . . . uh.

WLM: Would it be easier if I asked you some questions?

Woman: Yes.

WLM: Do you let him touch you with his fingers between your legs?

Woman: No.

WLM: Would you touch yourself in that area when you're with him?

Woman: No.

WLM: Sometimes a couple may not have intercourse but the partners find that they enjoy rubbing their genital areas against one another. For example, the man might rub his penis against the wet area between a woman's legs. Does something like that happen when the two of you are together?

Woman: Yes.

Comment: I again deliberately used the "permission" question (see Chapters 2 and 3) at this juncture, since I anticipated that this might be an area that she would be hesitant to talk about.

Comment: As described in Chapter 4, I obtain information from both partners about aspects of their sex response cycles that I do not already know.

Comment: There are times when allowing a patient to struggle through an answer is productive as, for example, in giving someone time to think through the answer to a question that had not been formulated previously in the patient's mind. This was not that kind of situation. Here, the patient knew the answer to the question but was embarrassed to reveal the information. Silence on my part would have been cruel if all that was accomplished was watching the patient squirm.

WLM: Do you come to orgasm when that happens?

Woman: Yes. Usually.

WLM: (to the man) Do you try to go inside when that's happening?

Man: I haven't for a long time.

WLM: Do you usually ejaculate when that's happening?

Man: Yes.

WLM: (to the woman) How do you feel about the wetness from his ejaculation . . . from his semen?

Comment: Attitudinal statements about sexual practices, body parts, and "sexual fluids", represent information that can be useful diagnostically and therapeutically.

Woman: It's not very pleasant.

WLM: How unpleasant is it to you?

Woman: Oh, it doesn't bother me. It's just messy, that's all.

WLM: Altogether, is it an enjoyable experience for you?

Woman: Yes. At least it's not painful.

WLM: I'd like to ask the two of you something else. (to the woman) How has this affected you . . . the fact of not being able to have intercourse?

Woman: It just makes you . . . like I feel like a freak . . . or . . . you know . . . you feel like you're abnormal.

WLM: How long have you felt this way?

Woman: Well, since . . . well, the longer your marriage goes on . . . as the years pass . . . at first you think, well, maybe a lot of people have this trouble . . . then my family doctor was sending me to a gynecologist and she wanted to operate . . . I told her the problem but she didn't want to talk about it . . . one thing I didn't like about her office . . . you could hear what other people were saying through the walls and so I didn't want to talk to her too much anyway.

Comment: Privacy in talking about sexual matters was obviously crucial to this patient, as it is for most. It was, clearly, one factor that inhibited conversation about this problem with her gynecologist.

WLM: (to the man) What about yourself? How have you felt about this?

Comment: The impact of the sexual problems on both partners has to be included in the assessment (see chapter 4). This also can have diagnostic and therapeutic significance. For example, information may be revealed about the relationship between the two people, their motivation to solve the sexual problems, and how damaging the difficulties have been.

Man: It's up to her. If she wants to do something about this, that's OK with me. I'm ready for some little ones to be running around.

WLM: We need to stop in a moment or two. We've talked about quite a bit today and I hope we can talk more but I wanted to ask you today if there's anything that we haven't talked about that we should have . . . that would help me understand the difficulties you've faced as a couple?

Comment: Among other things, this open-ended question allows the patient to raise issues that have not yet been discussed but nevertheless are of concern to her. Such matters may be etiologically significant.

Woman: I can't think of anything. You've certainly asked a lot of questions.

WLM: How do the two of you feel now about talking here today?

Woman: OK now. Not so good at first.

WLM: How were you feeling before?

Woman: Just . . . well, embarrassed about telling someone everything.

WLM: I think you've done very well. It's not easy to come in here and talk about what we've discussed today.

Comment: I often give this kind of reassurance. Patients usually seem grateful for this. Since this was (and usually is) an alien experience for which people don't have a frame of reference, a sincere statement from the interviewer represents useful feedback. In addition, I like to end a session on a positive note and saying something like this allows me to do so.

Woman: That's true. The more you put things off . . . and it builds up in your mind . . . it's usually not as bad as it seems . . . but try and tell me that months ago (laugh)!

WLM: (to the woman) Let me briefly explain what I think. It sounds as though you might have what health professionals who work in this area call vaginismus. That involves a spasm of the lower part of the vagina and prevents intercourse altogether or makes it painful.

Comment: Some explanation is reassuring. It helps to "hang your hat" on something that has a name and also allows the interviewer to be sincerely hopeful. Although a pelvic examination is extremely important in this situation diagnostically and therapeutically, pre-

Women are not able to control this spasm. There are several reasons for this spasm but fear is especially prominent in women who have never had intercourse. Fortunately, I see many couples each year who have this problem and seem to be of major help to the majority. To confirm the diagnosis of vaginismus, one of the things we need to do is to spend some more time talking. Are you feeling up to coming back and talking some more?

Woman: Oh sure.

Man: Yes.

WLM: As I mentioned when we began, it usually takes more than one visit to get a clear understanding about a couple's sexual difficulties. Have you done any reading about the treatment of sexual problems generally, or intercourse pain in particular?

Woman: No.

WLM: Are you interested in doing some reading?

Woman: Yes.

WLM: I like to suggest that you read a few chapters from a paperback book about sexual problems. I'll write down the title for you. We can talk about your impressions of the book when you are here next time.

Woman: Thanks.

WLM: I'd like to meet each of you separately as I mentioned when we started. Let's see if we can figure out some times to meet within the next week or two . . .

senting this idea now might make her needlessly apprehensive. While I never "spring" an examination on anyone without ample warning, it might be needlessly anxiety provoking to a patient to mention it on the first visit.

Comment: Readings are often helpful to people with sexual difficulties because people have so little knowledge about many sexual problems. Experience has taught me that people find the main benefit of readings to be not in the area of learning about the specifics of a treatment program, but rather understanding that they are not alone in having such trouble. That can be extremely reassuring: others have had similar problems and overcame them.

Appendix II

First Assessment Interview With A Solo Patient

(The following is a compilation of several taped and edited interviews with different patients, together with comments on what was said by me and why. Names and other identifying information have been changed for confidentiality purposes.)

Comment: The patient is greeted in the waiting room where there is an exchange of names and handshakes. I then usher the patient to my office. My first order of "business" is to explain the process; the second is to obtain some "identifying information" (see Chapter 6).

WLM: I'd like to meet with you today and for one or two more visits in the near future. Each visit will be for a bit less than an hour. The purpose of these first few appointments is to establish as clearly as possible the reasons for coming here, what sort of help you are looking for, and what I could do to be of some assistance to you. It generally takes more than one visit to accomplish that. When we get to that point, we'll put together the information and decide where to go from there. Is that OK?

Patient: OK.

WLM: I understand that you're here because of sexual difficulties but before getting to that subject I'd like to learn something about you. Tell me something about yourself such as your age, your living circumstances, and how you spend your days.

Comment: I ask people how they are spending their days rather than more directly (initially) about "work." I do this because some people are involuntarily unemployed and feel sufficiently badly about this without me making matters worse with a more direct question. Asking the question this way also circumvents the issue of whether the patient considers the domestic labor of a woman looking after children at home to constitute "work."

Patient: I'm thirty and in my time off during the winter, I'm an avid skier. Otherwise I work as an accountant.

WLM: Do you live on your own or with someone?

Comment: As well as finding out about relationships and other adults at home (e.g., grandparents), this is an indirect way of finding out about children. If necessary, a more explicit question about children can be asked later.

Patient: Now I live on my own. I was living with a girlfriend for 2 years, until we broke up 3 months ago.

WLM: Apart from her, have you had other relationships that involved living with the person?

Patient: No.

WLM: What about sexual relationships with other men? Has that been part of your experience?

COMMENT: I asked a question about his sexual orientation for several reasons: to signal that we could discuss such an issue if he wanted, to consider possible differences in his sexual function with opposite or same-sex partners, and to consider possible sexual practices that would make him vulnerable to STDs and HIV infection.

Patient: Never.

WLM: What's your health like generally? Do you have any major health problems?

Comment: In the context of an assessment of a sexual difficulty, I include questions about health, medications, alcohol, tobacco, and street drugs as part of an introduction, since any of these can have a major influence on sexual function.

Patient: Not really.

WLM: How about STDs or sexually transmitted diseases?

COMMENT: I don't ask this question when a partner is present, since it could pressure the patient into revealing information about past sexual liaisons that he/she might prefer to keep private. I do, however, ask this question when I see patients alone.

Patient: Only once. I got crabs when I was 15.

WLM: Do you take any medications on a regular basis?

Patient: No. Except for vitamins.

WLM: How about alcohol or street drugs, now or in the past?

Patient: Alcohol only once in a while at parties. I use marijuana a few time a year. I drank a lot more for a few years when I was in high school.

WLM: What about tobacco?

Patient: I stopped about a year ago but used to smoke . . . . smoked about 1½ packs a day.

WLM: Since?

Patient: Since I was about 17.

WLM: Have you ever seen any counselors because of sexual or other problems?

Comment: I often ask a patient to retrace the steps that led to a referral to me. A reasonable alternative is simply to ask the patient to state what the major sexual problem is now. The first method described is slightly less abrupt.

Patient: Nope.

WLM: Tell me how you ended up being referred here?

Patient: Dr. Fleming referred me here. He's my family doctor.

WLM: What did you say to him about sexual difficulties that ended up with you being referred here?

Patient: He referred me to a urologist who did some tests. The urologist talked about it being psychological.

WLM: What did you think about what the urologist said?

Comment: The patient never really answered the question that I asked so I quickly changed my approach and followed his replies. His answers had more to do with the process that he followed rather than providing a statement of the problem.

Patient: I don't know really. I didn't completely understand what he was saying. You know, I've been thinking about this for a long time. This problem goes back a long way.

WLM: When do you figure it started?

Comment: I generally start an inquiry about sexual difficulties by finding out what is happening now, (meaning the past month or so) and then comparing this to the "best ever" period in the past. Sometimes (and this was one such time) the flow of the interview is such that I start my questioning instead around the onset of the problem and work my way forward in time. My attitude about an assessment is that there is a *body* of information that I eventually want to have but that the *order* in which this information is obtained is not crucial. The order is determined more by art than by science. Rigidly following a specific interview formula usually means thinking more about the questions than the answers. This form of interviewing is more typical of TV interviews where follow-up questions take "a back seat" to the interviewer finishing a list of "first generation" questions (a process that is only superficially revealing and inappropriate to the health professional's consulting room).

Patient: Um. I don't know. Maybe eight years ago.

WLM: Eight years ago. What did you notice at that time?

Comment: I returned to asking him about the nature of his difficulty, anticipating that he was now ready to discuss what it was.

Patient: Not being able to maintain an erection, or having an erection and then it going away.

WLM: And you didn't have any problems before that time?

Comment: This is a leading question and also one that is negatively phrased (the worst kind of leading question in my opinion). The question would be better if phrased "and what were your erections like before that time"? One always knows a leading question has been asked when the patient is forced into answering only "yes" or "no". Since patients are often compliant (in the office), they are likely to answer "yes" to avoid offending the health professional, rather than answering candidly. The outcome might be that the interviewer becomes engaged in a circular conversation with him or herself.

Patient: Not that I can recall. That was so long ago. It was an ongoing thing and part of it was just being a man, a man with a macho image. You know, I didn't want to say . . . I didn't want to do anything about it because it was going to go away. Now, this time it cost me a relationship that really meant something to me. So I figure enough is enough.

WLM: I understand how you feel but I want to be sure that I get the time clearer in my mind. It started eight years ago. Did it begin gradually or suddenly?

Comment: It is essential to acknowledge his feelings but one must also obtain his history. Balancing both objectives is part of the art (rather than the science) of interviewing. An attempt to establish whether a problem is lifelong or acquired (Chapter 4) is not always easy. Sexual problems typically present after having existed for years (rather than weeks or months), and a patient's memory for sexual events many years before is often cloudy.

Similarly, sometimes the onset of the difficulty dates from a specific event but this kind of story is more likely to be the stuff of TV drama. More often than not, the beginning is gradual and the duration may be more accurately described in terms of a range of time, rather than a specific amount of time.

Patient: I'd say gradual but it's been so long I can't remember.

WLM: Looking back, what was the first thing you noticed?

Patient: I couldn't get an erection.

WLM: In any sort of situation?

Comment: I asked a leading question again. It would have been better to ask: "In what kind of situation?"

Patient: More or less. Well, no, not really. It would be there sometimes, and sometimes it wouldn't.

WLM: Did it follow any pattern?

Patient: No, not really.

WLM: What about your experience with erections recently. Are there times when you don't have problems?

Comment: I switched the time period about which I was asking questions, from the past to the present, partly because of the patient's lack of precision about the past but also to clarify what was occurring nowadays.

Patient: No. If I did get an erection it would be just like I was suffering from premature ejaculation.

Comment: I tried to determine whether the erection difficulty was situational or generalized (Chapter 4). In the process, the whole issue became more complicated with his statement that there was another sexual problem, this one relating to his ejaculation.

WLM: Please explain what you mean.

Patient: There were times we tried to make love and I wouldn't even be hard yet, and then when I did get an erection, it wouldn't last long at all before I'd ejaculate.

WLM: Are you saying that there were two different problems?

Patient: That only happened in the past year. But the main thing was . . . you know . . . sometimes you pass it off . . . you had too much to drink and all that. But that wasn't the case. I was living with this girl for two years and I'd get an erection and we'd go to bed and I'd lose it.

WLM: Within what period of time?

Patient: I don't know. We'd be going through the act of foreplay and during that, I seemed to lose it.

WLM: Gradually?

Patient: It wouldn't soften right up but it wouldn't be hard either.

WLM: Could you still have intercourse even if your penis became softer?

Patient: Sometimes.

WLM: So when was the last time you actually entered her vagina?

Patient: You mean successfully? Like coming inside?

WLM: OK. When was the last time you ejaculated inside her vagina?

Comment: The patient used the slang word "come." I chose to remain with the medical/technical language for reasons explained in Chapter 2.

Patient: About six months before we broke up. I managed to enter some other times but I'd usually fall out before coming.

WLM: When you talk about not having an erection with . . . can I ask you her first name?

Comment: These questions were an attempt to clarify what recently occurred in relation to intercourse with his partner. It is not so unusual for answers to be frustratingly unclear. An interviewer may have to accept that, especially in an initial assessment visit.

Patient: Jane.

WLM: On a 0 to 10 scale where 0 is completely soft and 10 is hard and stiff, what were your erections like when you'd be with Jane?

Comment: In establishing the erectile problem as generalized or situational (see Chapter 4), I ask about erections with a partner, masturbation, and sleep or on awakening in the morning. I also obtain a description of the fullness of the patient's penis when he's aroused using a 0 to 10 scale. These questions are quite specific, as are the answers.

Patient: About 5/10.

WLM: Was that at the beginning of a sexual experience or when you'd try to enter her vagina?

Patient: At the beginning. It got softer later.

WLM: What about when you masturbate? Is it any different then?

Patient: I don't do that very often but, no, it's just the same.

WLM: What about when you wake up in the morning? What is your penis like then?

Comment: I should have also asked the patient to specifically describe his present A.M. penis status using the same 0 to 10 scale.

Patient: I used to wake up almost every morning with an erection. Not anymore.

WLM: When did that change?

Patient: A couple or three years ago.

WLM: Do you wake up at night for any reason?

Patient: No, hardly ever.

Comment: If he had, I would have been able to include questions about sleep erections to what I had asked.

WLM: When your erections were full a few years ago, did you notice any bending to one side or another?

Comment: An infrequent problem causing erectile difficulties is Peyronie's Disease, where a growth of fibrous tissue in a particular area of the penis usually causes bending or pain (or both) when an erection occurs. Since patients are so often embarrassed to bring up problems such as this, I took the initiative in asking him this question.

Patient: No.

WLM: Have you noticed any problem with your sexual desire or interest since this trouble began?

Comment: I reviewed aspects of his sex response cycle that I didn't already know, and her's as well (see Chapter 4). These, too, are highly specific questions and the answers relatively easily formulated by patients.

Patient: No.

WLM: What about before?

Patient: No.

WLM: What about your ejaculation, apart from it being fast in the past year as you mentioned before?

Patient: No problems.

WLM: Is it the same as it was before?

Comment: I asked a leading question yet again. It could have (and should have) been phrased: "What was it like before?"

Patient: Yes.

WLM: Can I ask you some questions about Jane and how she managed sexually?

Comment: I used the "permission" technique for reasons explained in Chapters 2 and 3.

Patient: Yes.

WLM: Were there any difficulties with her sexual desire or interest?

Patient: No.

WLM: Any problems becoming vaginally wet when she was interested?

Patient: No.

WLM: Problems coming to orgasm?

Patient: Well, yes.

WLM: Tell me about that.

Comment: I asked this (and previous questions about the sex response cycle of his partner) to find out if *she* had sexual difficulties and the extent to which *he* might have contributed to these.

Patient: Whenever we had sex, I couldn't perform long enough.

WLM: Since?

Patient: The beginning.

WLM: Let me make sure I understand what you are saying. You felt there was a problem the whole time you were together?

Patient: Yes.

WLM: What were your feelings about all this?

Patient: I hated it. It didn't make me feel like a man.

WLM: Did the two of you ever talk about your sexual troubles together?

Patient: We did. At first, she thought it was her, and then I had to keep reassuring her.

WLM: Was there any one time together that sticks out in your mind?

Patient: One time she said "Oh, why do you bother?"

WLM: I don't know if you're a quiet sort of person ordinarily but you seem pretty much so today and not a man of many words. I was wondering if that's the way you usually are, or if it's because of the way you're feeling today?

Patient: I'm not usually loud, but I'm sure it's got something to do with my mood.

WLM: What's your mood been like?

Comment: I assumed he was talking about his ejaculation rather than his erection but I should have clarified that.

Comment: I temporarily side-stepped the details of her orgasm and his (presumed) ejaculation problem to talk to him about his present feelings, his reaction to his problems (see Chapter 4), and his communication about sexual issues with Jane, all of which seemed to be major areas of difficulty.

Comment: It is quite common to hear negative comments about masculinity from men with erection difficulties that are substantial enough to interfere with intercourse.

Comment: Sometimes, an interviewer must put aside the "sexual agenda" to discuss something else that takes priority. This was one such instance. I could have asked him about how he responded to Jane's comment and how he felt but sensed at that moment that his mood was sad. I chose to follow his feelings rather than obtaining more details about the encounter we were discussing.

Comment: I felt it important to find out about his present mood state and to search for some of the common accompaniments of depression, since he quickly let me know that he had experienced some aspects of a depressive syndrome. He seemed to have gone through a grief reaction to the loss of a relationship that he prized.

Patient: Down in the dumps for a long time.

WLM: Since?

Patient: Since we broke up.

WLM: Whose idea was it to break up?

Patient: Hers.

WLM: What did she say?

Patient: We had a big fight, and she said "my feelings for you are not the same as before." And that was it.

WLM: Did sex come into the discussion?

Patient: No.

WLM: What part do *you* think it played?

Comment: When a relationship has just ended, many solo men with sexual difficulties often blame this event on "sex." Clinical experience should make one skeptical of this explanation. Obtaining a more balanced perspective often becomes a therapeutic objective.

Patient: It was related.

WLM: You sound pretty sure about it.

Patient: No question about it. If I was with a woman and she didn't . . . I wouldn't like it either.

WLM: You said you were down in the dumps. Tell me a bit more about how that feels.

Patient: I think about her all the time and I think about the past. I think of her going with other people and that I'm never going to see her again.

WLM: You sound really sad. Sometimes when a person feels down, certain parts of their lives don't work the same as before. For example, some people find that their sleep has changed. Has that been your experience?

Comment: This is an example of the statement/question technique (see Chapter 2) used in a nonsexual context.

Patient: It's a lot better now, but it was really bad.

WLM: When?

Patient: For about a month after we broke up. I wasn't eating either. I lost about 20 pounds. My appetite's better so I've gained some of that back.

WLM: What was your energy level like then?

Patient: I've gotten back to playing sports, which I really love. For a while I wasn't doing anything. Not even seeing my friends.

WLM: Did it ever get so bad that you felt life wasn't worth living?

Patient: If you mean did I think about suicide, the answer is "no."

WLM: Sometimes a person in that situation feels that they wouldn't mind if something happened to them—not that they would do anything to bring about their own death. Did you feel that way?

Patient: I suppose so.

WLM: Feel that way nowadays?

Patient: Not in the past few weeks.

WLM: Did you ever do anything to try to kill yourself?

Patient: Never. I like life too much.

WLM: Just one other question about this. Has anything like this ever happened to you before?

Patient: No.

WLM: I'd like to go back to talking about sexual problems. Is that OK?

Comment: Having reassured myself that depression was not an issue that required my immediate attention as a matter of priority, I returned to questions about his sexual concerns.

Patient: Sure.

WLM: Were there times when the two of you agreed not to have intercourse but rather to engage in other sexual activities, since intercourse seemed always to be a problem?

Comment: Non-intercourse sexual activities are sometimes vital to couples when vaginal entry is difficult or impossible. Questions about this become indispensable in such a situation.

Patient: Well, yeah. Do you mean did she masturbate me?

WLM: That might be one thing that might happen, that you might stimulate one another to the point of orgasm using hands or mouths and without trying to put your penis inside her vagina.

Patient: She did it for me . . . using her hands . . . and her mouth . . . but I wasn't fully hard.

WLM: Never?

Patient: Never in the past three years. And she'd use her . . . what's the word for it . . . her female parts?

WLM: The wet area between her legs?

Patient: Right.

WLM: That general area is referred to as the vulva. Apart from that, what effect did that have on you?

Patient: None, erection-wise. It would be semihard. I'd ejaculate.

WLM: Were you ever fully hard then?

Patient: No.

WLM: Would you sometimes enter her vagina?

Patient: Yes.

WLM: Was it ever in your mind that you'd become hard but continue to stay outside?

Patient: Are you kidding?

Comment: It is important to establish what was taking place in the patient's *mind* in anticipation of having intercourse. Evidently, this was not the same as what he stated earlier about having planned times together when intercourse wouldn't occur. In his mind, intercourse was always an objective and so "performance anxiety" was always present.

WLM: Not really. But let's discuss the reasons for doing that later. I'd like to ask you more about your ejaculation. I'm a bit confused about how long the fact of you ejaculating quickly has been a problem for you.

Comment: Again, I used the statement/question technique described in Chapter 2.

For some men it's a problem right from the first attempt at intercourse. For others, it begins later. What's been your experience?

Patient: I used to have control over it. That's a long time ago though.

WLM: On the basis of time, how long would you usually last nowadays?

Patient: A couple of minutes. I was thinking in my mind, "Oh, I'm going to lose it."

WLM: What about with masturbation? Is there a problem with control of ejaculation when you're masturbating?

Patient: No.

WLM: If you judge by the number of pushes or thrusts when you're having intercourse, how many could you manage before ejaculating?

Patient: Oh, about 20.

WLM: Would you stop or rest along the way, or would you continue moving from the time you entered her vagina until you ejaculated?

Patient: Stop and go slower.

WLM: Who thought you were fast, you or Jane?

Patient: I did. But she did too.

WLM: What about before Jane? Was that a concern of other sexual partners?

Patient: To tell you the truth, I can't remember. There was this other girl I used to go out with. It didn't last long then either. We are talking way back. With Jane, I didn't have an erection all that many times. Time would go by. Weeks and months.

WLM: What would happen in those weeks and months?

Patient: Nothing. Like a normal life and then when we were in bed she didn't really want to try.

WLM: Are you saying that months would go by without any kind of sexual activity?

Patient: Right.

WLM: When you say months, how long are you actually talking about?

Patient: A month or two.

WLM: Would that include touching each other to the point of orgasm without having intercourse?

Patient: Yeah.

WLM: How would *she* feel about all of this?

Patient: If you're getting to the point that it was something to do with me and her, it's not that.

Comment: I was trying to establish what *her* reaction was to the fact of his sexual difficulties. He couldn't answer this since he didn't know. He was probably so troubled about his own feeling of responsibility for their difficulties that he was unable to be sensitive to her concerns.

WLM: People tend to look for explanations for things that don't go right in life. Have you tried to look for an explanation for your own sexual troubles?

Patient: I don't have one. I don't know what the problem is.

WLM: How much of these problems have you described to your family doctor?

Patient: Not much.

WLM: I would guess that you've been living with this without talking too much to anyone.

Patient: That's right.

WLM: Are there some important things that would help me to understand your difficulties that we haven't talked about today?

Comment: I was beginning to close the interview, and have found that this general question is useful at this point.

Patient: No.

WLM: How have you felt about talking here today? Some of my questions have been pretty explicit.

Comment: I think it is often useful to assess the level of nervousness someone feels after talking for some time. It is quite usual for this to diminish over the period of the first visit as the patient gains trust in the interviewer and the process. If initial anxiety does not decrease, the health professional has to think about the reasons. Likewise, if a patient claims not to feel nervous right from the onset of the interview, one has to be somewhat skeptical (given our cultural proscriptions against talking in detail about anything sexual).

Patient: Well, they have to be asked, don't they?

WLM: Yes. But that doesn't mean it's easy.

Patient: I realize that. It's a bit embarrassing but I need help so I guess I have to answer.

WLM: A bit embarrassing or a lot?

Patient: I realize it won't go past here. My feelings are that you have to open up. I want to get help. At first I was nervous. I feel better now.

Comment: I thought that the patient may have been implicitly asking for reassurance about the confidentiality of our discussion.

WLM: Indeed, what we talk about is quite confidential. I can't release any information about you without your permission. In addition, everyone's nervous when they come here. No one quite knows what to expect. It's normal to feel that way. I know it's a difficult subject to talk about. People don't usually talk about sexual matters with friends or relatives, much less a stranger like myself. You've done quite well today.

There was one question I forgot to ask you earlier. When was the last time you had a full, stiff, hard erection under any circumstances?

Comment: Almost always an interviewer forgets to ask something of importance during a first visit. There is usually no problem in stating candidly that a topic was unintentionally omitted. The one exception to this is raising an emotionally laden subject at the very end of the interview and having the patient depart from the office upset and possibly in tears. This is unfair to the patient and may result in that person becoming angry at the interviewer at some later time.

Patient: I can't remember. It's been so long.

WLM: More than three years ago?

Patient: Yes.

WLM: Over the past eight years, have you had sexual experiences with other women before Jane?

Patient: Two or three.

WLM: What were your erections like with them?

Comment: I previously asked about his ejaculation with other partners but (unfortunately) not his erections.

Patient: The same as with Jane.

WLM: And before that?

Patient: I had girlfriends but I could get it up without problem.

WLM: We've covered a lot of territory today. I'd like to meet with you again as I mentioned earlier. Is that OK?

Patient: Do you think you can do anything?

Comment: A fair question, and one that is on everyone's mind even when walking into the office of a health professional.

WLM: I believe that I can, but it's difficult for me to answer that question precisely now since I don't know you well enough or have a sufficiently clear idea of the history of your difficulties. I'd like to talk more with you and, perhaps, examine you and order some tests. Then, I'd be in a better position to answer your questions. I *can* say that erection problems are very common and that some very useful ways exist to help people with such troubles. Talking as we did today is usually helpful by itself, since there are so few opportunities for any one of us to talk as openly about sexual subjects as *we* have.

Patient: That's true. I do feel better about that part.

WLM: How much reading have you done about men and sex and sexual problems?

Patient: Not much.

WLM: What would you think if I suggest a pocket book for you to read?

Patient: I'd like that.

WLM: Good, I'll write down the title and author for you and maybe we can discuss the book next time.

Patient: OK.

WLM: I'd like to meet with you again next week. . . . .

Appendix III

Case Histories For Role-play Interviews

Health science students and professionals can practice sex history-taking and interviewing skills in a seminar format using the interviewing principles described in Chapter 2 and the topic model in Chapter 4. The case histories provided below are in the form of dialogue between "patient" and "professional" and can be used in role-playing. Preferably, each student should have the opportunity to be interviewER and interviewEE. Previously formulated case histories are used to save students and professionals the potential embarrassment of disclosing personal information.

Ground Rules For Role-Playing

1. The interviewer is given only *identifying information* and the *sexual chief complaint* by the instructor. All others in the seminar read the entire dialogue.
2. One of the main objectives of the seminar is for the interviewer to clarify the sexual problem declared by the patient (or discovered by the interviewer in the screening process) by using the model described in Chapter 4.
3. A second objective of the role-play is to practice using the interviewing techniques described in Chapter 2.
4. The interviewer is in the position of a generalist professional rather than a specialist in sexual disorders.
5. The duration of the "interview" is about 5 to 10 minutes.
6. Information about sexual issues should be elicited by the interviewer rather than volunteered by the person being interviewed. The purpose of this is not to apply more pressure to the interviewer but to reflect the reality of sex history-taking in that patients usually volunteer little information. The onus for acquiring this information rests mostly on the shoulders of the person asking the questions (see Interviewer Initiative, Chapter 2).
7. Some ad libbing by the patient is often necessary, since the case histories are incomplete.
8. Simulations are more "real" when done by individuals of the same gender as the patient described in the case history. Therefore, whenever possible, women and men should role-play a sexual problem manifested by someone of their own gender.

Case History "A"

IDENTIFYING INFORMATION: 32-year-old woman; married for three years; one child ten months old.

CHIEF COMPLAINT: "I'm not interested in sex"

HISTORY OF THE PRESENT ILLNESS

Diagnostic Topic #1 (lifelong versus acquired)
No problem with sexual desire (as manifested in her sexual activity or thoughts) in relation to two previous sexual partners, or with husband, until birth of child.

Diagnostic Topic #2 (generalized versus situational)
Not interested in sexual activity with husband. Does not masturbate. Does not have sexual thoughts involving other men. Has never been sexually interested in or had sexual experiences with other women. Has no dreams with sexual themes. Occasionally fantasizes about sexual activity with a (usually unrecognizable) man. Enjoys romantic stories in print or movies but is unresponsive to the sexual aspect of these tales. Her lack of sexual interest in men, greatly diminished sexual fantasy involving men, and unresponsiveness to erotica in books or movies all represent a major change from her past experience.

Diagnostic Topic #3 (description)
Sexual activity with husband used to occur two to four times each week. Now about once a month. Usually occurs on the initiative of her husband. Occasionally she will begin a sexual encounter because she feels that "enough time has gone by."

Diagnostic Topic #4 (patient's sex response cycle)
Does not get vaginally wet now and is not orgasmic. No problem with either in the past when sexually interested. Some vaginal discomfort associated with "prolonged" intercourse. No discomfort with vaginal entry.

Diagnostic Topic #5 (partner's sex response cycle)
No problem with husband's sexual interest, erections, ejaculation, and orgasm.

Diagnostic Topic #6 (patient and partner reaction)
She is concerned that husband will lose patience and will want to leave the marriage. He has not said so explicitly. He has, however, suggested to her that she see her doctor about this. He is irritable sometimes and she thinks that her lack of sexual desire is the reason. While she is seemingly unconcerned about the impact of the absence of sexual interest on herself (she says that she could live the rest of her life without sex), she does regard this as a problem and as abnormal. They have not talked about his feelings toward the changes in the level of their sexual activity.

Diagnostic Topic #7 (motivation for treatment when sexual problem not a chief complaint)
Wanting treatment because of concern about marriage disruption, which she does not want to happen. Says that she loves her husband.

Case History "B"

IDENTIFYING INFORMATION: 48-year-old man; married (second) 10 years; two children (from his first marriage)

CHIEF COMPLAINT: "I have trouble with my erections."

HISTORY OF THE PRESENT ILLNESS

Diagnostic Topic #1 (lifelong versus acquired)
Problems with erections only in the past five years.

Diagnostic Topic #2 (generalized versus situational)
Morning erections are full and stiff (i.e., no problem). No current sexual partners other than his wife. No erection problems in first marriage. Full erection with masturbation (a few times each month).

Diagnostic Topic #3 (description)
Erections full until intercourse attempted. Erection diminished (to about 60% of usual) in process of attempting vaginal entry. This pattern occurs on all occasions. On most attempts, is not able to gain vaginal entry.

Diagnostic Topic #4 (patient's sex response cycle)
Sexual interest and ejaculation unchanged compared to time before problem. Sexual interest, ejaculation, and orgasm also unchanged when masturbating.

Diagnostic Topic #5 (partner's sex response cycle)
Wife sexually interested. No problem with vaginal lubrication when interested. Usually orgasmic, and has no coital pain.

Diagnostic Topic #6 (patient and partner reaction)
Patient says that as a result of this problem, he feels that he is not "a man" anymore. Wife supportive. Says that her feelings for him have not changed.

Diagnostic Topic #7 (motivation for treatment when sexual problem is not a chief complaint)

Patient wants treatment. Has read about Sildenafil (Viagra) in the newspaper. Is interested in this for himself. He believes that his problem is "physical" (i.e., that it is "not in my head").

Case History "C"

IDENTIFYING INFORMATION: 30-year-old man; married 10 years.

CHIEF COMPLAINT: I've got Premature Ejaculation."

HISTORY OF THE PRESENT ILLNESS

Diagnostic Topic #1 (lifelong versus acquired)
Ejaculation fast with all sexual partners since first attempt at intercourse (including all four before marriage).

Diagnostic Topic #2 (generalized versus situational)
No current sexual partners other than his wife. Ejaculates quickly when masturbating but this is voluntary. He experiences no lack of control in this circumstance. When masturbating, he has warning that the feeling associated with ejaculation is about to occur so that stopping the further development of this sensation is entirely possible.

Diagnostic Topic #3 (description)
No warning before ejaculation when attempting intercourse. Ejaculation sometimes occurs before entry but usually after. Occurs within a few seconds (pushes or thrusts) after entry. Has tried several control methods (including distracting thoughts, anaesthetic creams, and condoms) but found that none of them were helpful. Neither emission nor orgasm is different compared to previous experience.

Diagnostic Topic #4 (patient's sex response cycle)
Interest is usual (high). Erections not a problem.

Diagnostic Topic #5 (partner's sex response cycle)
Wife interest unchanged. Usually experiences vaginal lubrication when interested. Orgasmic with touch. Non-orgasmic with intercourse, which she thinks is a result of him ejaculating quickly. No coital pain.

Diagnostic Topic #6 (patient and partner reaction)
Patient is concerned that wife wants to separate. He attributes this to sexual difficulties. Wife often angry. Says to patient that he is ejaculating fast purposely.

Diagnostic Topic #7 (motivation for treatment when sexual problem is not chief complaint)
Patient wants assistance, including immediate referral to specialist if necessary.

Case History "D"

26-year-old woman; married 2 years; no children.

CHIEF COMPLAINT: "It hurts when I try to have intercourse."

HISTORY OF THE PRESENT ILLNESS

Diagnostic Topic #1 (lifelong versus acquired)
Husband was first intercourse partner. Intercourse attempted first time on honeymoon. Did not achieve vaginal entry then or during subsequent attempts.

Diagnostic Topic #2 (generalized versus situational)
Never used tampons. Doctors have tried to do "internal" examinations but not able to. Never inserted own finger into vagina and also hurts when husband tries.

Diagnostic Topic #3 (description)
Pain located at vaginal entrance (versus deep); burning in character; not felt in particular area but rather all over; only occurs when vaginal insertion attempted and stops immediately after.

Diagnostic Topic #4 (patient's sex response cycle)
Before marriage was sexually interested, was wet when excited, and was orgasmic with husband's touch. Now, not interested, wet, or orgasmic with husband.

Diagnostic Topic #5 (partner's sex response cycle)
Husband usually sexually interested and does not have problems with erections, ejaculation, or orgasm.

Diagnostic Topic #6 (patient and partner reaction)
Patient feels incomplete as a woman and unfit as a wife. Is fearful of intercourse attempts. Husband quietly supportive.

Diagnostic Topic #7 (motivation for treatment when sexual problem is not chief complaint)
Referral to specialist previously suggested to patient but she was (and still is) apprehensive of what this would entail, especially if this involves a pelvic examination.

Case History "E"

IDENTIFYING INFORMATION: 23-year-old woman; single; has a sexual partner (male) of two years

CHIEF COMPLAINT: "I don't have an orgasm."

HISTORY OF THE PRESENT ILLNESS

Diagnostic Topic #1 (lifelong versus acquired)
Pattern has always been the same since the first intercourse experience at age 18. Does not experience orgasm during intercourse.

Diagnostic Topic #2 (generalized versus situational)
Has had orgasm with self-stimulation (masturbation) since age 15. Has not had orgasm with any sexual partner with intercourse or with touch.

Diagnostic Topic #3 (description)
Usual pattern with partner is brief genital stimulation before intercourse. Sexual arousal increases after entry but not to high level. Shy about giving directions to sexual partner. Usual pattern with masturbation is rapid arousal, vaginally wet, and orgasmic within a few minutes. Partner does not know that she is orgasmic when alone.

Diagnostic Topic #4 (patient's sex response cycle)
Often sexually interested, usually wet, and no coital pain.

Diagnostic Topic #5 (partner's sex response cycle)
Current male partner is sexually interested and does not have problems with erection, ejaculation, or orgasm.

Diagnostic Topic #6 (patient and partner reaction)
Patient feels her experience is not normal. Partner feels that patient is "missing something." She was previously pleased with intercourse experiences and unconcerned about not having orgasms with partner.

Diagnostic Topic #7 (motivation for treatment when sexual problem is not chief complaint)
Patient wants change. Is unsure what a referral involves.

Appendix IV

Sex-Related Web Sites For Patients/Clients/Consumers And Health Professionals

Internet resources are certain to change, since the medium is in its infancy. While the rapid speed of change presents a limitation in suggesting Web sites at any one time, those that are listed here are likely to remain in some form. (Like street addresses, locations may change when a move occurs but there is usually some indication of where the inhabitant has gone). At the current rate of change, Appendix IV need updating by the time this book is published. As new sites are created, health professionals will need to develop mechanisms for keeping information fresh for the benefit of their patients.

Rather than attempting to be comprehensive, the purpose in listing Internet sexuality resources in Appendix IV is one of suggesting a place to *begin* the process of investigating a particular topic. The focus is on the World Wide Web part of the Internet rather than e-mail, newsgroups, and chat rooms. Sites are selected for the information provided, for inclusion of links to other related Web sites, and for tasteful explanation and description of particular issues.

DISABILITY

National Rehabilitation Information Center (Naric)
http://www.naric.com/naric
Funded (not operated) for many years by the National Institute for Disability and Rehabilitation Research (NIDRR): a library and information center on these two subjects serving groups that include health professionals and the lay public. The Site operates some large databases covering published information on almost any aspect of disability and rehabilitation.

Roeher Institute
http://indie.ca/roeher
The Institute functions as a clearinghouse for information on disability issues in Canada and around the world. Services are used by many groups, including teachers, students, families, researchers, and government. Information obtained by contacting the Institute at it's e-mail address (info@roeher.ca) rather than on-line.

DYSPAREUNIA (see also Chapter 13)

Dr. Glazer's Vulvodynia Web site
http://www.vulvodynia.com
Dr. Glazer is a psychologist (PhD) with a special interest in biofeedback for vulvar pain syndromes. His Web site includes information about biofeedback in the treatment of vulvar pain, a discussion group for health professionals (password required), an e-mail 'list' for interested individuals, a vulvodynia bibliography, and links to related Web sites.

National Vulvodynia Association (NVA)
http://www.nva.org
A nonprofit organization dedicated to improving the lives of individuals with vulvodynia. NVA engages in educational activities for the public as well as affected individuals and their families, publishes a newsletter, encourages research, and is an active advocate for its members.

ERECTILE DYSFUNCTION   (see also Chapter 11)

htt://www.viagra.com
This Web site contains detailed product information for sildenafil (Viagra), the oral medication manufactured by Pfizer, and approved for distribution by the Food and Drug Administration in the United States for the treatment of erectile dysfunction.

GENDER IDENTITY (transgender, transsexual, transvestite, cross-dressing)(see also Chapter 8)

Transgender Forum
http://wwwtgfmall.com/
Offers an e-zine (electronic magazine) subscription after a free view edition online. Provides information about resources and links to other sites.

GENERAL/HEALTH

PubMed
http://www.ncbi.nlm.nih.gov/PubMed
"PubMed is a project developed by the National Center for Biotechnology Information (NCBI), located at the National Institutes of Health (NIH). It has been developed . . . as a search tool for accessing literature citations and linking to full-text journals . . . the database . . . is drawn primarily from MEDLINE and PreMEDLINE . . . MEDLINE . . . is the . . . NLM's premier bibliographic database covering the fields of medicine, nursing, dentistry, veterinary medicine, the health care system, and the preclinical sciences . . . the PreMEDLINE database provides basic citation information and abstracts before the full record are prepared and added to MEDLINE." (PubMed overview)

GENERAL/SEXUALITY

http://www.jagunet.com/~dgotlib/meanstreets.htm
The site was developed as a companion piece to a published article by D. Gotlib and P. Fagan for the Journal of Sex Education and Therapy, titled *"Mean Streets of Cyberspace: Sex Education Resources on the World Wide Web"* (vol 22, page 79-83, 1997). The site is information oriented and has direct connections to some sex-related Web sites on the following:

- General psychiatry (e.g., information on sexual side effects of psychotropic drugs)
- Comprehensive sexual resources (several of which have question and answer sections such as "Go Ask Alice!")
- Sexual dysfunctions (including erectile dysfunction, premature ejaculation, vulvar pain, and sexuality and cancer)
- Sexuality and disability; and gender dysphoria and transgender issues

HEALTH PROFESSIONAL AND SEXUALITY ORGANIZATIONS

Gay and Lesbian Medical Association
http://www.glma.org/
A 2000 member international organization (12 countries and 50 states in the United States) of gay, lesbian, bisexual, and transgendered (LGBT) physicians, medical students, and their supporters. It's mission is to combat homophobia, provide quality health care for LGBT and HIV-positive people, foster a positive professional climate, and support members discriminated-against on the basis of sexual orientation. The organization provides a newsletter (which one receives after becoming a member), promotes conferences, and supports projects (e.g., on Lesbian-related research).

The Kinsey Institute for Research in Sex, Gender and Reproduction
http://www.indiana.edu/~kinsey

Founded in 1947 by Dr. Alfred Kinsey, a major figure and pioneer in the field of sex research, the purpose of the Institute is to promote interdisciplinary research and scholarship in the fields of human sexuality, gender, and reproduction. The Institute has a specialized collection of resources for scholars, promotes programs in research and publication, organizes interdisciplinary conferences and seminars, and provides information to researchers. The Web site has an excellent list of links to other sex-related professional and public orgnizations.

The Society for the Scientific Study of Sexuality (SSSS)
http://www.ssc.wisc.edu/ssss/

SSSS is an international organization of over 1100 members devoted to the advancement of knowledge of sexuality. It is multidisciplinary in membership and is the oldest such group. SSSS promotes annual national and regional conferences, provides awards and grants, and publishes several periodicals.

World Association for Sexology(WAS)
http://www.tc.umn.edu/nlhome/m201/
colem001/was/wasindex.htm

An international organization of over 80 member organizations representing over 25 countries dedicated to "further the understanding and development of sexology throughout the world." WAS "brings individuals and organizations together to share scientific information, form networks, and promote international and intercultural exchange." WAS has sponsored 13 international congresses.

INTERSEX

Intersex Society of North America (ISNA)
http://www.isna.org

A peer-support, education, and advocacy group for individuals born with ambiguous genitalia, and their parents. The Web site includes Frequently Asked Questions, recommendations for treatment, information about hypospadias, and detailed bibliographies. ISNA promotes an approach that "is based on avoidance of harmful or unnecessary surgery, qualified professional mental health care . . . , and empowering the intersexual . . . to choose (or reject) any medical intervention."

MENOPAUSE

(see also Chapters 5, 9, and 13)
North American Menopause Society (NAMS)
http://www.menopause.org/

NAMS is the "preeminent resource on all aspects of menopause to healthcare providers and the public." The organization is multidisciplinary, international, and nonprofit. NAMS also provides information to the public and facilitates the exchange of information between members.

REPRODUCTION

Association of Reproductive Health Professionals (ARHP)
http://www.asrm.com/

APHP is an "interdisciplinary medical professional association" devoted to the education of health professionals and the public on family planning, contraception and other reproductive health issues, including sexually transmitted diseases, HIV, urogenital disorders, abortion, menopause, cancer prevention/detection, sexual health, and infertility."

Planned Parenthood Federation of America
http://www.plannedparenthood.org/

Provides sexual and reproductive health information on topics such as abortion, birth control, STDs, and safer sex.

SAFER SEX

The SaferSex Page
http://safersex.org/condoms.html

Information about aspects of condom manufacture and use.

SEX EDUCATION

Sexuality Information and Education Council of the United States (SIECUS)
http://siecus.org/
SIECUS is national, private, nonprofit, and devoted to advocacy, and the development, collection, and dissemination of sexuality information.

SEXUAL ASSAULT

(see also Chapter 8)
Domestic Violence Information Center
http://www.feminist.org/other/dv/dvhome.html
Connections to state coalitions in the United States and national organizations concerned with domestic violence. Provides hotline information about shelters, legal resources, health care centers, and counseling. Provides information on the Violence Against Women Act of 1994 and a list of Internet resources on domestic violence.

Men Assisting Leading & Educating (M.A.L.E.)
http://www.malesurvivor.org/
"A nonprofit organization dedicated to healing male survivors of sexual abuse." The goals of MALE are to help men "break the isolation" associated with their secrets; provide information and linkages to other sexually abused men as well as friends and family, to provide resources and services; raise awareness; prevention through public education; and advocating for treatment of victims and offenders.

The Sexual Assault Information Page (SAIP)
http://www.cs.utk.edu/~bartley/sainfoPage.html
SAIP is an information and referral service that provides information about acquaintance rape, child sexual abuse/assault, incest, rape, ritual abuse, sexual assault, and sexual harassment. The site includes a question and answer section.

Voices in Action
http://voices-action.org
Voices (Victims Of Incest Can Emerge Survivors) in Action is an international nonprofit organization designed to "help victims of incest and child sexual abuse become survivors, and generate public awareness of the prevalence of incest, its impact, and ways in which it can be prevented or stopped through educational programs." In addition, other goals include providing a clearinghouse for information and resources to help victims, facilitating research, and exchanging experiences.

SEXUAL ORIENTATION   (see also Chapter 7)

Gay Lesbian and Straight Education Network (GLSEN)
http://www.GLSTN.org
A United States based organization with chapters in many states. Provides such items as a bibliography of children's books with gay and lesbian characters, reference materials on gay and lesbian youth, information on youth suicide and violence prevention, and web links to other lesbian gay and bisexual teachers organizations.

The Lesbian's Mom's Web Page
http://www.lesbian.org/moms/index.htm
"This Web Site was designed to help those women . . . who want to have babies through non-traditional means, specifically lesbians." Provides information on Lesbian-friendly physicians and sperm banks, information to consider about donors, insemination, terminology, health factors, and insurance. First person accounts by Lesbian mom's.

National Gay and Lesbian Task Force (NGLTF)
http://www.ngltf.org/
"NGLTF is the front line activist organization on the national gay and lesbian movement" . . . and "serves as the national resource center for grassroots gay, lesbian, bisexual and transgender organizations . . ."

Parents, Families, and Friends of Lesbians and Gays (PFLAG):
http://www.pflag.org
PFLAG has chapters in all U.S. states and many other countries, including Australia, Canada, England, France, Israel, New Zealand, Russia, and South Africa. It is devoted to support, education, and advocacy.

Partners Task Force for Gay and Lesbian Couples
http://www.buddybuddy.com
Provides information and support on issues of interest to same-sex couples, including legal marriage, relationship safeguards, immigration, survey data on couples, and information lists. Also advocates for the right of same-sex couples to have the benefits of legal marriage.

Gaycanada.com
http://www.cglbrd.com/
Gaycanada.com is "the Internet arm of the Canadian Gay, Lesbian & Bisexual Resource Directory, a not-for-profit organization supported entirely by Canadian gay and gay positive businesses . . . ." The Directory "is . . . dedicated to the collection, compilation, and distribution of information important to or of relevance to the GLB communities across Canada."

Queer Resources Directory
http://planetout.com/pno/netqueery
Part of a large library of information on the Internet on gay, lesbian, and bisexual issues. Access is via the Yahoo search engine and the link to Society and Culture. The Directory is part of a larger Web site devoted to a variety of sexual orientation-related subjects.

Sexuality Information And Questions And Answer Services

Go Ask Alice
http://columbia.edu/cu/healthwise/about.html
Go Ask Alice is a service of Healthwise, the Health Education division of Columbia University Health Services. Topics addressed include: sexuality and relationship issues, health and fitness, emotional well-being, and alcohol and other drugs.

Sexual Health InfoCenter
http://www.sexhealth.org
Descriptive information that appears well delivered on a variety of topics, including: "better sex," "safer sex," STDs, aging, orientation issues, and problems. Also includes survey information (their own), a "sex tip," and a question and answer section.

Self-Help and Psychology Magazine
http://www.cybertowers.com/selfhelp/
"The largest self-help and psychology website in the world." The topics are varied but include a significant amount on sexual issues.

Dr. Ruth Online
http:www.drruth.com/
The online version of the popular Dr. Ruth

Dr. Marty Kline
http://SexEd.org
The site is operated by a sex therapist who is clinically active and teaches at Stanford University Medical School.

Sexology Netline
http://home.netinc.ca/F~sexorg/index/htm

Sexually Transmitted Diseases, Including HIV/AIDS

AIDS Research Information Center (ARIC)
http://www.critpath.org/aric
ARIC Inc. is a private, non-profit AIDS medical information service located in Baltimore, Maryland. ARIC provides the following services: a public outreach program through which the organization operates a mail, e-mail, and telephone hotline to answer questions from people with

AIDS or health professionals. ARIC also publishes an AIDS medical glossary for laymen, produces a quarterly newsletter, provides an information library on AIDS medical research and treatment, and has a resource guide for people with AIDS.

The American Social Health Association (ASHA)
http://www.sunsite.unc.edu/ASHA/
ASHA's mission is "to stop sexually transmitted diseases and their harmful consequences to individuals, families, and communities." The organization publishes educational materials; raises public awareness; operates National "hotlines" on AIDS (in English, Spanish and for the Deaf), STDs, Herpes, Resource Center, and Immunization information; and has several programs, including a Woman's Health program "to raise awareness of the disproportionate impact that STDs have on women."

The Body
http://www.thebody.com/cgi-bin/body.cgi
Described as "A Multimedia AIDS and HIV Information Resource." Provides information on "the basics" (e.g., testing and safe sex), treatment, conferences, quality of life, and government related information (e.g., CDC daily AIDS summary).

CDC National AIDS Clearinghouse
http://www.cdcnac.org/
This is a service of the Centers for Disease Control and Prevention and "designed to facilitate the sharing of HIV/AIDS and STD resources and information about education and prevention, published materials, and research findings, as well as news about related trends."

The STD Home Page
http://med-www.bu.edu/people/sycamore/std/
Located on the server of Boston University School of Medicine but not affiliated with that institution or Boston Medical Center. The site was created by a medical student, Tri D. Do, and carries an "Anti-Copyright (O) 1995 " symbol. The purpose of the site is . . . "to meet the needs of East Boston High School Students . . . ." The information is " . . . factually exhaustive for non-medical persons' level of understanding. . . . "

UNAIDS
http://www.unaids.org/
Co-sponsored by several UN organizations, including UNICEF, WHO, and UNESCO. Described as the main advocate for global action on HIV/AIDS. Provides extensive links to other HIV/AIDS-related organizations; information on conferences and press releases.

Appendix V

Medications & Sexual Function

Antihypertensive Medications

amiloride (Midamore)**
benazepril (Lotensin)
chlorthalidone (Hygroton, Thalidone)***
clonidine (Catapres)**
guanadrel (Hylorel)***
guanethidine (Ismelin)****
indapamide (Lozol)
labetalol (Normodyne, Trandate)*
lisinopril (Prinivil, Zestril)**
mecamylamine (Inversine)*
methyldopa (Aldomet) (men and women)***
metoprolol (Lopressor, Toprol XL)*
propanolol (Inderal) (men and women)**
reserpine (men and women)***
spironolactone (Aldactone) (men and women)***
timolol (Blocadren) (men and women)*

Antidepressants

amoxapine (Ascendin)*
bupropion (Wellbutrin)**
clomipramine (Anafranil) (men and women)****
desipramine (Norpramin, Pertofrane)*
doxepin (Adapin, Sinequan)
fluoxetine (Prozac)***
imipramine (Tofranil, Janimine)*

maprotiline (Ludiomil)*
nortriptyline (Aventyl, Pamelor)*
phenelzine (Nardil)*
protripyline (Vivactil)*
tranylcypromine (Parnate)*

Other Psychiatric Medications

alprazolam (Xanax)**
barbiturates
buspirone (BuSpar)**
chlorpromazine (Thorazine)*
clonazepam (Klonopin)*
diazepam (Valium, Zetran)*
fluphenazine (Prolixin, Permitil)****
lithium (Eskalith, Lithonate)*
lorazepam (Ativan)*
oxazepam (Serax)*
pimozide (Orap)*

Miscellaneous Medications

acetazolamide (Diamox, Ak-Sol)*
amiodarone (Cordarone)*
carbamazepine (Tegretol, Atretol, etc)
cimetidine (Tagamet) (men and women)*
clofibrate (Atromid-S)
cyclobenzaprine (Flexeril)
danazol (Danocrine)***
dichlorphenamide (Daranide)*
digoxin (Lanoxin)***

*Case report(s), package insert, or uncertain frequency.
**Infrequent side effect.
***Frequent side effect.
****Very frequent side effect.
Note: Medications and their accompanying side effects that are cited frequently as causing sexual disorders are in bold type.
Adapted from: Finger WW, Lund M, Slagle MA: Medications that may contribute to sexual disorders: a guide to assessment and treatment in family practice, *J Fam Pract* 44:33-43, 1997.

ethinyl estradiol (Estinyl)***
fenphluramine (Fastin) (frequent in women with large doses or long-term use)*
gemfibrozil (Lopid)
glycopyrrolate (Robinul)*
hydroxyzine (Atarax, Anxanil, Vistaril)
interferon
ketoconazol (Nizoral)***
medroxyprogesterone (Depo-Provera, Amen, Cycrin, etc)*
methadone (Dolophine)****
methazolamide (Neptazane) (men and women)*
metoclopramide (Reglan)*
metronidazole (Flagyl, Protostat)*
mexiletine (Mexitil)
morphine (MS Contin, Roxanol)
niacin (Nicolar, Niacor, Nicobid)***
norethindrone (Norlutin)
phendimetrazine (Adphen, Bacarate, Anorex, Statobex)*
phenobarbital
phenytoin (Dilantin)
primidone (Mysoline)
ranitidine (Zantac)

Illicit and Abused Drugs

barbituates
diazepam (Valium)
marijuana
MDMA**
methaqualone (in women)*
morphine (MS Contin, Roxanol)

Nonprescription Medications

cimetidine (Tagamet HB) (men and women)*
diphenhydramine (Benadryl, Genahist, Nordryl, etc)
niacin (Nicolar, Niacor, Nicobid)***
ranitidine (Zantac 75)

"Sexual Disinhibition"

propofol (Diprivan)*

"Changes In Sexual Desire"

prochlorperazine (Compazine)

"Sexual Desire Disorder"

alcohol (both acute and chronic effects)***

Increased Sexual Desire

amphetamines (may increase desire at low dose)
cyclobenzaprine (Flexeril)
danazol (Danocrine)***
ethosuximide (Zarontin)*
physostigmine (Antilirium)*
levodopa (Larodopa, Dopar)****
trazodone (Desyrel)

Erectile Disorder

Antihypertensive Medications

amiloride (Midamore)**
atenolol (Tenormin)***
benazepril (Lotensin)*
chlorthalidone (Hygroton, Thalitone)***
clonidine (Catapres)****
diltiazem (Cardizem, Dilacor XR)*
enalapril (Vasotec)**
guanabenz (Wytensin)***
guanadrel (Hylorel)***
guanethidine (Ismelin)****
hydralazine (Apresoline)*
hydrochlorthiazide (Esidrix, HydroDIURIL), Oretic)****
indapamide (Lozol)**
labetalol (Normodyne, Trandate)****
lisinopril (Prinivil, Zestril)**
mecamylamine (Inversine)*
methyldopa (Aldomet)***
metoprolol (Lopressor, Toprol XL)*
metyrosine (Demser)**
minoxidil (Loniten)*
nifedipine (Procardia, Adalat)**
phentolamine (Regitine)*

pindolol (Visken)*
prazosin (Minipress)**
propanolol (Inderal)****
reserpine***
spironolactone (Aldactone)***
timolol (Blocadren)*
trimethaphan (Arfonad)
verapamil (Calan, Isoptin, Verelan)*

Antidepressants

amoxapine (Asendin)***
bupropion (Wellbutrin)**
desipramine (Norpramin, Pertofrane)*
impramine (Tofranil, Janimine)***
maprotiline (Ludiomil)*
nortriptyline (Aventyl, Pamelor)*
paroxitine (Paxil)
phenelzine (Nardil)*
protriptyline (Vivactil)
tranylcypramine (Parnate)**
venlafaxine (Effexor)**

Other Psychiatric Medications

barbiturates
buspirone (BuSpar)*
chlordiazepoxide (Librium, Mitran, Reposans-10)
chlorpromazine (Thorazine)***
chlomipramine (Anafranil)****
clonazepam (Klonopin)
droperidol (Inapsine)*
fluphenazine (Prolixin, Permitil)****
Haloperidol (Haldol)*
lithium (Eskalith, Lithonate)***
meprobamate (Equanil, Miltown)*
mesoridazine (Serentil)*
pimozide (Orap)***
prochlorperazine (Compazine)
sulpiride (Supril, Sulpitil)***
thioridazine (Mellaril)****
thiothixine (Navane)

Miscellaneous Medications

acetazolamide (Diamox, Ak-Sol)***
amiodarone (Cordarone)*
atropine*
baclofen (Lioresal)

benztropine (Cogentin)*
biperiden (Akineton)*
bromocriptine (Parlodel)*
carbamazepine (Tegretol, Atretol, etc)***
cimetidine (Tagamet)***
clinidium (Quarzan)*
clofibrate (Atromid-S)***
cyclobenzaprine (Flexeril)
dichlorphenamide (Daranide)***
dicyclomine (Bentyl, Di-Spaz, etc)*
digoxin (Lanoxin)***
diopyramide (Norpace)**
disulfiram (Antabuse)
ethionamide (Trecator-SC)*
etretinate (Tegison)*
famotidine (Pepsid)**
fenfluramine (Fastin)**
furazolidone (Furoxone)*
gemfibrozil (Lopid)*
homatropine methylbromide (Homapin,
    Equipin, Lantro)*
**hydrochlorthiazide (Esidrix, HydroDIURIL,
    Oretic, etc)******
hydroxyzine (Atarax, Anxanil, Vistaril)*
indomethacin (Indocin)*
interferon*
ketoconazole (Nizoral)****
mazindol (Mazanor, Sanorex)*
meclizine (Antivert, Bonine)*
medroxyprogesterone (Depo-Provera, Amen,
    Cycrin, etc)*
methadone (Dolophine)****
methazolamide (Neptazane)***
methotrexate (Folex, Rheumatrex)*
methysergide (Sansert)*
metoclopramide (Reglan)*
mexiletine (Mexitil)*
morphine (MS Contin, Roxanol)
naproxen (Anaprox, Naprelan, Naprosyn)
nizatidine (Axid)
norethindrone (Norlutin)***
omeprazole (Prilosec)*
orphenadrine (Flexon, Flexoject, Norflex,
    Myolin)*
oxybutynin (Ditropan)*
phendimetrazine (Adphen, Bacarate, Anorex,

Statobex)
phenobarbitol***
phentermine (Fastin, Lonamin)
phentolamine (Regitine)*
phenytoin (Dilantin)***
primidone (Mysoline)***
probucol (Lorelco)
procarbazine (Matulane)*
prochlorperazine (Compazine)
procyclidine (Kemadrin)*
propantheline bromide (Pro-Banthine)*
ranitidine (Zantac)*
scopolamine (Transderm-Scop)*
sulfasalazine (Azulfidine)*
thiabendazole (Mintezol)***
trihexyphenidyl (Artane)*

Illicit And Abused Drugs

alcohol***
amphetamines**
amyl nitrite
barbiturates
cocaine***
MDMA****
methaqualone
morphine
tobacco**

Nonprescription Medications

antihistamines*
cimetidine (Tagamet HB)***
dimenhydrinate (Dramamine, Marmine, Calm-X, etc)*
diphenhydramine (Benadryl, Genahist, Nordryl, etc)*
famotidine (Pepcid AC)**
naproxen (Aleve)
ranitidine (Zantac 75)*

Orgasm/Ejaculation Disorder In Men: Delayed or Absent[†]

Antihypertensive Medications

clonidine (Catapres)**
guanadrel (Hylorel)***
guanethidine (Ismelin)****
labetalol (Normodyne, Trandate)****
methyldopa (Aldomet)***
metyrosine (Demser)**
phenoxybenzamine (Dibenzyline)***
prazosin (Minipress)
reserpine***
trimethaphan (Arfonad)*

Antidepressants

amoxapine (Asendin)*
desipramine (Norpramin, Pertofrane)*
doxepin (Adapin, Sinequan)*
fluoxetine (Prozac)****
imipramine (Tofranil, Janimine)
phenelzine (Nardil)***
sertraline (Zoloft)****
trazodone (Desyrel)*
trimipramine (Surmontil)*
venlafaxine (Effexor)***

Other Psychiatric Medications

alprazolam (Xanax)***
barbiturates***
buspirone (BuSpar)*
chlordiazepoxide (Librium, Mitran, Reposans-10)*
chlorpromazine (Thorazine)*
clomipramine (Anafranil)****
clonazepam (Klonapin)*
diazepam (Valium, Zetran)
fluphenazine (Prolixin, Permitil)*
haloperidol (Haldol)*
mesoridazine (Serentil)*
perphenazine (Trilafon)****
pimozide (Orap)*
prochlorperazine (Compazine)

[†]Information on orgasm/ejaculation is often not presented as gender-specific (versus information on orgasm in women).

thioridazine (Mellaril)****
trifluoperazine (Stelazine)*

Miscellaneous Medications

aminocaproic acid (Amicar)*
baclofen (Lioresal)**
isotretinoin (Accutane)*
methadone (Dolophine)**
methotrexate (Folex, Rheumatrex)*
naproxen (Anaprox, Naprelan, Naprosyn)*
phendimetrazine (Adphen, Bacarate, Anorex, Statobex)
phentermine (Fastin, Ionamin)
prochlorperazine (Compazine)
trimeprazine (Temaril)*

Illicit And Abused Drugs

alcohol: acute effects***
amphetamines: low dose*; **high doses and chronic use***
amyl nitrite*
barbiturates*
cocaine
diazepam (Valium)
MDMA**
methaqualone*

Nonprescription Medications

naproxen (Aleve)*

amphetamines*
clonidine (Catapres)**

diazepam (Valium, Zetran)* (cited frequently when abused)
imipramine (Tofranil, Janimine)*
methadone (Dolophine)**
methyldopa (Aldomet)*
phendimetrazine (Adphen, Bacarate, Anorex, Statobex)*
phenelzine (Nardil)*
phentermine (Fastin, Ionamin)*

Priapism

buspirone (BuSpar)*
chlorpromazine (Thorazine)**
clozapine (Clozaril)*
cocaine*
fluphenazine (Prolixin, Permitil)*
heparin*
hydralazine (Apresoline)*
labetalol (Normodyne, Trandate)*
mesoridazine (Serentil)*
molindone (Moban)*
omeprazole (Prilosec)*
perphenazine (Trilafon)*
prazosin (Minipress)*
prochlorperazine (Compazine)*
risperidone (Risperdal)*
tamoxifen (Nolvadex)*
testosterone*
thioridazine (Mellaril)*
thiothixene (Navane)*
trazodone (Desryl)*
trifluoperazine (Stelazine)*

†Information on orgasm/ejaculation is often not presented as gender-specific (versus information on orgasm in women).

Appendix VI

Selected Self-Help Books For Patients/Clients

The selected titles below are mentioned in various chapters in this book. They have been assembled here also so that the reader may easily see them at a glance. A more thorough list of self-help books is found in: Althof SE, Kingsberg SA: Books helpful to patients with sexual and marital problems: a bibliography, *J Sex Marital Ther* 18(1):70-79, 1992.

Aging
Brecher EM: *Love, sex, and aging*, Boston, 1984, Little, Brown, and Company.

Child Sexual Abuse
Danica E: *Don't: a woman's word.* Charlottetown, 1988, Gynergy Books.

Maltz W: *The sexual healing journey*, New York, 1991, HarperCollins Publisher, Inc.

Compulsive Sexual Behavior
Carnes P: *Out of the shadows*, Minneapolis, 1983, CompCare Publishers.

General
Michael RT et al: *Sex in America: a definitive survey*, Boston, 1994, Little, Brown and Company.

Chernick BA, Chernick AB: *In touch: the ladder to sexual satisfaction*, Huron Street, London, Ontario, 1992, Sound Feelings Limited.

Medical Illness
Schover LR: *Sexuality and fertility after cancer*, New York, 1997, John Wiley & Sons.

Men and Sexual Issues
Zilbergeld B: *Male sexuality.* Toronto, New York, 1978, Bantam Books.

Zilbergeld B: *The New Male Sexuality*, New York, 1992, Bantam Books.

Orgasm in Women
Heiman JR, LoPiccolo J: *Becoming orgasmic: a sexual and personal growth program for women*, revised and expanded edition, New York, 1976, 1988, Prentice Hall Press.

Barbach LG: *For yourself: the fulfillment of female sexuality*, New York, 1975, Anchor Books.

Blank J: *Good vibrations: the complete guide to vibrators*, San Francisco, 1989, Down There Press.

Premature Ejaculation
Kaplan HS: *PE: how to overcome premature ejaculation*, New York, 1989, Brunner/Mazel, Inc.

Safer Sex
McIlvenna T (ed): *The complete guide to safer sex*, Fort Lee, 1992, Barricade Books Inc.

Sexual Desire
Williams W: *Rekindling desire: bringing your sexual relationship back to life*, Oakland, 1988, New Harbinger Publications Inc.

Sexual Orientation
Isay R: *Becoming gay: the journey to self-acceptance*, New York, 1996, Pantheon Books.

Mondimore FM: *A natural history of homosexuality*, Baltimore and London, 1996, The Johns Hopkins University Press.

Women and Sexual Issues

Hite S: *The Hite report: a nationwide study on female sexuality,* New York, 1976, Macmillan Publishing.

Blank J: *Femalia,* San Francisco, 1993, Down There Press.

Bright S, Blank J: *Herotica 2: a collection of women's erotic fiction,* 1991, Down There Press.

Vaginismus

Valins L: *When a woman's body says no to sex: understanding and overcoming vaginismus,* New York, 1992, Viking Penguin.

INDEX